THE X FACTOR DIET

LESLIE KENTON

FOR AMELIA
I hope it was
worth waiting for

THE X FACTOR DIET

LESLIE KENTON

Vermilion
LONDON

First published in 2002 by Vermilion,
an imprint of Ebury Press, Random House,
20 Vauxhall Bridge Road, London SW1V 2SA
www.randomhouse.co.uk

Random House Australia (Pty) Limited
20 Alfred Street, Milsons Point, Sydney,
New South Wales 2061, Australia

Random House New Zealand Limited
18 Poland Road, Glenfield,
Auckland 10, New Zealand

Random House South Africa (Pty) Limited
Endulini, 5A Jubilee Road,
Parktown 2193, South Africa

The Random House Group Limited Reg. No. 954009

Papers used by Vermilion are natural, recyclable products made from wood
grown in sustainable forests.

Printed and bound by Mackays of Chatham, Chatham, Kent

A CIP catalogue record for this book
is available from the British Library

ISBN 0-09-1857457

Acknowledgements

There are so many people that have either helped me learn what I need to know in order to write this book, who have experimented with both programmes within the book and given me feedback, who have done the research that makes this new knowledge possible and who have painstakingly read the manuscript and have given me their comments and suggestions that it would be impossible to list them all. There are a few, however, who must be thanked by name: Dr Robert Jacobs, Dr Tony Edwards, Dr Gordon Latto, Nerena Leary, Stephen Eddey, Olly Nyberg and all of the participants of the TV documentary *To Age or Not to Age* who gave so willingly of their time, their energies and their creativity. I am also enormously grateful to Jeanette Stanley for her indefatigable hard work in typing every word, often three or four times, to Barbara Kisser for editing it, and to Denise Bates for working so hard to get it right.

Disclaimer

The material in this book is intended for informational purposes only. None of the suggestions or information is meant in any way to be prescriptive. Any attempt to treat a medical condition should always come under the direction of a competent physician – and neither the publisher nor we can accept responsibility for injuries or illness arising out of a failure by a reader to take medical advice. I am only a reporter. I also have a profound interest in helping myself and others to maximise the potential for positive health, which includes being able to live at a high level of energy, intelligence and creativity. For all three are expressions of harmony within a living organic system.

Leslie Kenton

BANKS PENINSULA, NEW ZEALAND

2002

Contents

THE X FACTOR IDIOTS' GUIDE

PART ONE:
WAKE-UP CALL

LEAN FOR LIFE

Perhaps once a century, a scientific discovery is made that has the potential to transform human life fundamentally. Less often a discovery is brought down to earth translated into the kind of information and practices you or I can use to change our lives for the better. This book is about such a discovery.

Pandora's Box

I am fully aware of what a huge statement this is. Yet it is true. The discovery is two-fold. First, there's the growing awareness that one of the most widespread epidemics ever to hit the Western world has moved into full swing, although few as yet even know of its existence. Known as *insulin resistance syndrome* or *Syndrome X*, this collection of troubles centres around your body's inability to handle the food you eat. It is almost certainly the reason why you, like literally millions of other people, have trouble losing weight and keeping it off no matter how hard you try. Syndrome X can be responsible for all sorts of other miseries, too – from chronic fatigue and anxiety to irritability, depression and a poor sense of personal worth. The second part of the discovery is that there's a way out. But first, let's take a closer look at Syndrome X.

Syndrome X affects the majority of us to one degree or another, even though we may not know it by name. We just imagine that the symptoms – aches and pains and the sense that something is 'just not right' in our body and life – are caused by something else entirely.

But what is it, precisely? Syndrome X is not one condition but a collection of them, all affecting our metabolism in one way or another. They include, among others, high blood pressure, high cholesterol levels and blood sugar disorders. Together they can make us vulnerable to overweight and obesity, and put us at increased risk of getting just about every age-related disorder you can name: eye problems, diabetes, heart disease, exhaustion, cancer and Alzheimer's, to mention only a few.

And as I've hinted, it's not caused by a virus or accident of nature. It's the result of the high-carbohydrate/low-fat, inadequate-protein way of eating which we have followed for a very long time, believing – as government directives still tell us we should – that such a diet constitutes nutrition for health.

Impeccable scientific research indicates that these directives are wrong. Eating this way screws up the human metabolism. It is contrary to what the human body, throughout the whole of evolution, has been programmed to thrive on – so contrary that it actually causes degeneration.

It happens like this. The hormone insulin helps the body turn the carbohydrates we eat into energy. But eating high-carbohydrate, low-fat food tends to flood cells with insulin. This leads to a cascade of problems. The cells lose sensitivity to insulin, which means even more of it is produced to redress the balance. Too much insulin causes the body to convert food into fat, yet prevents it from releasing the fat to use as fuel. It's not hard to see that the low-fat/high-carb diet can lead, directly or indirectly, to overweight, obesity, and the rest of Syndrome X's grim tally. So much for the bad news.

The good news is that all of these miseries can be reversed – not by popping a pill, but by shifting the way you eat and live. In fact, changing your way of eating and living is the only way to do this. Nothing else will work. No matter what your weight or age, or how long you have struggled with fat, you can transform your body into a radiantly healthy, fat-burning organism for life. Slowly and inexorably, the fat will melt away, you'll gain sleek, smooth, beautifully shaped muscles, and you'll reach levels of energy and vitality you may only have dreamed of until now.

The X Factor

How will this transformation happen? I've called it the X Factor Diet, because permanent weight loss doesn't happen until we deal with Syndrome X. Following any other kind of diet will mean the loss of lean body mass and an endless, tedious seesawing between losing weight and gaining it all back, with interest. In fact, making good use of the X Factor Diet puts an end to slimming diets forever – as well as the heartache, fatigue and sub-clinical nutritional deficiencies they cause.

The X Factor Diet redresses the balance by altering both the kind and ratio of the three fundamental nutrients – proteins, carbohydrates and fats. You'll eat only the best: slow-release, low-density carbohydrates, top-quality protein, vital plant nutrients, omega-3 fatty acids. Depending on your needs, you have two programmes to choose from – Ketogenics and Insulin Balance. Both are natural, scientifically validated programmes for a total and permanent physical metamorphosis.

Michelangelo once said that he never sculpted anything. All he did, he insisted, was take his chisel and remove extraneous marble to reveal the perfect form hidden within it. Ketogenics and Insulin Balance are your chisels, and a natural, healthy, lean body the perfect form which they can reveal. Both programmes work their health-giving wonders by altering the way you process food and creating more energy at the core of you – on a cellular level. Both are well supported by research which you'll find in the References section at the back of the book. These references and further reading are for you to study and to take further if you want to learn more, as well as for your doctor, who, with the inevitable busy practice, may as yet know little of these new discoveries.

Good For All

Insulin Balance is an excellent programme for anyone. In essence, it's a road to healthy living, and a superb way of controlling insulin and blood sugar levels and avoiding insulin resistance – all vital for avoiding conditions associated with Syndrome X, as we've seen. Insulin Balance is also an effective weight-loss tool and energy boost for a woman whose body fat is less that 35 per cent or a man who carries less than 22 per cent fat.

For women and men whose body fat percentage is higher, Ketogenics is the answer. This more dynamic fat-loss programme also counters the effects of Syndrome X, but works faster and goes deeper than Insulin Balance. It also requires more demanding changes in lifestyle.

People on Ketogenics usually switch to Insulin Balance once their body fat gets down to the appropriate level. Some people feel so well and are so delighted with the steady fat loss they experience with Ketogenics that they choose to remain on it until they have reached whatever body size and weight is appropriate for them. Both Insulin Balance and Ketogenics also make use of the right kind of physical activity – an essential ally in clearing fat from your body, as well as in protecting from and countering Syndrome X.

Help From My Friends

I have watched the information, tools and techniques which you will find within this book transform my own body and life and those of others. I am still watching and wondering – filled with fascination and gratitude. I see Ketogenics and Insulin Balance as great gifts of nature, now handed to all of us to use as we choose.

In formulating these programmes, I have been fortunate enough to work with doctors, nutritionists and biochemists at the cutting edge of research into Syndrome X. That has been fun and fascinating. In the process of researching and shooting a documentary on ageing, I have also had the pleasure of sharing both these programmes with wonderful people of all ages, and from all walks of life and a wide range of social and ethnic backgrounds.

These men and women, like me, wanted to see what Ketogenics and Insulin Balance could do to change their lives for the better. They were willing to invest the time and effort to learn how they work, and then to put them into practice in their own lives. These people, my new friends, chose to make this most exciting of journeys with me – a journey towards a leaner, healthier and more beautiful body.

Having them as travelling companions has continued to inspire my own passage. Witnessing profound changes happen to their bodies and their lives continues to remind me just how magnificent the human body is and how capable of transformation we all are – no matter what our circumstances. Many of them have shared recipes and comments with me, some of which I have incorporated into Part Five, 'Sheer Pleasures'. They join with me in wishing you the very best on your own journey through the discoveries of this book. May it be the journey of a lifetime.

HIGH-CARB MADNESS

In the so-called civilised world, human beings are fatter than ever. What's worse, we grow fatter still with each year that passes. Food manufacturers, government bodies and well-meaning doctors urge us to eat more low-fat-high-carb foods: masses of bread and cereals, rice and pasta. Fats, not carbohydrates, are supposed to be the villains of the piece.

Only they're not. Extensive research into the effects of the low-fat/high-carb diet on insulin resistance, obesity and the development of degenerative diseases shows quite clearly that these are precisely the foods which make us fat in the first place.

Ignorance Is Profitable

Apart from the fact that it usually takes 20 to 30 years for scientific research to have any impact on health, much of the refusal to recognise what low-fat/high-carb eating is doing to ruin our shape and our health comes not from the fact that 'ignorance is bliss'. Rather, it's that 'ignorance is profitable.' Food manufacturers, skilled in the art of increasing profits, have latched on to the notion that lots of carbs and low-fat foods are supposed to be good for you. They have been quick to translate *fat-free, low-fat,* and *reduced-fat* dogma into huge profits.

For 20 years, the convenience food market has been flooded with low-fat biscuits, muffins, cheeses, sweets, 'energy bars' – even entire low-fat meals for popping into the microwave. Virtually all of them are riddled with sugar – perfectly designed meals and snacks for anyone who wants to get fatter. The fat which food processors remove from these low-fat foods goes into making sweet treats and chocolate sold to us on TV as goodies which we should eat if we really 'love ourselves'.

The humourist P. J. O'Rourke has pointed out that the world is now full of 'masses waddling into airports, business offices and churches dressed in drooping sweats or fuchsia warm-up suits or mainsail-size Bermuda shorts, each with a mobile phone in

> 'The USDA Food Pyramid should be renamed "The Feedlot Pyramid". Its nutrient profile is the same as swine-fattening chow. And is fattening the population in the same way.'
>
> DRS. MICHAEL AND MARY DAN EADES

one ear and a Walkman in the other and sucking Diet Pepsi through a straw'. All thanks to low-fat-high-carb food.

Americans Go First

The United States led the way to the low-fat-high-carb revolution in 1988, when in a burst of enthusiasm the US Surgeon General officially directed all Americans to cut their consumption of fat – especially saturated fat – and increase the number of carbohydrates they eat. The rationale was simple: reduce fat intake to almost zero and you will leave behind heart disease, diabetes, obesity and most of the degenerative conditions plaguing modern man. It was based on studies which looked at animals and people who – for limited periods – were put on low-fat diets.

These groups showed better cholesterol levels, weight loss and improved health. But what wasn't seen at the time is that the studies had two major flaws. The first is that if you carry on eating such a diet for months or years, you develop fatty acid deficiencies that seriously undermine hormones, energy levels, skin and overall health. The second is that virtually no one – unless they happen to be a rat confined to a cage with no access to foods other than those provided – can live on such a diet long term. People get hungry and crave sugar and carbohydrate. Some even develop food sensitivities or food allergies. As a result, they gradually begin to eat more – and usually more of the wrong things. So they grow fatter and fatter.

Americans who, like the rest of us, embraced the advice wholeheartedly have been munching away in a low-fat-high-carb universe ever since. Meanwhile, health statistics get worse. In the 10 years following the US Attorney General's dietary directives, obesity in the US tripled. Adult-onset or Type II diabetes soared, while other degenerative diseases continued to mount. In fact, the only people to have benefited from the low-fat-high-carb revolution so far are food manufacturers. They whip up tasty low-fat products by adding lots of sugar and salt to cheap foodstuffs like flour and processed, or 'junk', fats, then sell them, often at inflated prices, as 'healthy' foods. So we grow fatter and become more obsessed with dieting and buy more and more of their concoctions, all to no avail.

Time To Quit

It is time to face facts: the low-fat-high-carb diet has proven itself a complete failure. It does not reduce cholesterol significantly unless it is followed religiously – that is, at a calorie count of something like 1000 to 1200 a day. But this level is impossible to maintain, for the average person, for more than a few weeks, and can create deficiencies in essential nutrients over time. Such a diet wreaks havoc with blood sugar levels and causes endless suffering to people with diabetes. It does not reduce high blood pressure either. That is, unless you are consuming very little food.

What's more, people who lose weight on a low-fat-high-carb diet cannot keep it off. Both their appetite and their metabolic biochemistry cry out for nourishment. In fact, some 95 per cent of people who go on a low-fat-high-carb slimming diet regain the weight lost within a year. Yet the myth persists. Go to your doctor to ask for help with losing weight. Unless he or she is among the few physicians who have been keeping up with leading-edge discoveries in the fields of biochemical nutrition, you are likely to get more of the same low-fat-high-carb advice, and be told to tighten your belt and try harder.

Banish Guilt And Failure
Such advice creates suffering for those of us who long to be lean, yet continually fail. We feel desperately that it must be our fault, when despite trying our hardest, we don't succeed. We chastise ourselves for not doing things right. We believe we have no willpower. We become riddled with guilt, low self-esteem and a sense of failure.

Now is the time to lay aside such self-accusations forever. The fact is – and it's a fact powerfully supported by revolutionary scientific evidence – it is the way you have been eating, not you, that has failed.

SOME OF THE NEGATIVE EFFECTS OF LIVING ON A HIGH-CARBS-LOW-FAT DIET:

- Raised serum insulin levels causing insulin resistance, resulting in metabolic distortions which undermine health and vitality
- Lowered basal metabolic rate leading to weight gain
- Increased fat tissue growth and reductions in lean muscle tissue
- Accelerated biological ageing
- Increase in common food allergies or sensitivities to grains and dairy food
- An over-active immune system which can eventually become immune failure
- Soaring incidence of heart disease, obesity and cancer.

Light Shines

At last we are beginning to emerge from this low-fat-high-carb madness. And it's all down to research on the drama's key player – insulin.

Knowing how insulin works for better and for worse in your own body, and learning how its effects can be influenced by diet alone, doesn't just make successful and permanent weight control possible. It also points the way to an understanding of how we can slow the ageing process and banish degenerative diseases. Middle-aged spread is an insulin problem. So, as we've seen, are obesity, compromised immunity, chronic fatigue and many emotional disorders. How insulin behaves in your body determines – probably more than any other single thing – whether or not you end up with hypertension, heart disease, Type II diabetes and many forms of cancer. Change the way you eat and you can have a lean, healthy, fat-burning body for life.

Do It Now

This is hot stuff – probably the most valuable discovery about human health in the last century. What I find especially exciting is that, armed with an understanding of how insulin works, you can begin steadily changing your life for the better. Right here. Right now.

The X Factor Diet has already changed my own life and the lives of many others for the better. Since puberty, despite eating a healthy diet, I have always been heavier than I felt right for my body. After menopause it got worse. Then I learned about the principles behind Ketogenics and Insulin Balance and began to apply them. Now, I feel better and look leaner than I did 20 years ago. It has been like tapping into a font of boundless energy. Now I have a sense that my brain and my body will support, with grace instead of strain, all the creative projects I want to take on now and in the future. Others on the X Factor freeway report similar experiences.

'Traditionally, a low-fat-high-carbohydrate diet was used to prevent CHD because it effectively reduces plasma cholesterol concentrations, but this dietary regimen increases plasma triglyceride concentrations and reduces HDL-cholesterol concentrations.'

ROCHE HMPROC NUTR SOC FEB 1999

So, I am inviting you to come on a journey with me to discover how the careful balance between the right kinds of carbohydrates, proteins and fats – coupled with an emphasis on fresh, organic, plant-based foods, many eaten raw – can not only help you shed excess fat forever. It can also rejuvenate and regenerate your body. It may well leave you feeling and looking better than ever. The best is yet to come.

SYNDROME X – FATMAKER

A sinister-sounding condition called Syndrome X is making news. However, it is not some recently discovered disease but a term used to describe a group of abnormal metabolic conditions that can dispose us to obesity, high blood pressure, diabetes and heart disease. Gerald Reaven, an endocrinologist at California's Stanford University, first described Syndrome X in 1988, after some 20 years of study. Although Reaven identified it, the work exploring Syndrome X since then, as well as the clinical experience of physicians trained in functional medicine, have taken our understanding of it way beyond Reaven's first assertions.

Beware Insulin Resistance

Some of the most significant implications of the syndrome centre around the way in which Syndrome X can contribute to the build up of fat stores in the body. And more and more researchers have recognised that the condition is a big health problem. How big? A few years ago, scientists estimated that Syndrome X affected one in four people. Now many insist it may be more like two-thirds of the adult population in the West.

It is no accident that another name for Syndrome X is *insulin resistance*. For the primary abnormality which links together this group of disorders is a mounting insensitivity to the hormone insulin at a cellular level. And there is a lot more to this powerful hormone than you might imagine. One of the great breakthroughs at the end of the last century was the discovery that insulin plays important roles in health and illness. Yet mention the word to most people – including doctors – and they immediately associate it with diabetes. Few are aware of the other essential roles insulin plays (see Box).

INSULIN: KEY TO ENERGY

Insulin is a hormone, secreted by an area in the pancreas known as the islets of Langerhans. The hormone plays one of its most compelling roles when your body is in the process of digesting carbohydrates. It works like this: say you've just eaten a bowl of cereal, a baked potato or a piece of toast. These so-called complex carbohydrates are converted into glucose very rapidly by the digestive process. The glucose is then absorbed into your bloodstream, and it's this sudden rise in blood sugar that triggers the release of insulin.

Part of insulin's job is to enable your body to make use of this glucose or blood sugar by binding to receptor sites on the surface of your cells. This process is very like a key (the insulin) fitting into a lock (the receptor). The insulin then 'escorts' the glucose into the cells, where it is burnt as energy. But if there's excess glucose in your blood, insulin turns some of it into glycogen, which is stored in your muscles and liver. Once there, glycogen, rather like a bank balance, can be turned back into glucose quickly and easily whenever you need energy. (Other metabolic fuels which your body can also use as energy include amino acids from proteins, dietary fats and ketone bodies produced from the breakdown of your body's fat stores.) If, after the stores of glycogen are all full, there's still glucose in the blood, insulin converts it into fat – a fact we'll be looking at in detail a little later on. Insulin's role doesn't stop there, however. It performs a lot of other metabolic and physiological tasks, too. It controls appetite. It tells your kidneys whether or not to retain fluid. It acts as a growth hormone which helps keep your body lean and young, and it regulates the liver's synthesis of cholesterol. All in all, it's an amazingly talented hormone, even orchestrating the flow of essential nutrients like amino acids and fatty acids, vitamins and minerals, into the 60 trillion microscopic cells of your body. That is, when it is working properly.

Diet Holds The Secret

Insulin's low profile hasn't kept it from being the focus of a lot of research. Back in the 1960s, researchers developed ways of measuring insulin levels. In the process they discovered that Type II diabetes is not just an abnormality involving soaring blood sugar levels. Diabetics also have high levels of insulin, compared to non-diabetics. Out of this discovery came an awareness of insulin resistance – and, over time, the realisation that it's not only diabetics who have this condition. Insulin resistance can also develop in people eating a diet rich in refined carbohydrates like white bread and sweets. The high levels of glucose triggered by such foods mean that your body cells are frequently flooded with insulin, causing them to become jaded and non-responsive to the hormone. So your pancreas just keeps secreting more and more of it in an attempt to get energy into your cells.

The amount of insulin released in your body is determined (wait for it…this is the big surprise) by *what you eat*. There's worse to come. Say you've just eaten a classic high-carb meal such as pizza and ice cream. The high insulin levels your body produces in response to that meal stimulates *lipogenesis*. What this means is that your body fails to burn the glucose as energy in your cells the way it is meant to do, but instead stores it as fat. Over time this process produces more and more body fat. So in the long term, a high-carb diet means more and more fat – and less and less energy.

In the past 30 years, a growing number of people have experienced an alarming breakdown in most of the metabolic processes which insulin controls. Over half the population of English-speaking countries are now overweight. In the United States alone, 50 million people have chronic high blood pressure. The same number have elevated cholesterol levels. And what lies beneath these abnormalities is Syndrome X – insulin resistance. It is now considered a prime cause – what is known as a 'risk factor' – for heart disease. It is also the bête noir behind cholesterol imbalance and elevated triglycerides, hypertension and some kinds of cancer.

Knock Knock – No Joke

With Syndrome X, insulin is knocking at the door but no one is answering. The pancreas, as we've seen, secretes yet more insulin, and in some cases the cells do not respond even to high levels of it. Glucose builds up in the blood to the point where Type II diabetes can result. Only recently has insulin resistance begun to make news specifically in relation to how fat our bodies are becoming and why we have so much trouble losing weight. In most countries, people are not only getting fatter, but they're also becoming less active. Insulin resistance produces obesity. It also makes people disinclined to move. This creates a vicious circle, as people who have it often lack the energy to exercise. If they are not processing energy from their foods, they are only laying down more fat. And both obesity and physical inactivity only aggravate insulin resistance, further compounding the problem.

Silent Killer

It's not just body fats that Syndrome X promotes either. It boosts dangerous blood fats too – total cholesterol and triglycerides – while depleting high-density lipoprotein (HDL), or 'good' cholesterol, increasing your risk of heart disease. You don't have to be overweight or have all of the symptoms associated with Syndrome X to suffer from unhealthily high insulin levels either. Thin people can experience Syndrome X as well. And it can remain undetected for years – bringing with it such experiences as chronic fatigue, fluid retention, intense craving for sweets, an inability to concentrate or think clearly and many other problems which are all too often blamed on other conditions. So insidious is Syndrome X that it often goes unnoticed for 30 or

40 years – until serious health issues begin to surface.

The Culprit

Are there factors other than diet that trigger Syndrome X? Yes. Growing older is one. Insulin resistance can be both a cause and an effect of ageing – a finding that has been seen in animals as well as humans. Research has shown that elevated insulin together with increased glucose, cholesterol and triglyceride levels, obesity, and heart disease, also occur in a number of animals as they get old as well. But by far the greatest culprit is an excess of certain kinds of carbs – particularly the refined kind – and sugar. For although the human body runs on glucose as its principal fuel, it was never designed to deal with a diet of convenience foods in which most of the calories we eat come from high-density carbohydrates that rapidly pour sugar into the bloodstream when we eat them. Even the so-called 'good' carbohydrates, such as whole-grain breads and brown rice, can cause insulin resistance if eaten to excess. The mix can get more dangerous if you also have nutritional deficiencies, generally eat too much, ingest too many highly refined and processed foods, drink too much alcohol, smoke, and/or have a sedentary lifestyle.

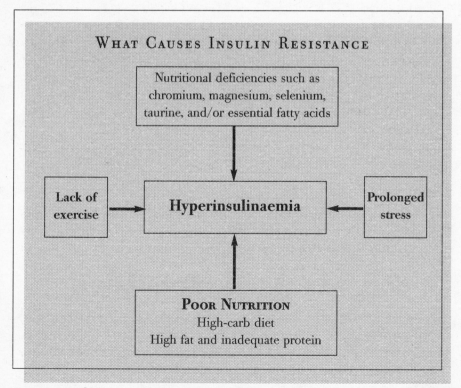

WHAT CAUSES INSULIN RESISTANCE

Nutritional deficiencies such as chromium, magnesium, selenium, taurine, and/or essential fatty acids

Lack of exercise → **Hyperinsulinaemia** ← Prolonged stress

POOR NUTRITION
High-carb diet
High fat and inadequate protein

If you are fat, or are constantly battling to stay lean, there is a 95 per cent chance that insulin resistance is the culprit. Banish it and you not only stop fighting the battle of the bulge, you help prevent numerous degenerative diseases, slow the rate at which you are ageing and quite literally regenerate your energy and rejuvenate your body.

Endless Cravings

Compulsive eating and carbohydrate cravings seem to be endemic in the West. These, too, are rooted in insulin resistance, as ongoing high levels of insulin can create constant feelings of hunger. This happens because insulin 'tells' the hypothalamus, the gland in the brain responsible for letting you know when you are hungry and thirsty, to send out hunger signals. But if your insulin levels are very high, the hypothalamus is getting too much of the message. As a result, you can find yourself eating a meal, yet feeling hungry soon afterwards. You can even begin to feel that no matter what you eat, nothing will satisfy you. And all of this is made much worse for your health by what has come to be known as the Randle Effect (see Box).

THE RANDLE EFFECT: FATS VS CARBS

In the standard Western diet, a lot of fats and carbohydrates are eaten together. This is bad news, as the fats effectively reduce cells' ability to use the blood sugar released by the carbohydrates. So while the fats are being burnt as fuel, there's more excess glucose swirling around in the bloodstream and ultimately ending up as fat. This is the Randle Effect, and it throws any overweight insulin-resistant person into a terrible vicious circle, in which hunger and carbohydrate cravings lead to overeating, followed by an inevitable increase in blood sugar and insulin levels as well as body fat deposits and more cravings. When your body is unable to use the foods you are eating for energy, it only knows how to store glucose as fat in your belly, hips and thighs. *The irony is that for a long time we have been blaming dietary fat for all this when this phenomenon is actually caused by a high carbohydrate intake in the presence of fats.*

Eaten on their own or together with protein but without an abundance of carbohydrates, the right kind of fats – we will be looking in depth at these soon – do not cause the laying down of fat in the body. This is perhaps the most difficult thing for those of us who have been highly schooled in the low-fat-high-carb approach to weight loss to grasp, yet it is absolutely essential to understand.

Enter The Heroes

Ketogenics and Insulin Balance reduce insulin levels by limiting the kind and the amount of carbohydrate foods that you eat. In someone who's overweight, lowering high levels of insulin enables your body to burn its fat stores as energy. It maximises permanent fat burning and weight loss in a number of ways, as shown in the Box below.

KETOGENICS AND INSULIN BALANCE:

- Switch your body from carbohydrate burning to fat burning
- End carbohydrate cravings – usually within a few days
- Stabilise blood sugar and eliminate the ups and downs of energy which result in fatigue, mood swings, brain fog and emotional roller-coastering
- Help break addictive eating habits and cravings such as a continual longing for chocolate, sugar, coffee, wheat, corn-based foods or alcohol
- Show you quickly how easily your body can burn fat while eating delicious, satisfying foods, many of which you may have been avoiding for a very long time in the belief that they would make you fat

---

Stop Blaming Yourself

Take heart. It is not your lack of willpower or a curse from the gods that is making you fat. It is the fact that you have been eating food for years which your body was *never* genetically designed to cope with. You, like me and millions of other people, may also have inherited the *thrifty gene*, a trait of many peoples whose ancestors lived in harsh environments (see page 24).

DO YOU HAVE THE THRIFTY GENE?

The thrifty gene is a survival mechanism which enables the body to store energy long-term, and to make the most of any food that's eaten. It made it possible for ancient humans to live through times of famine, while those without it died. In paleolithic times, the thrifty gene was one of the greatest gifts a child could inherit from its parents. Now, in the face of an onslaught of convenience foods replete with high-density carbohydrates, thrifty-gene people constantly struggle to get lean and stay that way.

Enough of the bad news. The good news is that it is possible both to prevent and to treat insulin resistance as well as to shed the fat that results from it without ever going hungry again, simply by following the X Factor Diet, and changing the kind of foods that you eat. A new lean life can begin for you right here and now.

FORGOTTEN MAGIC

The low-carbohydrate diet is as old as recorded history. Yet until recently we had all but forgotten its power. When the king of Ethiopia met a delegation from the Persian court in the 5th century BC, Herodotus tells us, he asked two questions: 'What does the Persian king like to eat?' and 'What is the greatest age Persians attain?' The oldest Persians, he was told, lived to be around 80. The Persian ruler loved bread most of all. On learning this, the Ethiopian king expressed surprise that Persians were so short-lived. In Ethiopia, he said, where people ate mostly meat and milk, many lived to be 120.

The French Connection

Until recently, when research began to show how high-carbohydrate diets contribute to rapid ageing, Herodotus's tale might have been considered apocryphal. Now the scientific evidence to back it up is filling medical journals. When people ate only moderate amounts of low-density carbohydrates, such as green leaves and plants, together with wild, protein-rich foods, their bodies aged more slowly than ours do today. And they were never overweight.

We'll look at the prehistoric menu in detail in the next chapter. For now, let's take a leap to Europe at a time of great historic ferment, when the high-carb tale started to become a decidedly grim one. By the end of the 17th century, high-carbohydrate diets had become the norm among corpulent European aristocrats, for it was primarily the wealthy that could indulge their cravings for sweet, fluffy foods. Concern over their degraded health was widespread, so it's no accident that this was when experiments with low-carbohydrate diets first began in Europe.

Anthelme Brillat-Savarin, a judge in the French supreme court during the 18th century, was fascinated by physiology, chemistry and medicine. Brillat-Savarin also wrestled with obesity. Eventually, in 1825, he wrote a book on how to counter it – *Physiologie du goût*. In it he describes 'an infallible method both for preventing excess corpulence and for reducing it'. He then goes on to give the magic formula for fat loss: 'A diet based upon the most reliable principles of physics and chemistry and suited of the desired end. Such a diet must take into consideration the most common decisive causes of obesity. Since it can be taken as proven that fat formation in man and animals is due to flour and starch, the logical conclusion to be drawn is that more or less complete abstinence from flour – and starch-containing foods – will lead to a reduction of growth.'

The programme worked both for Brillat-Savarin and for his rich, overweight readers. But we would have to wait until the end of the 20th century before science had any hints as to why.

In England in the mid-19th century, overweight undertaker William Banting consulted a Dr Harvey because he was losing his hearing. Harvey advised Banting to refrain from eating carbohydrates. When Banting did so, not only was his hearing restored, but his weight dropped by nearly 50 pounds in a year. Until then, Banting had only been able to walk downstairs backwards. In 1864, overjoyed by the results of his no-carbohydrate diet, he wrote and published a booklet recommending a low-carb diet to all sufferers of excess weight. In it, Banting says, 'the items from which I was advised to abstain from as much as possible were bread, sugar, beer, and potatoes which had been the main and, I thought, innocent elements of my existence, or at all events they had for many years been adopted freely. These, said my excellent advisor, contained starch and saccharin matter, tending to create fat, and should be avoided altogether. I can now confidently say that *quantity of diet may be safely left to the natural appetite; and that it is the quality only, which is essential to abate and cure corpulence.'* Harvey knew what he was talking about.

Dense And Artificial

The work of Dr Weston Price, an American dentist who journeyed the world with his wife studying so-called primitive populations in the 1920s and 1930s, was a revelation. Price pioneered the study of the insidious degeneration that occurs in people who gradually abandon low-carbohydrate diets in favour of high-carb Western fare. Although this shift began with the coming of agriculture, it has been much exacerbated by the advent of high-tech food manufacture and by our increasing reliance on nutritionally inadequate convenience foods made from refined flour, sugar and junk fats. These concentrated, high-density 'artificial' carbohydrates are whipped up from formulated foodstuffs. When we eat these ersatz foods regularly in large quantities, over time they produce insulin and blood sugar disorders and make those with an inherited tendency for storing fat grow fatter.

Weston Price found again and again all over the world that, after introducing high levels of starch products into a peoples' diet, only one generation was needed to bring about dental caries, crooked teeth and jaw malformations. He discovered that sugars, pastries, bread and processed foods of all kinds are the dietary components which underlie the widespread deterioration of human health worldwide. As far back as the 1930s, he was warning that unless a shift took place soon within the eating habits of humankind, and unless we reverted to a diet more in keeping with our ancestors, we would continue to deteriorate as a species. His words have proved prophetic.

The Fat Of The Land

More revealing research was carried out by the physician and anthropologist Vilhjalmur Stefánsson, the Canadian-born son of Icelandic immigrants. Stefánsson spent 15 years travelling on foot and horseback and by dogsled from one village to another studying the Inuit of Canada. Stefánsson marvelled at their diet and the high level of well-being these people seemed to enjoy. Except for a few berries which they preserved in whale oil and a bit of moss they took from the stomachs of animals they hunted, the Inuit peoples lived entirely upon animal foods. Their diet was high in fat and virtually devoid of carbohydrates. Yet heart disease, strokes, cancer and elevated blood pressure remained unknown among them. The Inuit were never overweight, even though they ate huge quantities of food – especially fats – devouring far more calories each day than we do now. Nor did the women suffer from the reproductive difficulties we do today – from PMS to osteoporosis. These people lived in relation to each other and to the land itself in great harmony, with no evidence of emotional disturbance or mental illness.

Not Bread Alone

When Stefánsson completed his studies of the Inuit, he wrote a number of books about his experience including: *Not by Bread Alone* and *The Fat of the Land* as well as *Cancer, Disease of Civilisation*, in which he presented documentary evidence that Eskimos had been cancer-free before contact with American civilisation and its high-carbohydrate foods. Western carb-based foods entered the lives of these peoples at the turn of the last century. By the time they were eating large quantities of them, the diseases of civilisation began to appear, from high blood pressure to cerebral strokes.

Impeccably documented, Stefánsson's work was highly esteemed, yet when his books were published they were greeted by the scientific community with incredulity. He was even openly accused of publishing uncritical scientific reports and of fabricating his statistics.

Intent on refuting these accusations, Stefánsson, together with fellow researcher Karsten Anderson, decided to carry out an experiment at Bellevue Hospital in New York City. The experiment was overseen by the highly esteemed metabolic expert Eugene Dubois. In 1928, both men checked themselves into hospital and began living on a diet of nothing but fresh meat and fat, to find out what the outcome would be.

The experiment made headlines all over America. Physiologists, immersed at that time in their investigations of vitamins, were certain that many symptoms of deficiency, such as scurvy, would develop. Although Stefánsson and Anderson stayed on a meat diet for months, no sign of illness was ever detected. Stefánsson occasionally left the hospital on various work assignments. Anderson remained under constant surveillance in the metabolic unit of Bellevue for a whole year. During this time he neither became ill nor developed any deficiencies, and reported that he felt extraordinarily well. He shed all the excess weight he had been carrying and many minor complaints he had previously experienced completely disappeared. When the experiment ended, metabolic expert Dubois commented that 'the most remarkable thing about the experiment was that nothing remarkable occurred'.

Dubois was only partly right. In truth, a number of remarkable things happened. Both men lost weight and felt extraordinarily well. They looked younger. Their vitality increased. They were cured of all ailments. Why? Because the health benefits of a low-carbohydrate diet go far beyond its ability to make a fat body lean. But while this was the first time the scientific community began to take seriously the way a low-carbohydrate diet reduces excess weight, they did not accept the rest of the results. Only Stefánsson and a few scientists who looked at his work remained convinced that the value of a low-carbohydrate diet lies not just in helping people get leaner, but also in preventing and curing many of the diseases of civilisation.

Eat Fat

In the 1950s, the British psychiatrist Richard Mackarness revived interest in low-carbohydrate eating. Richard was a close friend of mine and a remarkable man. His expertise lay in the field of food allergies and mental illness. He had long suffered from a weight problem and, fascinated by the work of Stefánsson, Brillat-Savarin, Banting and others, he began to experiment with a low-carbohydrate diet. Not only did it solve his weight problem forever, it also cleared up many ailments he suffered from which at that time had no remedy.

In the course of his psychiatric clinical work, Richard also discovered that a low-carb diet that included adequate protein significantly improved the mental health of his patients, too. In 1959, he wrote a popular book called *Eat Fat and Grow Slim*, which became a best-seller. The low-carb diet he propounded worked wonders for readers. Yet just as they had with Stefánsson, the medical community largely ignored Richard's work. His diet was treated as some kind of fad – at most, only marginally useful as weight control for a few people. Most doctors and government advisors on health still did not grasp the significance of what was going on: that the human body is healthiest on a low-carbohydrate diet. We are, in fact, genetically programmed to thrive on such fare, rather than masses of carbohydrates. Yet that is what we continue to eat.

Good Business – Bad Health

Carbohydrate foods are cheap to manufacture and easy to manipulate into saleable items. They are also highly addictive. Eat them and you want more. Great for business – bad for health. Called carbohydrate craving, it's a constant or intermittent hunger that people on a high-carb diet know only too well. You eat one biscuit and suddenly find yourself scoffing the whole packet. Such behaviour is not the consequence of a lack of willpower, but the result of significant imbalances in the body caused by a high-carb diet.

With every month, more evidence surfaces that more than any other single factor, a high-carbohydrate diet – still promoted by most governments and official advisory bodies – results in obesity, degenerative diseases and early ageing. And as we've seen, high-carb eating is harmful because it triggers distortions in hormonal functioning and balance, insulin resistance, hyperinsulinaemia (the overproduction of insulin), and blood sugar problems – yes, it's Syndrome X again.

Proof Of The Pudding

But there are encouraging developments. We now have hard clinical evidence showing that when you make a shift away from high-carb eating towards a healthy, low-carb diet with adequate protein and essential fatty acids, you not only alleviate many of these conditions, you often completely reverse metabolic imbalances.

Many have already taken the plunge and used the research, with remarkable results. Dr Wolfgang Lutz is one of them. For almost half a century he has been helping patients in Europe achieve perfect weight control and optimum health the low-carb way. In 1967, Lutz published a book about his work in which he presented clinical evidence that low-carbohydrate nutrition is a powerful force for healing disease. Sadly, this book, now in its 14th edition, remains unknown to most of us – it was published only in German. Sad, too, is the fact that most of the books which have been published since about low-carbohydrate nutrition ignore Lutz's work. In 2000, however, a paperback by Lutz appeared in English, co-written by an American, Christian B. Allan. Called *Life Without Bread*, it is well worth reading.

Rule Of 20 Years

While Lutz was busy with his European clients, British surgeon T.L.Cleave was hard at work charting global dietary change as director of medical research at the Institute of Naval Medicine. In 1974, Cleave published a brilliant study called *The Saccharin Diseases*. It is certainly one of the most important books on health in our time. He carried out meticulous studies of hospital records of many countries, particularly in West Africa. He found that not one person native to these nations experienced classic diseases of the West – obesity, colon cancer, gallstones, diverticulitis, heart disease or diabetes.

Cleave discovered that these diseases do not exist in people who've never eaten refined, high-density carbohydrates. But almost exactly 20 years after introducing these foods, the diseases appear. Within another 20 years, all of them become widespread. Cleave dubbed this phenomenon the 'rule of 20 years'. Recently, Cleave's discourses have been validated by other studies, for example one on Arizona's Pima Indians, and another in Saudi Arabia. India, Mexico, Japan and many other countries are all seeing his theory borne out. However, Cleave's book is now out of print – another fine researcher whose work is still largely ignored, to the detriment of human health throughout the world.

Sugar – Pure, White And Deadly

In 1972 John Yudkin, a British professor of nutrition, wrote *Sweet and Dangerous*, another important milestone towards understanding the relationship between high-carbohydrate diets and degeneration. In it Yudkin examines the links between disease development, weight gain and sugar intake. Since then, a number of books on weight loss have appeared that all, in one way or another, make use of the low-carbohydrate diet, from *Dr Robert Atkins's Diet Revolution* and Herman Tarnower's *The Complete Scarsdale Medical Diet*, to *The Zone* by Barry Sears and *Protein Power* by Michael and Mary Dan Eades. Atkins is the most widely known and successful writer in the world about low-carbohydrate weight loss. He has been using low-carb diets in the treatment of tens of thousands of overweight patients, despite great opposition from the medical community – for he too has been continually attacked for what is considered his unconventional approach to the treatment of obesity. Yet Atkins has shown that 90 per cent of the time, overweight is the result of malfunction on a hormonal level which occurs when a person eats a high-carbohydrate diet over a long period.

Go For The Best

Each of the low-carb gurus has a slightly different approach. The one thing they have in common is that when it comes to weight loss, most of the low-carb diets work. But cutting carbohydrates just to lose weight, while continuing to eat convenience foods and ersatz breads, does not go far enough. Like a growing number of people who have tried one or more of these popular diets, I am not happy with the idea of filling my belly with cream, rich cheeses, fatty meats, phoney muffins and artificial sweeteners. I want low-carbohydrate nutrition that doesn't just restore my normal weight and proportion of lean body mass to fat. I want more. I want to eat in a way that improves my looks, regenerates my body and rejuvenates my brain, skin and flesh. And to achieve these goals, you need to go further and look deeper.

You need a way of eating and living that fulfills the criteria for optimal energy and well-being and breeds ongoing health, no matter what your age or condition when you begin it. You need to know how specific fatty acids can be used to enhance weight loss and improve overall metabolism, while balancing emotions and strengthening nails and hair. You need to find out about the newly discovered plant factors, which can not only help in regulating your body mass ratio, but also function as antioxidants and strengthen the immune sytem to prevent – even reverse – the ageing process. You need to make use of the power of life energy itself, carried in the enzymes of raw living foods. Finally, you need an approach to nutrition capable of raising your body to new levels of radiance and well-being.

Since, as they say, necessity is the mother of invention, and since I have always wrestled with a tendency to gain weight even on the very 'best' diets and lots of exercise regimes, I went looking for the very best. That is how the X Factor Diet came into being. Its power for transformation is virtually unlimited. But to understand how and why, we will need to go back to the future.

BACK TO THE FUTURE

There has long been a belief, even among scientists, that throughout the ages human beings have been vegetarian. Just where this notion came from I've never been quite sure. Countless studies in palaeopathology and archaeology show without doubt that our primitive ancestors – going back a million years and more – lived on a diet of flesh foods and fat, together with herbs, seeds, roots, berries and whatever fibre-rich vegetables and herbs they could gather.

Go Wild, Go Free

Scientists estimate that from 60 to 90 per cent of the calories paleolithic man and woman took in came in the form of large and small game animals, eggs, birds, reptiles and insects. Vegetables and grains were still in their wild form and had not been cultivated to create the starchy potatoes, rice and other crops we know today. An examination of these prehistoric hunter-gatherers' remains show that they had superb bone structure, flawless teeth and heavy musculature. And, whether our political and religious leanings like it or not, it's their protein-oriented, flesh-based diet that remains the healthiest for us. For it is on such a diet that the forces of natural selection have refined and moulded us to function best. To put it another way, we have been genetically programmed to eat this way for at least 100,000 years.

The physiology of the body has changed little over the millennia. We are still genetically adapted to wild foods, not to the refined and processed foods we now consume. A hard look at the skeletons of those early hunter-gatherers revealed that pre-agricultural people were not just robust, but about the same size as us. Their diet was three times higher in protein than ours and usually – although not always – lower in fat. Not only was their protein-to-carbohydrate ratio much lower than ours, their fibre intake was much higher – around 100g a day. The foods they were eating were, of course, fibre-rich, unprocessed and unrefined. Their calcium intake was also higher than ours, even though dairy products as we know them did not exist. They also managed to consume more potassium than we do, and their vitamin C intake, estimated at 400mg, was several times

'99.99 per cent of our genes were formed before the development of agriculture.'

DR. S. BOYD EATON, MD, MEDICAL ANTHROPOLOGIST

higher than our government-recommended daily requirement. And their intake of phyto-nutrients – the amazing plant factors, from flavonoids to carotenoids, that sport powerful antioxidant and immune-enhancing properties – was a whopping 300 times greater than ours. Even their ratio of polyunsaturated to saturated fat was different from ours. For the beasts they hunted, including small animals, birds, fish and insects, were themselves high in polyunsaturated fats – in marked contrast to the meat from grain-fed animals we eat now, which is full of saturated fat.

Come The Revolution

The agricultural revolution began some 10,000 years ago, although it did not peak until 2000 BC. Our art, craftsmanship, science and great religions would never have been possible without the high degree of urbanisation that growing grains and vegetable hybrids and domesticating livestock made possible. Collect people together en masse and you need to feed them within a small area. This meant relying heavily on carbohydrates – mostly in the form of starchy vegetables like potatoes, and cereal crops like rice and wheat, which came to be seen as 'the staff of life'. Gradually cereals, fruits, and starchy vegetables came to play a big part in human nutrition, and lifestyles became relatively sedentary. And our bodies suffered for it.

By 4000 years ago, when the agricultural revolution was in full swing, an enormous amount of degeneration had already taken place. Men and women had shrunk in height. Dental decay and malformation of the jaw had become widespread. Disease epidemics shortened the human lifespan. This moment in history marks the beginning of what we nowadays call the diseases of civilisation, including obesity. At the time, however, the growth of such distortions in human health were looked upon as evils sent by God rather than the consequence of a less-than-optimal diet. A few cultures even came to value the fat that grew on people's bodies – believing it to be a sign of abundance and power. It's hard to imagine a more different scenario from the healthy, nomadic ways of the ancient hunter-gatherers.

Secrets Of The Mayans

Anthropological studies carried out on the ancient Mayan Indians in what are now Mexico and Guatemala demonstrate just how costly, in terms of physique and health, the switch to an agricultural existence can be – especially for slaves and peasants who cannot afford to eat scarce flesh foods. During the early period of the Mayan civilisation, meat was plentiful. At that time the average male skeleton was 165 centimetres tall. Later on, as the availability of meat became limited and as agriculture developed, the height of the average male of the lower classes – now subsisting mainly on corn and beans – declined to 150 centimetres. Yet the stature of his ruling-class cousins, who could still afford to supplement their diet with animal protein, increased to 170 centimetres.

A Modern Look

In the 1930s, when Weston Price was travelling the world searching out peoples largely untouched by civilisation, his travels took him from the mountains of Switzerland to the plains of Africa and the frozen tundra of the Eskimos. Everywhere these isolated communities were living on primitive diets of natural, unrefined foods, and were free of chronic disease. Although the specific foods in them varied greatly from one area to another, all the diets had certain things in common.

Nearly all contained liberal quantities of protein from seafood, game, meats and dairy products. The people also believed foods played an important part in their diet and were essential for good health. They ate vegetables, legumes, nuts, seeds and whole grains, in a fresh, unrefined state. And every one of the diets boasted good quantities of raw foods – both of animal and vegetable origin. Price reported that those who consumed a high-protein diet showed virtually no dental decay and suffered little mental illness. Unlike 21st-century man with his heart disease, diabetes, arthritis and gout, these were sturdy, strong people who produced healthy children generation after generation. Throughout his travels Price had many opportunities of comparing the bone structure, general health and longevity of these isolated peoples in relation to the kinds of natural foods they ate. Those whose diets consisted largely of legumes and grains, although much healthier than modern men in cities and developed areas, nonetheless had more dental problems and were shorter and unhealthier than those whose diets centred around protein foods such as fish and meat, together with herbs and seeds and non-starchy vegetables.

Secrets Of The Cave Man

In the past two decades, Price's reports have been substantiated by studies of paleopathologists who have examined the remains of prehistoric peoples living in pre-agricultural times. They report that early human skulls were largely free of dental caries and abscesses – that is, until the advent of agriculture when the levels of carbohydrates they ate went up. After the agricultural revolution dental problems began to develop. So did bone problems and chronic illnesses.

So, gradually, the 'ideal' diet for human health has emerged, based on our biological inheritance and our genetic makeup. It is a diet higher in protein than the one we eat now and much lower in carbohydrate – a way of eating based on non-starchy, low-glycaemic carbohydrates (we'll hear more about this in later chapters), which do not readily cause insulin and blood sugar problems. It is also higher in vitamins and minerals, antioxidants, and other phyto-nutrients, with a ratio of the essential fatty acids omega-3 (found in fish and flaxseed) and omega-6 (found in sunflower and sesame seeds) very different from today's norm.

Genes change slowly – over many millennia. The forces of natural selection have been shaping and moulding our genetic makeup and biochemical functioning over thousands of centuries. We have only been exposed to large volumes of high-density carbohydrate foods like bread and rice for the last four thousand years. Anthropologist Kathleen Gordon at the Smithsonian Institute in Washington DC puts it rather well when she says, 'Not only was the agricultural "revolution" not really so revolutionary at its inception, it has also come to represent something of a nutritional "devolution" for much of mankind.'

The Way Forward

What does all of this mean in relation to our overall health and weight control? A lot. It means it is time to go back to the future. We need to make major shifts in both the ratio of proteins to carbohydrates and fats that we are taking, as well as the kinds of foods that we are eating. That is what the X Factor Diet does. It is this that enables a person using them to shed excess fat, heighten vitality, and look and feel great. Ketogenics and Insulin Balance give your body what it needs to make the changes – naturally. At the very core of natural health and healing you find the belief that when you provide the body with a diet and lifestyle to which it has been genetically adapted, you're giving it what it needs to restore balance where it's needed, as well as healthy form and harmony. To reap the greatest benefits of Ketogenics and Insulin Balance, it is important to understand the important roles that phyto-nutrients in fresh raw foods play in creating radiant health. We need to look at the major components of diet – the macronutrients – protein, carbohydrates and fats. We need to examine the optimal balance between these according to our genetic inheritance.

Before beginning either programme, there's essential information in the following chapters that I strongly urge you to follow. If you can't wait to start, then turn to Part Three and jump right in. Later you can go back, explore the whys and wherefores and delve into deeper issues.

PART TWO:
INSIDE STORY

COLOUR OF ENERGY

Both Ketogenics and Insulin Balance look to the source and origins of life to gather power for the life-transforming gifts they bring. These programmes not only make use of an optimal balance between the best proteins, carbohydrates and fats, based on the diet of our early ancestors. They also call on an abundance of immune-supporting, energy-enhancing, anti-ageing phyto-nutrients from fruit and vegetables. Finally, they draw on life energy itself carried in fresh, organic, raw foods. This is the one factor 21st-century nutrition has only just begun to quantify, but which natural health and healing have used since the beginning of time.

Bright Idea

Together, this creates an unbeatable combination for fat loss, and the highest levels of energy, well-being and protection from ageing. Later we'll be looking in depth at the macronutrients – proteins, carbs and fats – and the role they play. But first, let's explore the gifts that phyto-nutrients and life energy bring.

Remember the old saying, 'An apple a day keeps the doctor away'? Eat several portions of brightly coloured vegetables along with that apple and you'll be in the peak of health. Ketogenics and Insulin Balance show that the phyto-nutrients from vivid red, green, yellow and orange vegetables pave the way to optimum health. Why the rainbow hues? We'll find out a little later. In the meantime, we have some catching up to do – our paleolithic ancestors ate 300 times as many phyto-nutrients as we do today.

What exactly are these amazing substances? Everyone knows that fruits, vegetables and herbs are storehouses for vitamins and minerals – nutrients necessary for the healthy working of our bodies. But the contents of your salad crisper and fruit bowl also boast high levels of *phytochemicals* (*phyto* being Greek for 'plant'). Also known as *phyto-nutrients* or *nutriceuticals*, these microscopic powerhouses are not essential nutrients – we won't die if we don't manage to get them, or even experience symptoms of deficiency such as scurvy. They are, however, important active compounds that play a number of roles in the body – they may help regulate the immune system, stabilise vitamins in body tissues, or protect from serious illness.

In fact, eating substantial amounts of phyto-nutrients can stave off colon, breast and skin cancer, as well as slow the growth of cancerous cells. They are also being heralded as a way of helping to prevent macular degeneration, a loss of vision that can happen in middle age when sight-sensing cells in a region of the retina malfunction. And they help minimise the risk of developing heart disease and degenerative conditions associated with ageing, such as inflammation of the joints, loss of memory and concentration. Many scientists now believe they can slow the ageing process itself. In the following pages we'll be looking at a number of these wonder workers in detail.

Mysterious Plant Factors

In the early 1980s my daughter Susannah and I spent several years investigating the healing properties of raw foods – especially fresh fruit and vegetables. A diet rich in these foods has long been used to heal both acute illness and degenerative conditions and to rejuvenate the body. At that time we were aware that certain plant chemicals played an important part in our Raw Energy Diet, in which 50 to 75 per cent of food is eaten raw – particularly in the sometimes miraculous way it enhances health and beauty. At that time there was very little research on the health-enhancing properties of plant-based chemicals. So at the time we wrote *Raw Energy*, science could only partly explain why such a diet is so powerful a means of transforming health and good looks. Now, a lot of research later, we are beginning to understand more. While phytochemicals may not be essential nutrients, they are equally important. Without them you can survive, but it's unlikely that you will thrive.

Colour Has Clout

You don't have to look much further than your fridge or store cupboard to find many of these remarkable plant factors. Berries, citrus fruits, grapes, broccoli, cabbage, spinach, carrots, soy beans, red pepper, onions, garlic and tomatoes are packed with them. They also occur in spices and herbs – basil, oregano, parsley and mint, to name only a few. Phyto-nutrients are often grouped within the same plant, and act in tandem to heal the body at deep physiological and biochemical levels. You'll notice that nearly all of these fruit and veg blaze with colour. Colour is the key to content, in fact: the pigments actually contain the phyto-nutrients. In this context it's easy to see what's missing from the average Western diet of bland, manufactured, neutral-hued convenience foods. So when it comes to choosing fruits and vegetables, aim to pick a full spectrum, and get your phyto-nutrients at their source rather than from supplements.

Protect And Survive

How do phytochemicals interfere with, or block, specific disease processes? Some inhibit the enzymes which promote the development of diseases like cancer. Others clear our cells of toxic substances such as herbicides and pesticides we take in from our environment.

Still other phytochemicals protect us by acting as antioxidants and fighting free radicals. Free radicals are chemical compounds arising from sources of combustion – radiation, cars burning petrol, even the frying of food – which can damage cells and cause serious diseases and conditions such as cancer and damage to the arteries. Not long ago at Tufts University in the United States, scientists developed a method of quantifying the antioxidant power of specific fruits and vegetables by measuring their ability to quench free radicals in a laboratory test tube. In other words, they discovered how to test a food's *oxygen radical absorbance capacity*, known as the ORAC test. Scientists are now beginning to categorise a fruit or vegetable according to its overall antioxidant power. Fruits such as blueberries, blackberries, strawberries and raspberries are at the top of the list, along with vegetables like kale and spinach, Brussels sprouts and broccoli. I find it fascinating that all these foods are low-density, low-glycaemic fruits and vegetables as well. That means fruits and veg that don't turn into sugar in your bloodstream too quickly, and that are non-starchy.

Flavonoid Synergy

Berries, grapeseeds, cherries and citrus fruits are excellent sources of water-soluble phytochemicals known as flavonoids. Vegetables can be a good source too: green peppers, tomatoes, red and yellow onions and cucumbers are rich in them, and yams and buckwheat contain good quantities. Flavonoids guard the integrity of collagen within the body. Like many of the phyto-nutrients, they enhance the positive effects of the antioxidant vitamins A, C, E and betacarotene in the body, improving the function and condition of capillaries, the tiny blood vessels that deliver nutrients and oxygen to our cells. This not only raises overall energy, it also helps create smooth and elastic skin and protects against bruising, enhancing memory and improving eyesight. Many phytochemicals carry weird names like *catechin, quercetin* and *hesperidin*. Among the more than 20,000 known, hesperidin, rutin, quercetin, catechin and pycnogenol are especially important. Catechin reduces allergic reactions by calming histamine release in the body. Rutin helps guard the health of capillaries, veins and arteries as well as the skin itself.

Green Liberation

By now practically everybody has heard what a wonder broccoli is. This dark green vegetable is a treasurehouse of nutrients, including anti-tumour phytochemicals like sulforaphane, which encourages the formation of enzymes that have the ability to process and remove cancer-causing substances from our cells. Cauliflower, brussels sprouts, collard greens and kale, as well as other green vegetables, are all rich in sulforaphane.

Cabbage also has a bounty of phyto-nutrients, each with the ability to improve health and good looks in its own unique way. Take the isothiocynates – watercress is particularly rich in these. They inhibit the production of a group of highly destructive enzymes in the body known as Phase 1 enzymes, which change harmless chemical compounds into cancer-causing ones. Their presence also boosts the numbers of other enzymes, known as Phase 2 – intermediate compounds which can then be further broken down and bound to certain protein molecules that have the ability to escort them from the body to the kidneys or faeces. This helps reduce the level of cancer-causing chemicals in the body altogether.

In one animal study isothiocynates reduced the incidence of cancer by over a half when animals were exposed to the carcinogenic chemicals in cigarette smoke. Indoles, phytochemicals in turnips, cauliflower, broccoli, brussels sprouts and other vegetables, also encourage the activity of enzymes that break down harmful substances and minimise the risk of cancer.

Let's Pick Orange

Another main group of players in the plant-factor symphony is the carotenoids. These pigments are found in the protein complexes of brightly coloured fruits and vegetables, and include lutein, lycopene, alpha carotene, zeaxanthin and beta-carotene. Carotenoids live in green plant tissues as well, but in this case they tend to be covered by chlorophyll so that their presence only becomes evident after the green pigment has degraded – as it does when you cook the plant – or when it begins to die in the autumn. Carotenoids also bring natural colour to organisms which themselves do not produce them, such as salmon, lobster and shrimp. When such creatures are deprived of carotenoids from the plants which they normally ingest, they lose their wonderful colour. This is why the flesh of farmed salmon turns grey unless special carotenoids are added to the food.

A number of epidemiological studies have shown that the more we eat of fresh fruit and vegetables rich in carotenoids, the more our risk of cancer is diminished. Part of this is due to carotenoids' powerful antioxidant activity, which as we've seen protects the body from free radical damage. Scientists estimate that there are probably more than 600 naturally occurring carotenoids in our foods, making them the most widespread pigments found in nature.

Here are some of the ways carotenoids keep us healthy:

▨ They improve the flow of electrical or life energy from cell to cell in the body, enhancing what is known as *gap junction communication*. This means that small molecules bring nutrients to the cells with much greater ease.

- They have anti-tumour properties, helping to protect us from cancer and probably from many other degenerative illnesses as well.
- They act in the human body very much as they do in plant cells. They offer protection as a cellular screen against photo-oxidative damage from the sun as well as from other kinds of free radical damage. They also help protect the skin from ageing.
- A high intake of both beta-carotene and the other carotenoids is associated with a significantly reduced rate of skin cancer, lung cancer and cancer of the cervix.
- They intensify the protective properties of interferon, a protein that we make in our body partly to inhibit the replication of viruses.

The wider the variety of fruits and vegetables you eat, the greater will be the protective benefits from carotenoids. Eat more spinach and leafy greens such as silver beet, kale or collards, for instance, and you tap into a rich supply of zeaxanthin and lutein to protect the eyes and brain from degeneration.

The Eyes Have It

In one study of 356 older people reported in the *Journal of the American Medical Association*, research has discovered that when older people eat good quantities of leafy green vegetables – the equivalent of a large spinach salad each day – this reduces the risk of macular degeneration by 43 per cent. Another study published in the *Journal of Neuroscience* showed that eating a good portion of spinach each day delays the onset of age-related memory loss as well. Not only do leafy greens bring protection, broccoli and Brussels sprouts, rich in sulforaphane and indoles, help protect DNA from damage. Tomatoes, like many colourful fruits and vegetables, counter premature ageing too, thanks to their phyto-nutrient content.

Scientists estimate that of the 60 trillion cells in the human body, each one suffers 10,000 free radical 'hits' each day. And with rising levels of chemicals in our environment, it's getting worse. Phyto-nutrients help protect us from oxidation damage. So make friends with the colourful vegetable kingdom. Build your daily meals around them by eating salads, and by cooking them in ways that preserve as much of their innate life-enhancing properties as possible. Here are a few of the fruits and vegetables now being widely studied and praised for their powers. There are many more discoveries yet to come.

Sunlight Quanta

Just as important to weight loss as these amazing plant chemicals is the quality of life energy a plant carries. Our universe was born 15 billion years ago – an event the Russian-born physicist George Gamow christened the Big Bang in

1948. In a single moment, a titanic bestowal of free energy burst forth from a mix of particles compressed into a tiny volume. As this primeval mixture expanded and cooled, hydrogen, helium and lithium emerged, gradually condensed into gas clouds and, half a billion years later, formed the galaxies. In 1965 Arno Penzias and Robert Wilson measured the cosmic background radiation of the universe – and realised this was the afterglow of the Big Bang. Amazingly, this radiation from the moment of creation makes up almost all the light energy in the universe at this very moment.

Our sun is, of course, also emitting light and heat – radiant energy that has made life on earth possible. Not surprisingly, this energy has a direct, life-enhancing effect on us. The famous Swiss doctor Max Bircher-Benner, who early in the 20th century became famous for healing many 'incurable' diseases using high raw and all raw diets, dubbed this light energy *sunlight quanta* – 'quanta' being another name for energy units. And although the working of sunlight quanta remains a mystery, just as phytochemicals were 20 years ago, they play a central role both in weight loss and in healing and enhancing physical, mental and spiritual well-being. This life energy, which is destroyed when foods are cooked or processed, is the second powerful force in Ketogenics and Insulin Balance. Both programmes make use of lots of fresh, raw foods full of this ineffable yet powerful energy. Bircher-Benner's sunlight quanta bring *aliveness* to the body – yet defy chemical analysis.

So far, the world of nutrition has confined itself almost exclusively to the analysis of foods through chemistry. Few scientists have yet investigated the energetic influences of living foods on living bodies – something which can only be done with the help of high-level physics. When we eat fresh plants or animal foods from clean and healthy stock in their pristine, uncooked form, this special energy becomes part of our own physical make-up. Fresh, uncooked, organic foods impart to the body a high level of energetic and biochemical *order*. This living order increases our ability to resist illness, obesity and degeneration, or what one of the two great laws of physics – the second law of thermodynamics – refers to as *entropy*.

Phyto-nutrient-rich plants

Plant	Phyto-nutrients	Benefits
garlic and onions	*allyl sulfide (allicin)*	You will find potent antiviral and antibacterial properties in these vegetables. *Allicin* decreases the risk of stomach cancer and colon cancer, lowers LDL ('bad') cholesterol, encourages the production of glutathione S-transferase – an enzyme that helps eliminate cancer-causing toxins from the body. These foods also offer many more useful anti-ageing and health-promoting properties.
green leafy vegetables: spinach, turnip, beet tops, collard greens, kale; also in yellow marrows or squashes	*lutein*	A big-league carotene antioxidant which resides in the fatty pigments of plants, *lutein* keeps carcinogens from binding to DNA, and in doing so protects against degenerative diseases including eye diseases. It is the primary *carotenoid* present in the macula of the human retina. It also protects cells all over the body, including the skin, from premature ageing.
crucifers: broccoli, Brussels sprouts, cabbage, other leafy green vegetables	*indoles* *sulforaphanes*	*Indoles* prevent cancer-causing hormones from attaching to cells by increasing the body's supply of the enzymes that weaken cancer-producing xeno-oestrogens. They also eliminate toxins and enhance immunity. *Sulforaphanes* remove carcinogens from cells and, in animal studies, even slow cancer growth.

Plant	Phyto-nutrients	Benefits
soya products	*isoflavones such as genistein, saponins, and phytosterols*	*Isoflavones* – powerful antioxidants – protect against cancer, including breast cancer, and early ageing. In addition, *genistein* is a plant oestrogen which helps prevent dangerous chemical oestrogens from being taken up by the body's receptor sites. Among Japanese women who eat large quantities of soya-based products like tofu, the incidence of breast cancer is only one-fifth that of American women. *Saponins* enhance immune functions and bind to cholesterol, limiting its absorption into the intestines. *Phytosterols* in soya products lower elevated cholesterol.
tomatoes	*lycopene P-coumaric acid coumarins*	A carotenoid, of the same family as beta-carotene, *lycopene* is one of the most potent antioxidants of all. It has great antioxidant power. Where it is high in the diet, colon and bladder cancer are low. It also helps lower the risk of cardiovascular disease. *P-coumaric acid* (which you find in strawberries and peppers as well) inhibits the production of cancer-causing nitrosamines in the body. *Coumarins* reduce inflammation.

Plant	Phyto-nutrients	Benefits
citrus fruits: oranges, tangerines, grapefruits	*limonene* *glucarase*	*Limonene* increases the body's production of anti-cancer enzymes and enhances immunity. *Glucarase* inactivates cancer-causing degenerative chemicals that get into the body and eliminates them.
orange vegetables and fruits: mangoes, pumpkins, carrots, sweet potatoes, squash marrows	*alpha-carotene* *beta-carotene*	These vegetables get their colour from carotenes – antioxidants with a major capacity to boost general immunity and decrease the risk of many kinds of cancer as well as other degenerative diseases and premature ageing. (Other carotenoids in other foods such as *lycopene, lutein, zeaxanthin* and *cryptoxanthin* may be equally important or even more valuable.)
berries, red grapes, red wine, artichokes, yams	*polyphenols*	*Polyphenols* lower the risk of heart disease and flush out cancer-causing chemicals. This group of phytochemicals includes the *flavonoids*, which fight cell damage from oxidation, strengthen blood vessels, decrease the permeability of capillaries, protect the integrity of skin and improve the health of the eyes.

Plant	Phyto-nutrients	Benefits
flaxseed or linseed	*lignan precursors*	*Lignans* are *polyphenol* antioxidants. Linseed (or flaxseed) is chock-full of lignan precursors – chemicals the body turns into lignans through its metabolic processes. They help prevent cancers, including breast cancer, by binding to oestrogen receptor sites inhibiting oestrogen's cancer-producing activities. Flaxseeds are also an excellent source of omega-3 fatty acids, which are important for the production of hormones.

Life Is Unique

Entropy is a word used in physics to describe the measure of the disorder at atomic levels which takes place as energy is degraded in any living or non-living system. According to the laws of physics, in each system of the universe, all motion eventually comes to a standstill where differences in electrical or chemical potential are equalised and temperatures become uniform by heat conduction until finally a permanent state is reached where the whole system fades until it becomes an inert lump of matter. This state of thermodynamic equilibrium is what physicists call *maximum entropy*.

What makes living systems unique is that, so long as our body is alive, it avoids decaying into this inert state of equilibrium through metabolism – eating, drinking and assimilating energy from the outside.

The Austrian physicist and Nobel laureate, Erwin Schrödinger, puts it rather well – although in terms that the nutritional world still tends to ignore:

'What then is that precious something contained in our food which keeps us from death? That is easily answered. Every process, event, happening – call it what you will – in a word, everything that is going on in Nature means an increase of the entropy in the part of the world where it is going on. Thus a living organism continually increases its entropy – or, as you may say, produces positive entropy – and thus tends to approach the dangerous state of maximum entropy, which is death. It can only keep aloof from it, i.e. alive, by continually drawing from its environment negative entropy...What an organism feeds upon is negative entropy...which is in itself a measure of order. The device by which an organism maintains itself stationary at a fairly high level of orderliness (= a fairly low level of entropy) really consists in continually sucking order from the environment.'

So, to stay healthy the body has to quite literally 'drink order'! When you include plenty of fresh, raw foods in your diet, in effect you are drinking this energetic order from living foods. And that, in turn, implants energetic order into your own living system.

We need to eat fresh, living matter which not only carries the highest-quality nutrition from a chemical perspective, but in which the sunlight quanta – that light energy at the basis of the universe – has not been debased by oxidization, spoiling, processing or cooking.

Thanks to the phyto-nutrients and sunlight quanta in fresh foods, the X Factor Diet can take you to places of energy, radiant health and well-being that you may have longed for but not known how to reach. Our bodies need to live by the genetic rules we've evolved by. And to stay fully alive we also need to eat the right kinds and balance of the macronutrients – protein, carbohydrates and fats – and to stay active and on the move.

CARBS IN CLOSE-UP

In the scientific context, carbohydrates are just organic compounds made of carbon, hydrogen and oxygen. Ideally – that is, if in a beneficial form and eaten by someone who's young and healthy – they're turned into glucose to supply fuel for most of the organs of the body. But throughout the history of human civilisation, as we've seen, carbohydrates have been manipulated, used and abused in a number of ways, all of them pointing down a road that ends in premature ageing, physical degeneration and obesity. In this chapter we'll be taking a much closer look at how carbs came to this pass.

The Dope On Carbs

Nutritionists divide carbohydrates into two categories – simple and complex – despite the fact that all of them are made up of simple sugars called monosaccharides: fructose, glucose and galactose. Monosaccharides, in turn, link together into chains of two called disaccharides and then into longer chains called polysaccharides or simple starches, which can contain hundreds of thousands of glucose molecules.

Simple carbohydrates are also called 'refined' carbohydrates. These include not only sugar, honey and other obviously sweet foods, but snack foods like breads, as well as any form of sweetener which, digested and assimilated quickly, leads to a rapid increase in insulin and blood sugar. Complex carbohydrates are made up of more complicated sugars and starches as well as various types of fibre. These include whole-grain breads and cereals, brown rice, some vegetables, beans and legumes, and certain fruits like apples and berries. Complex carbohydrates are richer in fibre than their simple cousins, so your body assimilates them more slowly. They cause a more moderate insulin and glucose response and – provided you do not eat too many of them – help protect from high insulin levels, energy swings and Syndrome X. But simple or complex, all the carbohydrates you eat get into your bloodstream as glucose and raise your blood-sugar levels. Each gram of dietary carbohydrate from your foods appears in the bloodstream as 1g of glucose. As we've seen, in healthy people, glucose can either be burned right away for energy or stored as glycogen – a longer chain of glucose molecules that's stored in the muscles or the liver for you to use later. But if you're eating more carb-rich foods than your metabolism can use as energy, the glucose in your blood can be converted into fat in your liver, or shunted directly into the fat cells to make you fatter.

Meet The Glycaemics

To make matters even more complicated, carbohydrates are not only separated into complex and simple carbohydrates, they are also categorised according to their *glycaemic index* (GI). The GI is a measure of just how much a specific carbohydrate food will raise your blood glucose level, and how fast. A food's glycaemic rating will tell you whether it will cause a sharp rise in blood sugar and insulin levels, or whether it will enter your bloodstream more gradually. What might surprise you is that foods with a high GI – which you want to avoid – include not only honey and table sugar, but all sorts of snack foods like corn chips, breakfast cereals and most grain products such as bread (both wholewheat and refined white) and pasta. Finally, to make it even more complicated, it is not only the *kind* of carbohydrates we consume that affects insulin and blood sugar, but also how much fibre we take in and how much protein we eat at the same meal.

But while it sounds convoluted, eating in this way is not as difficult as you might imagine, especially when you go back to first principles and ask those same old questions: 'What did our ancestors eat?' and 'How can we adjust our own diet to supply the *kind* of carbohydrates, in the *quantities* and *balance* to support our genetic inheritance, enhance our health, and restore normal weight and body composition?'

Golden Oldies

In the light of all this, let's take another look at prehistoric eating habits. Their carbohydrates came from wild herbs and vegetables that they gathered by foraging. These plants bore little resemblance to the highly cultivated vegetables and fruits that we eat today. They were more like kale and silverbeet, a leafy green vegetable similar to spinach which few people eat now. Our ancestors ate little fruit. In the northern latitudes it was virtually never eaten – except for very small and wild fruits which looked more like rosehips than those on our supermarket shelves. The plants our ancestors ate had much more fibre than our modern plants do, so paleolithic humans ate about five times more fibre a day than we do.

There's a lot to be said for fibre. First, foods high in fibre take time to eat and demand a lot of chewing. This in itself gives a sense of satisfaction and fullness which we don't get from eating refined carb convenience foods. Fibre also slows the digestion of plant starches and buffers the sugars they contain. In this way, fibre-rich foods help minimise sharp rises in glucose and insulin. Virtually all of the paleolithic plant foods were fibre-rich. Our early ancestors rarely ate grains or cereals, which in any case were gathered from wild grasses and other plants and bore little resemblance to today's top-heavy, carb-rich cultivated varieties.

Today, most convenience foods are manufactured from grains in highly refined form. They are shunted into the bloodstream very quickly, and can, as we've seen, wreak havoc with our insulin and blood-sugar levels, producing peaks and troughs of energy, cravings, chronic fatigue, insulin problems and weight-gain.

Goodbye Fibre

What's the inside story on the agricultural revolution? As you'll recall, around 10,000 years ago human beings started to eat foods much higher in carbohydrate, like legumes and whole grains, as they shifted away from a high-protein diet. This switch of emphasis from protein to carbohydrate compromised human health. Once the agricultural revolution was in full swing, people began using grinding stones to grind their grains into flour. This was the beginning of food processing. The basic technique made a big leap forward (or backward, depending on how you look at it) in mid-19th-century Europe, with the introduction of roller milling. Before that, only aristocrats ate fibre-stripped white flour, for it was very labour-intensive to produce. After all, some peasant had to sit with a winnowing basket tossing the ground flour into the air to separate out the bran from the white stuff.

With the introduction of roller milling, it became easier and cheaper to produce large quantities of white flour. The steel roller mill refined wholewheat grains and sugar cane quickly and cheaply. These white products produced from refining held a fascination for the masses. They were not only pleasant to taste, they also had cachet. As people began consuming more carbohydrates and as these carbs became ever more processed, the degenerative conditions of the rich and the royals, such as heart disease, diabetes and obesity, began to spread.

Refined flours obviously have most of their fibre stripped out. We've already met T.L. Cleave, the researcher who devised the 'rule of 20 years' to chart the spread of disease that follows a culture's introduction to a high-carb diet. Cleave also recognised the importance of fibre in the diet, and his work in the 1970s almost singlehandedly changed attitudes to it. Until then, fibre was something considered to be of no nutritional value whatsoever simply because the body does not burn it as calories. After Cleave published his discoveries, the medical community began to recognise that fibre plays an important role in protecting the body against degenerative illnesses such as colon cancer and diverticulitis.

Steps Towards Degeneration

In the wake of Cleave's work, the British medical researchers Dennis Burkitt and Hugh Trowell carried out their own extensive studies. Burkitt and Trowell carefully documented the exact sequence of events that happens when a people switch from a hunter-gatherer style diet to the typical Western one. Most all of these changes revolve around shifts in the kind and ratio of carbohydrates eaten:

- **Stage 1:** The primitive unprocessed diet of plant eaters complete with large quantities of unprocessed wild low glycaemic carbohydrates and whole foods is eaten. There are very few examples of degenerative disease.
- **Stage 2:** The Western diet is introduced, including refined and high-glycaemic carbohydrates. Obesity and diabetes become common among privileged groups able to afford foods of commerce.
- **Stage 3:** Diet becomes moderately Westernised. Obesity becomes more widespread, as do constipation, haemorrhoids, varicose veins and appendicitis.
- **Stage 4:** The Western diet is now widespread. Excess weight and obesity are common in all social groups. So is heart disease, high blood pressure, diverticular disease, hiatus hernia, cancer and other Western diseases.

Enter Food Manufacturing

For more than half a century, food manufacturers intent on making profit have been producing a great variety of palatable foods by fragmenting and reducing the raw materials of food – grains and seeds, fats and sugars, vegetables and legumes – to simple 'nuts and bolts' – the chemical compounds and substances they are made up of. These nuts and bolts are then whipped up into the manufactured convenience foods that we find on our supermarket shelves – from meals ready to eat in a minute, to candy bars, cakes, breads and cereals – in short, the stuff that makes up some 75 per cent of what people eat these days. White flour- and sugar-based convenience foods full of denatured fats have an ultralong shelf life, which suits food purveyors intent on making a profit. Yet convenience foods are really junk food, often devoid of any nutritional value other than calories. The processed fats they contain, along with the masses of artificial chemicals used as flavourings, colourings and preservatives, are far removed from the foods we genetically need for health. It is little wonder many human beings today – even those in economically privileged countries – do little more than survive.

As far back as the 1930s health professionals had begun to notice that people who used white bread as a staple in their diet tended to suffer from conditions related to nutritional deficiencies – especially a lack of vitamin B1,

B2, B3, calcium and iron. This led to governments insisting that white bread be 'enriched' – namely, that some of the nutrients lost in refining flours had to be added back before the bread was baked. Except the nutrients that were added back were vastly inferior to the nutrients lost in the processing. For example, calcium was added to white bread in the form of chalk, which the body cannot absorb. The synergy of nutrients characteristic of natural, unrefined foods – where the way the whole works together is greater than the sum of its nutrient parts – had also been destroyed. You cannot take one, two, three or four nutrients lost in processing and expect, by adding them back, to restore real nutritional value to a food.

Sweet Hell
Take sugar – a highly refined substance which provides nothing but empty calories. We in the so-called civilised world eat between 150 and 200 pounds of the stuff per head per year. Both sugar and white flour are devoid of magnesium, chromium and zinc. These three minerals are absolutely essential if your body is to be able to process carbohydrate foods properly. When you do not have adequate levels of these three, insulin resistance, obesity and degenerative diseases develop at an accelerated rate. The more industrialised and commercial in orientation our societies become, the more processed carbohydrates we eat. And the more processed carbohydrates we eat, the more our blood sugar and insulin levels get screwed up.

Tinned vegetables raise insulin and blood sugar more than fresh vegetables do. Concentrated fruit juices raise insulin and blood sugar more than fresh fruit does. Ever since paleolithic times, our carbohydrates have become increasingly *dense*. This means that our foods have more and more grams of carbohydrate per serving in them and less and less fibre, as well as lower levels of some essential nutrients. All of these changes have played a central role in the widespread development of obesity and the rise of Syndrome X. All of these issues need to be addressed if you are going to shed excess fat from your body forever and improve your overall health. Let's take a closer look at glycaemics and carbohydrate density, as well as dietary fibre, all of which play an important role in encouraging fat loss and enhancing health.

GOOD, BAD AND UGLY

A major ally in combating Syndrome X is the glycaemic index. The GI, the result of many years of research, is a rating system for carbohydrates that enables you to choose the foods which offer a gradual conversion into glucose. In doing so, you help your body release insulin more slowly and keep your levels of insulin lower. And the benefits are enormous. Once you improve insulin control using the GI, you help burn away body fat, reduce serum cholesterol, prevent and even reverse hypertension, improve your overall health and increase your energy. Good glycaemic control also slows the formation of cross-linking collagen in the skin – which causes wrinkles and discourages free radical damage, so that you age more slowly.

Health By Numbers

This is how it works. The index is a long list of different carbohydrate foods, all given a numeric value ranging from 0 to 150. Each value shows the rise in blood sugar in a healthy person after eating a measured amount of the food in question. Just to complicate matters, there are two standard glycaemic indexes. One, the glucose-standard index, assigns a value to glucose of 100 on the glycaemic table. The other assigns a value of 100 to white bread. It doesn't matter very much which of the two standards you work with, because the values are only relative – and that's what makes them valuable for our purposes. For instance, on the chart where the GI of glucose is 100, the GI of brown rice is 50, so you'll know that eating brown rice produces only half the rise in your blood sugar that glucose does.

How Low Can You Go?

The lower the glycaemic rating of a carbohydrate, the more desirable will be your body's glucose and insulin responses to that food. Eating foods high on the index are more likely to create blood sugar problems and insulin resistance. These are the foods you'll want to eliminate from your diet by following either Ketogenics or Insulin Balance. After normal weight is established, you will want to eat them, if at all, only very occasionally. Your diet should always emphasise foods with a moderate to low rating on the index to help protect you against obesity and premature ageing.

Getting fat starts with eating high GI foods – refined bread, potatoes, cakes and candies, cereals and sugars. These foods all cause rapid glucose absorption, raising insulin and blood sugar levels, and screwing up blood fats. They also boost levels of adrenalin. Researchers have found that after eating these foods, teenagers frequently demonstrate bingeing behaviour – the result of insulin spikes, carb cravings and adrenal stimulation, all of which trigger an increase in appetite.

Low Glycaemic Diet Regulates Lipid Metabolism And Fat Distribution

Slightly overweight men were allocated to either a low glycaemic index diet or a high glycaemic index diet for five weeks. These men were then crossed over in the double-blind study. The low glycaemic index diet induced:

- **Lower post-prandial glucose**
- **Lower area under the curve for glucose**
- **No change in body weight**
- **Total fat mass decreased by 500g (mostly abdominal)**
- **Lower total plasma cholesterol**
- **Lower area under the curve for triglycerides**

Bouche C. *et.al.* American Diabetes Association 60th Scientific Session June 9-13, 2000.

Don't Be Deceived

When you first come upon the GI, you might be inclined to conclude that all refined, or simple, carbohydrates have a high GI, while complex carbohydrates – the so-called natural foods like whole-grain breads and rice – have a low GI. This is not actually true. Some vegetables such as carrots and potatoes have an amazingly high GI. They produce a more rapid rise in blood glucose than ordinary table sugar. Almost as surprising is the fact that certain simple sugars like fructose – found in fruit – are lower on the index than a number of common grains, vegetables and legumes. That doesn't mean that you should eat masses of fructose. For although fructose is low on the index, it can still encourage fat storage. Consuming a great deal of fructose has also been shown to have a number of other degenerative effects on the body, including an increase in oxidation damage and the cross-linking of collagen. In case you are in the habit of having a glass of orange juice between meals, it would be wise to go for a cup of herbal tea instead.

The Low Down

Low glycaemic foods are the ones to make good use of when following either programme in the X Factor Diet – Ketogenics or Insulin Balance. These include all of the non-starchy vegetables like broccoli, cauliflower, courgettes, tomatoes, celery, sprouts, spinach and other leafy greens. Foods which are fundamentally protein or fundamentally fats, such as butter and meat or fish, are not even rated on the GI as they are virtually devoid of carbohydrate. As such, they are excellent foods for both programmes.

Glycaemic Index of Common Foods Using Glucose as the Standard Of Comparison

Food	GI	Food	GI
Glucose	100	Potato crisps	51
Baked potato	98	Green peas	51
Cooked carrots	92	Ice cream	50
Honey	92	Whole-grain cereal	44
Instant white rice	91	100% whole-grain rye bread	42
Cornflakes	84	Pasta	41
White bread	72	Apples	39
Bagels	72	Tomatoes	28
Mashed potatoes	70	Plain yoghurt	38
Whole-wheat bread	69	Chickpeas	36
Table sugar	64	Skimmed milk	32
Beetroot	64	Strawberries	32
Raisins	61	Kidney beans	29
Oatmeal	61	Peaches	26
Pita bread	57	Cherries	24
Popcorn	55	Fructose	20
Buckwheat	54	Soya beans	15
Banana	53	Peanuts	13

Ketogenics emphasises foods which have a rating of less than 20 on the glucose-standard GI – from red-leaved rucola, cos lettuce and romaine to spinach, kale, endive, collard greens, beet greens, cabbage and bok choy, as well as alfalfa sprouts, broccoli, Brussels sprouts, cauliflower, celery, green beans, mushrooms, courgettes and turnips, as well as herbs like oregano, parsley, sage, mint, onion, fennel and dill. Their low GI makes them especially valuable for shedding excess fat from your body. When following Insulin Balance, you can use the glucose-standard GI to choose foods with a rating of 60 or lower. These include chickpeas, apples, strawberries, whole-grain rye bread, pasta, plain yoghurt and pinto beans.

If ever you find yourself eating foods that are too high on the GI you can, in part, mitigate their effect on your insulin and blood sugar levels by eating only small amounts of them, and making sure that you eat them with proteins, fats and plenty of fibre. These three help buffer the glucose-elevating effect to some degree. So long as you want to shed fat from your body, avoid high glycaemics altogether. And never assume that just because you find something in a health food store, or because a food is labelled 'natural', that it is necessarily going to be healthy. Most snacks you find displayed as 'healthy' contain foods like honey and grains, which have a GI that's far too high to benefit your health or your efforts to lose weight. By now many studies have shown that a simple shift towards eating foods low on the GI improves both insulin functions and glucose tolerance. You will find a useful list of foods on page 56 which you can follow in selecting the best carbs.

Dense Carbs, No Way

To make things even more complicated, there are quite a few foods that don't rank too badly on the GI, yet which should be avoided, especially when following Ketogenics. These include some whole-grain cereals and certain starchy vegetables. Although they do not cause the rapid rise in blood sugar and insulin that really high glycaemic foods do, they can be *carbohydrate dense.* Carbohydrate density is a measure of useable carbohydrates – the amount of digestible carbohydrates calculated from the total carbohydrate content of food, which includes fibre. The equation looks like this: total carbohydrate content minus fibre equals carbohydrate density (TC – F = CD). When you eat too many carbohydrate dense foods this also encourages the production of high levels of insulin, speeds up weight gain and increases carbohydrate cravings. Again, to avoid these things it is important to eat mainly low carbohydrate dense foods like non-starchy vegetables and fruits such as strawberries and pink grapefruits.

Carbohydrate density of common foods

Food	Serving Size	Carbohydrate Density in Grams (Usable Carbohydrate)	Total Carbohydrate in Grams	Fibre
Baked potato with skin	10 x 5 cm	47	51	4
Low-fat yoghurt with fruit	1 cup	43	43	<0
Chickpeas (cooked)	1 cup	35	45	10
Cornflakes	28 g	24.9	25.2	0.3
Banana	15cm	24.8	27.6	2.8
Tomato sauce	1 cup	14	18	4
Milk	1 cup	11	11	<1g
Blackberries (raw)	1 cup	10.7	18.3	7.6
Tomatoes	1 cup	6	8	2
Brussel sprouts (raw)	1 cup	4.5	7.8	3.3
Carrots (raw)	1 medium	4.4	6.2	1.8
Whole almonds	28 g	4	6	2
Cauliflower (raw)	1 cup	2.7	5.2.	2.5
Celery (diced)	1 cup	2.3	4.3	2.0
Chinese cabbage	1 cup	.3	3	2.7

Generally speaking, the more carbohydrate dense foods you eat – that is, legumes, whole grains and starchy vegetables – the more insulin you will produce. The more insulin you produce, the more weight you will tend to gain – particularly if you have any genetic tendency to store energy as fat in your body (see Do you have the thrifty gene?, page 24). By contrast, low carbohydrate dense vegetables like broccoli, spinach and Chinese leaves have 4 to 10 times less carbohydrate than grain-based foods, legumes and starchy vegetables. That means you can eat a lot of low carbohydrate dense foods without having to wrestle with insulin-related health problems. Carbohydrate density is equal to the amount of usable carbohydrate a food contains. Above is a listing of many common foods giving their carb density. Usually, the best carbs rate low on both the GI and the carbohydrate density scale.

Fruits generally rank lower on the GI and are lower in carbohydrate density than most starchy vegetables, whole grains and legumes. But not all fruits. Fruit juices, for instance, dried fruits and bananas have high GIs and are carb dense too. You will want to avoid these. In any case, on either Ketogenics or Insulin Balance, while you are losing weight, limit fruits drastically – even cut them out altogether for a time.

All this might seem a lot to take on at first – in fact, enough to make your head spin. But don't worry. When you get to Part Three you will find lists of 'good' and 'poor' carbs that are easy to follow. What is particularly important to understand is just how drastically the kind of carbohydrates we now eat have deviated from what out bodies need for high-level health and leanness.

Fibre Matters

We got an inkling of how important fibre is in the last chapter. Dietary fibre does play a special role in weight loss and health. Made up of the components in plant cells and cell walls which are not broken down by digestive enzymes, fibre is by no means one single substance. It is made up of many different ones – cellulose and hemicellulose, pectin, lignins, gums and mucillages, as well as the polysaccharides found in algae and seaweeds. Except for lignins, all the components of fibre are considered carbohydrates. But they are carbohydrates with a difference – they pass through your body without yielding energy.

Good quantities of fibre in your diet improve insulin and glucose responses. Regardless of whatever total carbohydrates you are eating, a high-fibre diet improves blood glucose control as well. The soluble fibres act favourably on insulin concentrations in the blood. This is not only because they slow down the rate at which the stomach empties and therefore the rate at which glucose is absorbed, but also because they inhibit the degradation of starch in the small intestine. A plant food may contain many kinds of fibre all in different proportions. A typical plant fibre, for instance, can have 45 per cent polysaccharides, 35 per cent cellulose, 17 per cent of the woody lignins, 3 per cent protein and 2 per cent mineral ash. Each component exerts a different positive health-promoting and lean-preserving effect on your body.

Psyllium husks are fine for adding fibre on Ketogenics. To get the right amount of fibre on Insulin Balance, use psyllium husks or flaxseeds. Best of all would be a good mixture of rice bran, beet fibre, oat fibre, apple juice and cellulose, but be sure to get one with no sweeteners added, and read labels carefully looking for hidden carbs. You may also find you want to add extra fibre to your protein drinks both on Ketogenics and Insulin Balance.

The convenience foods that fill our supermarkets are extremely low in fibre. We all need more of it. High-fibre foods even help alter brain chemistry in a positive way to stabilise emotions and bring a pervading sense of calm. Eat plenty of them.

PROTEIN POWER

When it comes to shedding excess fat, transforming the texture of your skin, slowing down the ageing process, and enhancing overall health, no food is more important than protein. The word protein itself comes from the Greek *proto*, meaning 'holding the first place'. And it is essential for life. But the 19th-century Swedish chemist Jacob Berzelius, who coined the term, actually named protein after the Greek sea god Proteus.

Lean And Lively

Proteus, of course, had the ability to change shape to suit any occasion, and this is exactly what eating the right kind of protein in the right balance will do for your body. The trouble is, very few people – including some who are considered the 'experts' in nutrition – know much about what kind of protein works and what doesn't. So bear with me while we look at this remarkable macronutrient. What you learn may transform not only the way you look and feel, but your whole experience of power and energy on a mental, emotional and spiritual level too.

The single most important *biomarker of ageing* – the measurement by which an expert in physiology determines your biological (as opposed to chronological) age – is your *lean body mass to fat ratio*. Your body is made up of two basic components: lean body weight, which is basically your muscle tissue, bones, nerves, tendons, circulatory system, ligaments, skin and all your organs; and fat.

Lean body weight is also referred to as lean body mass. Your lean body mass demands oxygen. It uses nutrients from your food, it moves, grows and repairs itself. Paleolithic humans had a very high percentage of lean body mass to fat, much like wild animals today. This is what gave these early people their ease of movement, stamina, and firm, sleek bodies. That is what gives wild animals and young, healthy human beings their vitality and power. And – this is stunning news – the key to aliveness in any body, no matter what its age – lies not just in burning excess fat but also in increasing your lean body mass. More specifically, it means increasing muscle. For your muscle is the engine which turns calories from food into energy. Muscle tissue also burns fat, as we'll see later on. And it creates feelings of simple joy in movement, supplying life energy for you to think, to move and to feel. The power of the horse, the rhythmical gait of the wolf, able to run on and on with ease, the wild playfulness of the dolphin – all these depend on good strong muscle. So does your ability as a human being to experience passion and excitement in your life. A good lean body mass to fat ratio helps prevent the decline in hormones which limit sexual drive and the intensity of orgasm as people get older. Enhance the quality of your muscle and you enhance the vitality of your whole body. And remember: every molecule of muscle in your body is made from the proteins you eat.

Protein For Transformation

Half the dry weight of your body – that is, when water is removed – is protein. Of this, one-third lies in the muscles, one-fifth in the bone and cartilage, one-tenth in the skin and the rest in your blood, body fluids and tissue. Your brain cells, your genes and the haemoglobin which transports oxygen throughout your body are all made from protein. So are the thousands of enzymes which orchestrate your body's metabolic functions – from the growth of nails and hair to the digestion and assimilation of the foods you eat. And, like Proteus, no protein structures in your body are fixed. Each is constantly being broken down and reshaped. In fact, the whole structure of your body is continually rebuilt, day by day, entirely from the proteins you eat. Ninety-eight per cent of your body's molecules, including your teeth and bones, organs and muscles, are replaced each year. You've grown a new skin just within the last month. Within the last three months, you have received a whole new blood supply. And within the last six months, just about every molecule of protein in your muscle has been replaced. What is exciting about all this is that, when you shift your protein consumption to better quantities and quality, you can completely transform, regenerate, and rejuvenate not only the way your body functions, but also the way it looks.

Unique Stuff

Protein is unique among the three macronutrients. Unlike fats and carbohydrates, the chemical structure of protein not only includes the elements carbon, hydrogen and oxygen, but also nitrogen. In fact, the content of nitrogen is the key element in determining the crude protein content of foods. Experts calculate protein content by multiplying the number of nitrogen atoms in a food by 6.25. This figure is based on an average nitrogen content in protein of 16 per cent.

Talking about protein is misleading, in a sense: it's actually a kind of umbrella term used to describe 22 biological compounds called amino acids. Because your body has the ability to synthesise 13 of these, the remaining eight are generally considered *essential amino acids* – meaning we must get them from what we eat. These eight are called isoleucine, leucine, lysine, methionine, phenylalanine, threonine, tryptophan and valine. (Two extra amino acids, arginine and histidine, are considered essential for human infants and animals.)

So where are all these essential amino acids found? Meat, primarily, although mixing together some vegetables and grains can also provide the full spectrum of them, allowing our bodies to build new proteins.

Only it's not quite as simple as this. It is time to lay aside the notion of essential and non-essential amino acids because, although your body can turn non-essential amino acids into essential ones, it can do so only if there are enough of the specific amino acids needed. High-quality proteins – the kind of proteins you need to grow a lean, powerful body – are found in foods which offer not only the essential amino acids but good quantities of the rest as well. That cyberworld saying, 'Garbage in, garbage out,' is absolutely true when applied to protein foods. For your body cannot build a strong immune system, blood, skin and muscle if you are not supplying it with proteins of the very highest biological value.

Make Way For The Good
Most of the existing books and government guidelines about protein are dinosaurs. Two officially accepted terms for measuring protein quality, the Protein Equivalency Ratio (PER), a measure of growth, and the Net Protein Utilisation Index (NPU), a measure of nitrogen retained in the body, still appear in numerous articles, but they're based on an obsolete science which depends on how much protein you *eat* rather than the amount of protein you *absorb*. The biochemist Michael Colgan, a nutritional expert in sports medicine, puts it rather well. He says, 'relying on the obsolete science of the amount of protein consumed, rather than the amount of protein absorbed, they are about as accurate at assessing human needs as the Victorian practice of phrenology (feeling the bumps on your skull)'. The reason these measurements are still around, by the way, is that the meat marketing industry keeps pushing them as a way of trying to convince people that meat is a high-quality source of protein, and that we should eat more of it.

The only measure of protein quality worth paying attention to is Biological Value (BV). This determines the amount of protein actually *retained* within your body per gram of protein you absorb. The BV measurement was developed a long time ago when eggs were still believed to be the highest biologically assimilable protein in the world and were therefore rated at 100 per cent. Within the last 20 years, thanks to some pretty remarkable, health-oriented developments in food technology, a number of microfiltered whey products and whey peptide blends with biological values higher than a whole egg have appeared on the market.

The development of microfiltered whey proteins has rendered the whole concept of BV percentages meaningless. However, while percentages may be meaningless, the biological value measurements still work. If we retain a BV of 100 for a whole egg, the BV of lactalbumin, a form of microfiltered whey protein, would be 104 and the BV of the whey peptide blends vary from 110 to 159. Here is a chart of the BV of common dietary proteins.

BIOLOGICAL VALUE (BV) OF COMMON PROTEINS

Whey Peptide blends and microfiltered whey	110-159
Lactalbumin (whey protein concentrate)	104
Egg	100
Cows milk	91
Egg white (albumin)	88
Beef	80
Fish	79
Chicken	79
Soya	74
Rice	59
Beans	49

Protein Denatures

It may surprise you to see that meat and fish, which we've always been told are the top-quality proteins, are rated much lower on the BV scale than many other protein sources. There are a number of reasons for this. First of all, the BV of meat, fish and other common protein foods is measured in these foods after they have been *cooked.* When proteins are heated, some of their amino acids become so *denatured* – changed in their molecular structure – that they're useless, since the digestive enzymes in the gut have difficulty processing them onwards. A few amino acids can even be destroyed by cooking. Grill a steak at 239° F, and the amino acids cystine and lysine are lost. Glutamine, one of the important amino acids in the prevention of arthritis and the regulation of appetite, can also be destroyed by heat. There is evidence that cooked milk proteins, as well as cooked meat, poultry and egg proteins, can chemically bind with vital nutrients too, making them unavailable for use by the body in building the new protein molecules it needs. The meat, game, shellfish and small insects paleolithic humans ate were nearly all uncooked, so the BV of those proteins was much higher than those of the animal sources of protein we eat now.

Look To The Ancestors

Our distant ancestors ate varying amounts of protein, depending upon the region they lived in and the season. On average, they consumed about 35 per cent of their total diet as protein. This is almost three times the amount the average person eats today. The wild animals hunted by paleolithic people moved freely about, eating an enormous variety of grasses and herbs – a very different life compared to that of our domestic animals, which are kept in pens and fattened for market. So the meat eaten by our ancestors was much higher in muscle, and significantly lower in both total fat and saturated fat content than the meats that we eat today. Along with lakefish and shellfish, which many early humans ate in large quantities, these meats were also very rich in omega-3 fats, healthy fatty acids that protect against insulin resistance, heart disease, obesity and Syndrome X.

All Change

When agriculture kicked in and our ancestors began to eat more cultivated foods – grains and cereals, as well as higher carbohydrate vegetables – their protein intake decreased. With this decrease came the upsurge in bone malformations, osteoporosis, tooth decay and heart disease we have looked at. In ancient Egypt, for instance, the spread of the high-carbohydrate, low-protein diet led to a marked increase in early-onset cardiovascular disease.

Yet in the West, cardiovascular disease, diabetes and other degenerative diseases were still uncommon at the start of the 20th century because about 30 per cent of the average diet came from dairy products, meat and eggs. Half the population of North America lived on farms and raised domestic animals for food. These chickens, pigs, cattle and sheep were given no hormones or chemicals to fatten them. They were simply put out to pasture and left to graze. So at the turn of that century, Westerners were eating more or less the same type of protein as their paleolithic ancestors, except that the meats were not as lean or as rich in omega 3 fatty acids. The other difference was dairy products – cheese-making was not a skill of ancient humans. But both groups fished in lakes, rivers and the sea, and both hunted for wild game.

It Gets Worse

Before long, however, farmers began to fatten their livestock on soya beans and corn instead of letting them graze on natural grasses. The problem with this practice is that some grasses contain high levels of beneficial omega-3 fatty acid, while corn and soya beans are high in carbohydrates and the less healthy omega-6 fatty acid. Nor were the animals allowed to roam as widely as before. The decrease in exercise and grain-based diet made them grow fat and significantly altered the quality of protein and the fatty acid profile of their meat. People began to eat less fish and more beef and dairy products. Hormones and antibiotics began to be added to feeds to increase meat production. Herbicides and pesticides began to pollute the environment, and animals fed on crops treated with them ended up with pollutants in their flesh which we, in turn, ate and took into our own bodies.

With the coming of convenience foods, more and more preservatives, as well as sugar and salt, were added to our foods in an attempt to give them a longer shelf life. Pretty soon, housewives were buying more and more ready-to-eat meat products instead of going to the butcher to buy a steak from a recently slaughtered, healthy animal. These products are vastly inferior nutritionally to the animal protein on which we are genetically programmed to thrive. So it is not only shifts in carbohydrate consumption that have that undermined human health over the centuries. Changes in protein foods have also contributed to the development of obesity, Syndrome X and related health problems.

One of the most important principles of the X Factor Diet is to eat good-quality protein with a high biological value at every meal and in every snack. This practice helps keep insulin and glucose within healthy ranges. Eating protein foods raises insulin levels only gently, and helps protect the body from runaway weight gain. It is time to think of protein in new ways. It needs to form the core and centre of your diet for life.

THE RIGHT STUFF

When you consider that the average person in the West only eats about 12 per cent of their calories as protein, and paleolithic people were eating at least 35 per cent, it is not surprising that we need to eat more protein if we are to re-establish metabolic balance and restore normal weight. Because not only does protein provide the essential building blocks for the immune system, muscles and cells. It also encourages the production of *glucagon* (see Box).

GLUCAGON: BURN THAT FAT

Glucagon is a hormone that has the opposite effect from insulin. Insulin enters the picture when blood sugar levels are high, and then escorts it into cells. Glucagon gets in on the act when levels are low, and helps release stored glycogen as usable blood sugar. It encourages your body to burn stored fats for energy as well. Glucagon also balances excess insulin production and stabilises blood sugar so you don't go through mood swings. If you want to reverse insulin resistance as well as prevent it, if you want to feel good, if you want to shed excess fat from your body, you need enough really good-quality protein throughout the day to support your body's production of glucagon.

Where do you get the best-quality protein? The highest-value proteins come from microfiltered whey, as we saw in the last chapter. This stuff, which comes in powder form, is great for drinks, snacks and desserts. Next are the animal foods – eggs, fish, seafood, game meats, turkey, chicken, red meat and low-fat cheeses. A good serving size of these protein foods for most people is 100 to 125g, which will give you something between 28 and 35g of protein. This is good, but not an enormous quantity when you consider that only 40g of a good-quality microfiltered whey protein powder mixed with water can provide as much as 36g of pure protein.

The Palm Method

When eating meat, fish or other protein foods, an easy way to measure how much is enough at a meal is to use what is known as the *palm method.* Although using the palm of your hand is not as accurate a method for determining minimum quantities of protein per serving as actually weighing the food, it works pretty well. It also keeps you from getting neurotic about the whole thing. This is how it works: place a piece of protein food in the palm of your hand so that it covers the palm, although not the thumb and fingers. It should also be about the same thickness as your palm. That's about right for a piece of fish, for instance. You are not going to go very far wrong in determining the size of portion you need. (See page 176 for how to use this method in Ketogenics, and page 187 for how to use it with Insulin Balance.)

Whenever you can, choose game meat such as rabbit, venison, partridge and wild duck instead of farmed meat. They are not only high in protein, but low in overall fat and rich in micronutrients. The next best meats come from free-range animals raised organically, without antibiotics or steroids or other hormones. The best chickens are those that have been fed on flaxseeds or fishmeal, both rich in omega-3. In many countries of the world, however, this practice is not yet widespread. Whatever kind of meat you choose, stay away from processed meat products like sausages and hotdogs, most bacons and artificially smoked fish and meats. Eat fish as often as you can, especially the deep-sea fish such as wild salmon, tuna, sardines and mackerel. They are rich in the omega-3 fatty acids that encourage fat burning. If you are going to eat cheese, choose it carefully. Most are much higher in fat than they are in protein. Small quantities of low-fat cheeses are not a bad source of protein, provided you are not allergic or sensitive to milk products. Cheeses like low-fat or fat-free cottage cheese, feta and mozzarella have more protein than fat. However, if you are watching your carbohydrate levels very carefully – especially at the beginning of Ketogenics – leave cheese out of the equation until you have lost the weight that you need to lose and have moved into Insulin Balance.

The Vegetarian Way

What about vegetable proteins? These have many health attributes, but eating vegetable protein alone isn't the way to build the healthiest possible body. First, you have to eat masses of soya proteins and beans to get the same kind of levels that even a reasonable amount of animal-based proteins brings. Secondly, eating beans together with grains to create a 'complete protein' makes problems of its own, not the least of which can be more food sensitivities and cravings. Both are anathema to anyone wanting to shed excess fat permanently and keep it off. Eating a lot of beans means you are ingesting a high concentration of the sugars they contain – *raffinose* and *stachyose.* These are carbohydrates your body doesn't need. They are hard to digest and often ferment in the gut. And they are all too high in carbs for Ketogenics. So if you are going to choose a vegetarian way of eating, I would strongly suggest that you eat the lion's share of your proteins as microfiltered whey.

Go For Whey

In truth, this is good advice for anyone on Ketogenics. The best whey protein concentrates – and note that you need to look for them, as there is a lot of junk on the market – are nothing less than transformative for your overall health and life. They are convenient to carry with you when you are on the go, at work or when travelling. You can use them to make delicious low-carbohydrate shakes. You can also cook with them and make great ice creams from them. You can even use them as a substitute for flour in some recipes. I like to make desserts from them using the herb stevia as a natural method of sweetening. So excellent are whey-based desserts in terms of health and weight loss that you could literally sit down and eat a whole meal of them. Microfiltered whey protein concentrates and whey peptide blends are great allies for 21st-century life. They keep you full of energy and stave off premature ageing, thanks to their high biological value and capacity to protect the immune system. I don't know now how I ever managed my life without them.

The Power Of Whey

These space-age foods, carefully manufactured to preserve nutritional value, are the result of more than 20 years of research and dozens of international studies. They have been shown to help decrease body fat, stimulate immune function, help prevent cancer, reduce total cholesterol and improve bone health as well as enhance lean body mass. Microfiltered whey is a superb way to help bring about cell renewal and new tissue growth, which is exactly what you are after when transforming how your body looks and functions.

Not so long ago, whey was considered a worthless by-product of cheese manufacturing. Not only was it not given to humans, there was a long time in which it wasn't even used for animals. Then farmers began to employ it as a spray-dried powder to enrich animal feeds, and it was used as a bulking agent in ice cream and yoghurts. Before long, technology stepped in to change the course of events – much to our benefit. Using highly specialised processing equipment, technicians gradually learned how to process whey at low heat without solvents, turning it into a protein with a very high biological value. Microfiltered whey contains not only all of the essential and non-essential amino acids, but more of the important branch chain amino acids than any other food. This type of amino acid is central to building a lean, powerful, strong body, which is why it's often used by athletes. And, of course, anyone following Ketogenics or Insulin Balance.

In a preliminary study carried out at the University of Nebraska in the US, researchers showed that whey protein concentrate significantly improved strength as well as their ratio of lean body mass to fat. They took 40 athletes and divided them into two groups. One group received whey protein concentrate and the other group received a placebo based on carbohydrate. All 40 athletes were put into the same weight training programme for four days a week. After a month, their weight and lean body mass to fat ratios were measured. Researchers discovered that the group fed on whey proteins were significantly leaner and stronger than the placebo group. They had also lost more than double the amount of body fat within this very short period.

Better Immunity

Whey protein does wonderful things for the immune system, too. It affects immunity directly thanks to some of its active ingredients, known as *subfractions*. These include *isolactoferrin*, a potent antioxidant with both antiviral and antimicrobial properties, as well as *alpha-lactalbumin, beta-lactoglobulin* and *immunoglobulins* (IgGs). Thanks to these subfractions as well as other ingredients, whey protein has the remarkable ability to increase the body's level of glutathione (see Box).

GLUTATHIONE: PRIME PROTECTOR

Glutathione is hot stuff when it comes to preventing premature ageing and protecting you from illness. It's an antioxidant with protective properties. It neutralises toxic residues in the body from exposure to pesticides, herbicides, heavy metals and peroxides. It helps protect many physiological processes related to immune functions. It also enhances enzyme activities and protein synthesis, and protects your DNA. You cannot rely on taking oral supplements of glutathione since your body breaks it down before it can be used. Eating microfiltered whey protein is pretty much the only way to increase your levels of this substance.

Anti-Ageing At Its Best

Whey protein concentrate brings other health and beauty benefits as well. There is growing evidence that it activates the activity of osteoblasts, the cells in your bones that are responsible for building new bone. There is every indication that it can play an important role in increasing bone density as well as improving the quality of collagen in the connective tissue and skin. There is even some evidence that it may prevent or reverse the cross-linking of collagen that comes with ageing, and creates wrinkles in the skin.

Whey protein is even being studied for its ability to help protect against cancer and other tumours, both in animals and humans. It is already used to boost the recovery of cancer patients. Finally, research shows that whey protein concentrate helps lower cholesterol levels even better than soya. In one study which compared soya beans, casein and whey protein concentrate, whey showed itself to be 20 per cent more effective than casein and 38 per cent more effective than soya beans. In another, whey protein concentrate demonstrated its ability to lower high blood pressure 10 per cent more effectively than soya does.

MICROFILTERED WHEY PROTEIN CONCENTRATE:

- Helps build lean body mass
- Enhances immune functions
- Improves the quality of collagen
- Helps build new healthy collagen
- Enhances skin, nails and hair
- Encourages fat loss
- Protects against free radical damage
- Strengthens bones
- Increases glutathione
- Helps eliminate many food sensitivities.

End To Food Allergies

Another wonderful thing about these products is that many people with food sensitivities find they're no longer troubled by them once they eliminate high carbohydrates from their diet and add good quantities of whey protein concentrate. Just why this is so I am not sure, except that I think we may have been labelling certain reactions to foods 'allergies', when they may have more to do with Syndrome X. Whey protein concentrates even work well for many people who have a known milk allergy.

Big Tub – Big Scam

The best whey protein concentrates – and the only ones that you should ever consider using – are processed at very low temperatures to create a virtually undamaged product with all the important subfractions (parts that are unprocessed and have immune-enhancing properties) biologically active. These proteins are not cheap, although ounce by ounce they are a cheaper source of protein than most meats. When buying them, you get what you pay for. Because they are expensive to produce, manufacturers wanting to sell them, yet keep costs low and profit margins high, sometimes blend them with cheap soya proteins or milk proteins and then pretend that they are selling the real thing. There are a lot of products out there – particularly those that you find in sports stores, pharmacies and even most health stores – which are not worth the weight of the containers that hold them.

Michael Colgan, the biochemist we met in the last chapter, is a man determined to help the world's top athletes reach their highest possible levels of performance, strength and well-being. Colgan has examined in depth the whey products on the market. He warns against buying any whey protein products which list in their contents a 'proprietary blend' of protein. This is a way of masking the fact that the bulk of the product they are selling is likely to be worthless. He says:

'The worst blends we've found are less than 10 per cent good proteins, and over 90 per cent cheap milk casein (BV 77), soya isolate (BV 74) or cheap whey. Unlike pure whey protein, which is heavy and dense, all these powders are light and bulky because they are loaded with lactose (milk sugar) and other unwanted components. So you seem to be getting more for your money. A good rule of thumb is, the bigger the tub, the bigger the scam. The giant plastic tubs of these products sent to the Colgan Institute for testing make such great trash cans you can see right away that that's what they were designed to hold.'

There is also a lot of bad labelling on whey protein products. Not long ago the Canadian Health Protection Branch tested eight protein supplements sold in Canada and the United States. Two of them were labelled 100 per cent pure crystalline free-form amino acids, while the other six were presented as products derived from protein hydrolysates. What the Canadian Health Protection Branch discovered was that not one product fulfilled the promises on its label. The total protein/amino acid content in these products ranged from 30 to 82 per cent. Four of them appeared to be nothing more than cheap gelatin powder. Two contained only a single amino acid, lysine, as well as large amounts of ammonia.

Buy The Best
When choosing whey proteins, go for those produced without heat or acid extraction. For both of these methods destroy bonds between the di-peptides and tri-peptides which your body needs to be able to build protein. Otherwise, what you're putting in your body is simply not going to be used. The chemical

keys that come from di-peptide and tri-peptide bonds – your body's locks – are recognised and absorbed by the body much better than single amino acids. This enables your body to hold onto and make use of twice the protein you would get from high-quality ordinary protein foods like meat and fish. The proteins to look for are microfiltered and ion-exchange whey proteins. Denatured whey proteins are simply no good. Only buy from companies who have built a solid reputation in nutrition (see Resources). Another thing Colgan warns against is any whey protein that gives you an upset stomach. Get rid of it.

Help From Soya

Although soya protein is much lower in biological value than many other proteins, it's still a remarkable food – numerous scientific studies round the world have shown that the humble soy bean has masses of anti-ageing, anti-disease, anti-obesity properties. If you are not using soya foods in your life, you are definitely missing out. Eating even small quantities of soya – a mere 25g of soya protein, or about half a cup of tofu, a day – reduces your risk of heart disease, lowers cholesterol levels, helps alleviate Syndrome X, helps prevent osteoporosis, decreases PMS and menopausal symptoms and reduces your risks of many types of cancer.

Much of soya's health-enhancing power comes from a group of phytochemical compounds it contains called isoflavones, which we have already encountered in the chapter 'Colour of Energy'. The isoflavones include genistein, diadzein, and glycitein. Each has its own unique benefits, but like many things in nature, they act together in synergy. This is probably why soya can be beneficial in reversing insulin resistance, obesity and Syndrome X. The isoflavones decrease insulin levels and bring about beneficial changes in blood lipid profiles and a decrease in arteriosclerosis. Soya has been shown to significantly reduce total cholesterol, low-density lipoproteins (LDL) or 'bad' cholesterol, and triglycerides, although it only minimally affects the high-density lipoproteins (HDL) or 'good' cholesterol.

For many years researchers have been pointing out that Asian populations, where a large number of soya products are eaten, have a statistically lower rate of death from heart disease than people who get little or no soya protein in their diet. Many believe that post-menopausal women – whose levels of oestrogen are considerably lower than their pre-menopausal sisters – can especially benefit from adding soya to their diet. In one study of menopausal and peri-menopausal women, each was given 80mg of isoflavones a day for five to 10 weeks. The researchers discovered that the improvement in blood pressure was dramatic, and close to that on hormone replacement therapy. Soya isoflavones also have a beneficial effect on women's reproductive systems. They are often recommended for PMS, oestrogen imbalances, endometriosis, breast cancer and menopausal problems, all of which may improve when women add soya foods to their diet.

The Amazing Oestrogen Paradox

Soya isoflavones, like so many health-enhancing phyto-nutrients, help restore some of a living system's balance when it has been lost. Many of soya's protective and health-enhancing influences have to do with its oestrogen-like activity. Isoflavones – themselves weak oestrogen-like plant chemicals – bind together with the body's oestrogen receptors and help protect it from damage. But here is a paradox. Although isoflavones are oestrogen-like themselves, they are not dangerous, unlike oestrogen drugs or oestrogen-mimicking chemicals from the environment. For they are very weak in their oestrogenic activity. And when they hook up with the body's oestrogen receptor sites, they actually exert a beneficial anti-oestrogenic effect. They block the uptake of the dangerous oestrogen-like chemicals – known as *xenoestrogens* – carried in herbicides and pesticides in the environment as well as oestrogen drugs such as the Pill, all of which have been linked with cancer.

Post-menopausal Japanese women who regularly eat soya foods seldom suffer menopausal symptoms and rarely use hormone replacement. Eating a little soya protein also helps strengthen bones. In one study, a mere 45mg of soya isofavone increased the bone density of post-menopausal women in only 24 weeks. Studies carried out on older Asian women who eat soya foods over a lifetime suggest that isoflavones not only improve bone integrity, but protect against bone loss and reduce the risk of osteoporosis and fractures.

Nowadays many women, when advised to turn to synthetic hormone replacement on the understanding that it may help protect them from osteoporosis, decide that the benefits promised are not offset by the risks implicit in putting their bodies under long-term drug treatment. More and more women are turning to soya as a safe alternative. Isoflavones improve bone mass because, like whey protein, they trigger activity in the osteoblasts – cells responsible for the formation of new bone tissue. They probably also increase your body's ability to absorb and retain calcium from the foods you eat.

SOYA FOODS CAN:

- Help reverse Syndrome X
- Reduce risks of some cancers
- Rebalance sex hormones
- Help prevent osteoporosis
- Lower LDL ('bad' cholesterol)
- Build stronger bones.

The Down Side

Not all soya is worth using – far from it. Almost 75 per cent of the soya beans grown now come from genetically modified beans. In the opinion of many well-informed scientists, eating such foods is like drawing a wild card in poker. You quite frankly do not know what you are getting. There have been no long-term studies to show the effects on human beings of eating genetically modified crops. Some soya foods carry high levels of aluminum in them as well – the result of the way the beans were grown. Rather than gamble with the unknown, I choose soya products that are made only from organic soya beans.

By weight, soya beans are 42 per cent protein, 33 per cent carbohydrate, 20 per cent fat and 5 per cent fibre. Products made from them include soya protein isolate, which is about 90 per cent protein. When buying soya protein isolate, make sure that it says 'water processed' on the label, as this practice leaves most of the valuable isoflavones intact for your body to use. Other soya foods include tempeh, miso, tofu, lecithin, textured vegetable protein and soya milk. Be careful when choosing soya products, especially when following Ketogenics. Read labels carefully and make sure they do not contain too many carbohydrates. Once you move onto Insulin Balance this is not of great concern. The best-tasting soya milk often contains malt extracts – sugars that are far too high on the glycaemic index. As always, it pays in terms of health to eat the very best.

EAT FAT

Did you ever begin a weight loss diet only to discover you were overcome by chronic fatigue and constant hunger? This is probably because you were following a low-fat regime. Low-fat diets are notorious for being virtually impossible to keep to for long, since low-fat foods just do not satisfy. These diets can also be dangerous. Since so many of your body's tissues, hormones and all of its cells are dependent on a good supply of essential fats, a low-fat regime undermines your overall health. And it doesn't enhance your good looks – those fatty acid deficiencies also cause your body to age prematurely.

Throw Out The Junk

It may seem bizarre to lose weight by eating fat. Yet that's how it works – as long as you're eating the right essential fatty acids, in the right proportions. We'll be looking at all that in detail below, but first, an overview of the ones to avoid on the X Factor Diet.

Diets high in the wrong fats are just as harmful as low-fat regimes. Margarines and the golden vegetable oils you see lined up on supermarket shelves are claimed by many gourmets to be good for us. Yet in the Western world, where 45 per cent of our calories come from fats, fatty acid deficiencies are rampant. Why? Because all those oils and 'healthy' margarines are actually junk fats that the body can't use. And if the body isn't getting the fats it needs, the results can be horrendous:

- Obesity
- Dry skin and eczema
- PMS
- Arthritis
- Emotional and behavioural problems
- Raised cholesterol levels
- Suppressed immunity
- Premature ageing
- Heart disease
- Sterility in men.

For generations we have been told that fat is unhealthy. In part, this is just a marketing strategy to sell more carbohydrate-loaded foods. In part, it is simply misguided. Fats are surrounded by false beliefs. A major one is that the Western diet has increased dramatically in saturated fat over the last century. In fact, the reverse is true. From 1910 to 1970 in the United States, the proportion of saturated animal fats in the American diet declined from 83 to 62 per cent, while butter consumption went down from 18lb a year to a mere 4lb.

Fat Fears

What *has* increased is the percentage of fats we are taking in in the form of refined vegetable oils, margarines and junk fats through processed foods. Consumption of these has increased 400 per cent during the same period. The famous Framingham heart study is often cited to prove that fats are bad for you. This was a huge study that began in 1948 and involved some 6000 people in Framingham, Massachusetts. Two groups of people were compared every five years – those who consumed little cholesterol and saturated fat and those who consumed large quantities. After 40 years the director of the study admitted that 'in Framingham, Massachusetts, the more saturated fat one ate, the more cholesterol one ate, the more calories one ate, the lower the person's serum cholesterol…We found that people who ate the most cholesterol, ate the most saturated fat, ate the most calories, weighed the least and were the most physically active.' Similar large-scale studies in Britain and elsewhere substantiate his observations.

While these findings should never be taken as an imperative to eat more animal fat, they suggest it is time to banish our fear of fats. It is also time we became more aware of the fats that can help Ketogenics and Insulin Balance work their wonders, and the fats you need to avoid. This is a complex issue, for each fat is unique. A few even have a capacity to spur fat burning. So bear with me as we wind our way through the labyrinth of fat biochemistry. It is a valuable side trip on your journey towards a lean body.

What Is A Fat?

Fat is a macronutrient which exerts little effect on insulin levels, but which strongly decreases appetite. Provided you are getting the right kind of fats in your diet, they can rebalance hormones and re-orient how you look and feel, thanks to their effects on important regulatory chemicals in the body called prostaglandins, which we'll look at later. All fats are organic compounds scientifically known as triglycerides, composed of a glycerol molecule with fatty acids connected to it. Chemically, a fatty acid consists of a chain of carbon and hydrogen atoms to which one oxygen atom is attached. Although carbohydrate molecules also consist of carbon, hydrogen and oxygen atoms, a molecule of fat is very different because it contains a lot less oxygen. This is what makes fat highly concentrated and calorific: there are 9 calories to each gram of fat, and only 4 calories to each gram of carbohydrate or protein.

Saturated And Unsaturated

Fats can be divided roughly into two groups – saturated and unsaturated. In a molecule of saturated fat, each carbon atom is connected to a hydrogen atom in such a way that none of the carbon can connect with other atoms. Because of this, saturated fats – found in meat, dairy products like cheese, ice cream, milk and tropical oils like palm kernel oil and coconut oil – are stable, relatively inactive and virtually inert in your body. There are exceptions to this, however, and we'll look at these later. The *raison d'être* of most saturated fats is to provide energy which can be stored in the body's fat cells and used later.

Unsaturated fats are very different. They are found in foods of vegetable origin like nuts, seeds, grains and vegetables, although some of the most health-giving oils are also found in fish and game. Unlike saturated fats such as butter, which are solid, unsaturated fats come in liquid form. According to classical nutrition, only two unsaturated fatty acids are necessary for human health – linoleic and alpha-linolenic acids – so these are called 'essential' fatty acids. These two types of fatty acid are actually families – our old friends omega-3 and omega-6. Alpha-linolenic acid is head of the omega-3 family, while linoleic acid is head of the omega-6 family. Out of these two, your body is supposed to be able to make all of the other fatty acids it needs. The trouble is that many people, having lived for years on processed foods, lose their ability to make conversions. They need to get their fatty acids in a more direct way, which we'll discover in a minute.

ESSENTIAL FATTY ACIDS PREVENT RAPID AGEING. THEY:

- Ensure insulin sensitivity and good blood glucose control
- Reduce excessive inflammation
- Regulate
  - Cholesterol levels
  - Triglyceride levels
  - Blood pressure
  - Fibrinogen level
- Maintain cellular hydration.

They are the fundamental nuts and bolts that your body uses to structure the brain, eyes, ears, reproductive organs and cell membranes that surround and protect every cell in your body. Without them, you would not be able to move a muscle. You could not think, see or hear. Essential fatty acids are also needed for your body to make hormone-like chemicals called prostaglandins. Critical to cellular functioning in the body, a good balance of prostaglandins helps your body resist illness – from arthritis and ulcers to migraines and cancer. It also supports the working of your immune, reproductive and central nervous systems and your heart. Finally, prostaglandins regulate brain chemicals – neurotransmitters – which are themselves created out of essential fatty acids.

The Good And Bad Prostaglandins

THE GOOD
Series one prostaglandins:
Act as vasodilators
Act as immune enhancers
Decrease inflammation
Decrease pain
Increase oxygen flow
Increase endurance
Prevent platelet aggregation
Dilate airways
Decrease cellular proliferation

THE BAD
Series two prostaglandins:
Act as vasoconstrictors
Act as immune suppressors
Increase inflammation
Increase pain
Decrease oxygen flow
Decrease endurance
Cause platelet aggregation
Constrict airways
Increase cellular proliferation

Keys And Caterpillars

To understand how fats work, think of them as chemical keys. I like the way the Canadian expert in fat metabolism Udo Erasmus describes a fat molecule. He says it looks something like a caterpillar, with a fatty head and body and an acid tail. The way fats differ from each other on a molecular level depends on the length of their carbon chains and the number of arrangements of hydrogen atoms along their caterpillar 'bodies'. These differences are enormously important. They are the chemical keys that determine whether a particular fat fits into a particular lock in your body so you can use it to build hormones, cell walls and prostaglandins and carry out the other important duties that fats perform.

Omega-6 and omega-3 essential fatty acids – in the right balance – can help your body shed fat stores in at least three different ways:

- They increase metabolic rate and fat metabolism so more of your stored fat can be burnt as energy.
- They influence the production of prostaglandins in subtle but powerful ways favourable to fat burning.
- They increase your cells' sensitivity to insulin, which allows it to do its job of regulating blood sugar.

Fat Burners

At the Garvin Institute of Medical Research in New South Wales, Australia, Dr Leonard Storlien and his team discovered that the omega-3 fatty acids – prevalent in fish oils and also in flaxseed – improve insulin levels and increase your body's ability to use both fats and carbohydrates as fuel. So dramatic was the effect of the omega-3s on insulin that they are now used to prevent insulin resistance and diabetes in animals prone to both conditions.

Your body needs a balance of omega-3 and omega-6 to maintain health and normal weight. Paleopathologists have determined that our distant ancestors consumed omega-6 and omega-3 fatty acids in a 1:1 to 2:1 ratio. In other words, these essential fats were eaten in relatively equal quantities.

Out Of Balance

In today's Western diet the balance between these two has become completely screwed up. We consume omega-6 and omega-3 fatty acids in a ratio of about 22:1 – far too high for optimal health and fat loss. So you'll eat more omega-3s when following either programme in the X Factor Diet. Omega-3s spur fat burning, and help protect from inflammation. People with Syndrome X can be especially prone to this condition, as can those who convert omega-6 oils to arachidonic acid in the body (see page 228-9). Since omega-6 oils are readily available in the modern diet, we don't need to add more of them when following Ketogenics and Insulin Balance. Omega-3s can be harder to come by. Cold-processed flaxseed oil is a good source, and can be eaten on salads. Supplements of omega-3 fish oils rich in DHA and EPA are an alternative. Both can be a great asset to your health and fat loss (see Resources, page 339).

Studies which show the benefits of DHA and EPA-rich fish oils now number in the thousands. We know now that adequate omega-3s decrease insulin resistance, improve cardiovascular health, counter both chronic and acute inflammatory conditions from arthritis to a hyper-reactive immune system and help protect your body from degeneration. Many large-scale epidemiological studies have turned up evidence that when the diet of a group of people is rich in omega-3s, their risk of heart disease is dramatically lowered compared to the average Western diet.

The Cis Have It

In Ketogenics and Insulin Balance, the essential fatty acids used to help ensure health and reduce overall body fat are all *cis* fats. (Hydrogen atoms can be arranged in two different ways in fatty acid molecules. One way is known as cis, the other trans.) Cis fatty acids are unprocessed and natural, the only form that your body can use for anything except for making you fatter. Omega-3 and omega-6 cis fatty acids are destroyed by modern processing procedures like bleaching, hydrogenation, heating and deodorising, which turn corn, peanuts, safflowers and sunflower seeds to those shimmering, golden oils you see on supermarket shelves – the kind of oils that go into mass-produced foods. These are the trans fats, and they are not good for you.

Cis fatty acids, the good-guy fats, are keys which fit perfectly into your locks – that is, the molecular fat receptor sites – and help your metabolic processes work properly. Trans fatty acids are the bad guys. Not only do they not fit into your metabolic machinery, their presence in your body gums up your metabolic works and can make your life miserable. Avoid them.

Fats Beat Addiction

If you have struggled with your weight, you'll know all too well the results of eating a high-carb/low-fat diet – especially carbohydrates which are high on the glycaemic index. Recall that the more of these foods you eat, the more insulin your pancreas produces to control blood sugar levels. As soon as the insulin lowers your blood sugar, energy falls, sending out messages to your brain that you need to eat more carbohydrate to get more energy. In fact, high levels of insulin produced in response to large quantities of carbs block that other pancreatic hormone, glucagon, from operating effectively. Glucagons help unlock stored body fat, allowing it to be burnt as fuel. Too much insulin blocks glucagon from doing this. Excess carbs, in effect, slam the doors to fat release shut. Eating healthy fats improves the ratio of insulin to glucagon, slows down the release of sugar from carbohydrate foods you do eat and empowers glucagon to get on with its job. So does the right kind of regular exercise.

When you produce enough glucagons, they unlock your fat storage banks and begin the process of converting your body's fat stores into energy. In effect, you kill two birds with one stone. You eliminate addictive hunger and cravings since blood sugar is controlled and insulin secretion is lowered. Also, since fat is metabolised slowly, you experience satisfaction rather than hunger.

Neither programme in the X Factor Diet places a restriction on how much fat your eat, and this is why. You will find, once you get into these new ways of eating, that your own appetite will make those decisions for you. What matters is not so much the quantity of the fats you eat but what kinds of fats and in what kind of balance you eat them.

Natural Appetite Control

When shedding stored fat from your body, the omega-3 fats are particularly good at leaving you feeling satiated. These natural appetite suppressants work in an interesting way. After you've eaten them they release a hormone called cholecystokinin, or CCK, from your stomach. CCK signals your brain, letting it know that you feel satisfied. When you reduce the level of fat in a meal your brain does not receive the same message and, although your stomach may be filled with food, you still want to eat more. Many of us have experienced this – sitting down to a meal and, no matter how much we eat, still craving food at the end of it. For although your body may be registering a feeling of fullness, that does not mean satisfaction, so you are left wondering what is wrong with you. This phenomenon can even lead to eating disorders and a real mistrust of your body and yourself; you can end up feeling you have to watch yourself carefully to keep your eating under control. Add essential fatty acids to your diet and you gradually begin to feel full and satisfied. You also learn that you can trust your body's messages.

Essential fats – those curvy caterpillars – matter a lot when it comes to shedding fat from your body and keeping it off. What makes these molecules curvy is that, unlike saturated fats whose carbon atoms, as we've seen, are all linked up with hydrogen atoms, unsaturated fats lack hydrogen atoms at various places along one side. These empty spaces, called 'double bonds', make the molecule curved. It's also what makes them cis fatty acids. I've only hinted at the wonderful things these fats do for the body. They transfer oxygen into the alveoli, or air sacs, of the lungs, and from there into your red blood cells to be carried throughout the body. At the level of every cell membrane, it is the essential fatty acids that draw out the oxygen from the haemoglobin in your blood and bring it into the cell so it can be burnt for energy. Eat plenty of these, especially the omega-3s.

LEAN MEANS ENERGY

The next time you have a chance, watch an animal move. The rhythmic lope of a wolf, whose body almost becomes the motion. The horse in a field, tossing its mane, pounding its hooves and charging about for sheer pleasure. The dolphin who leaps high in the air, twisting its powerful body before disappearing into the waves to emerge a minute later with yet another joyous leap. For many years I wondered why after childhood most of us no longer experience this kind of explosive, rhythmical freedom and energy, grounded in the physical body. Why do we often feel only half alive?

Muscle Magic

And why do those of us who are women tend to look upon our bodies as something separate from ourselves, to be criticized, judged, or pushed and shoved into shape, instead of celebrated for its power and joy in movement. For too many human beings, the primary experience of life is one of lifelessness. And since none of us is able to live with this dead feeling for long, we are forced to seek extreme stimuli – drugs, alcohol, compulsive work or sex – just to make us feel alive again. The trouble is, none of these ever seems to work for very long. Where does the real key lie?

The answer to this question may surprise you. It stunned me when I first came upon it, because it is so simple. The key to aliveness is found in the body itself. It lies in muscle. When the engine of your muscle is at work, you're turning food calories into energy, burning fat – and creating a feeling of ongoing, simple joy. Muscle creates the life energy for you to think, to move and to feel. To create a firm, beautiful, lean body for yourself, begin to listen to, nurture and develop your muscle. The better your muscle, the greater your sense of being alive.

Animal bodies, like ours, are made up of two basic components – *lean body mass* (LBM), which encompasses muscle tissue, and *fat*. Lean body mass is the part of you which is most alive. It consists of organs such as the heart, the liver, the pancreas, bones and skin, as well as your muscle tissue. Your LBM demands oxygen, uses nutrients from your food, thinks and feels, moves, grows and repairs itself. Wild animals have a high percentage of LBM. That is what gives them their power, their ease of movement, their stamina and their sleek bodies.

The rest of you is fat. The hardest thing to understand for most of us who have been brainwashed by low-calorie slimming nonsense is that it is your body's *fat* stores that need dealing with, not your weight as measured by the scales.

Fat tissue is very different from muscle. It does not need oxygen, does not create movement or activity, and cannot repair itself. In fact, body fat is just about as close as you can get to dead flesh within a living system. Dr Vince Quas, an American expert on body change and fat loss, says it better than anyone else I have ever met: 'Your lean body mass *is* you,' he says. 'Your fat is *on* you.'

Finding Yourself

With the X Factor Diet it is the muscle portion of your LBM you will be working with, through both dietary change and exercise. For it is your LBM that transforms your shape and energy. It is a fascinating metamorphosis to go through. It does not alter you in any intrinsic way, nor does it turn you into someone else's idea of the perfect body. It only makes you what, in essence, you really are. What happens is that your LBM slowly but inexorably begins to transform your body – which may have become distorted over the years by stress, poor eating and lack of movement – into the true form that is hidden within it. People sometimes talk about the body as if it were a machine. In reality, it's nothing like a machine. A machine wears out.

The right kind of exercise will help you rid yourself of the tendency to gain weight, as well as help prevent degenerative diseases such as cancer and heart disease. An eight-year study which followed more than 10,000 men and 3000 women, reported in the *Journal of the American Medical Association* not long ago, looked at the long-term effects of physical fitness. It found that sedentary women – women who are not fit and therefore have a low LBM to fat ratio – were 460 per cent more likely to die of degenerative diseases than those that took exercise more regularly. Men in the low fitness category were 340 per cent more likely to die of them. Being a lounge lizard is a major risk factor, not only for becoming overweight but also for degeneration and disease.

In fact, the finest diet and all the best nutritional supplements in the world won't make up for a lack of physical activity. For our bodies inherited not just a genetic makeup that demands the right balance and the best quality of proteins, carbohydrates and fats, complete with essential nutrients, but also a need to move. Your body was designed to be active. The more you use it wisely, the stronger and more beautiful it will become – regardless of your age.

By now, thousands of research projects have been carried out into the effects of exercise on health, leanness and age prevention. The conclusions are unequivocal. If there is one thing which improves insulin sensitivity, energy, emotional balance and a capacity for experiencing simple joy in life, it is regular exercise. Our ancestors were in continual movement. They trekked long distances in search of food. They ran in short bursts when hunting animals and being hunted. Simple walking took up a large part of the day.

A New Attitude

If you consider exercise a chore – something you are 'supposed' to do even though you hate every moment of it – it's time to shift the way you think. In fact, why not get rid of the word 'exercise' and replace it with 'physical activity', on the understanding that the more you use your body, the more power, energy and expansiveness of spirit you experience in your day-to-day to life. Robert Ornstein and David Sobel put it rather well in their book, *Healthy Pleasures*. Exercise, they say, is a 'usually deliberate, sometimes odious, sweat-soaked endeavour that can take away from your life, whereas physical activity can be any daily undertaking, work or play, that involves movement.' When you begin to think of movement as physical activity instead of exercise, you may find you can make a lot more space for it in your life. Once you do, the benefits are almost boundless.

REGULAR WORKOUTS WILL:

- Help you burn calories to control or lose weight
- Build muscle and increase muscle strength
- Lower body fat
- Increase glucagon
- Increase insulin sensitivity
- Boost immunity, helping you fend off illness and disease
- Build bone density in people under 30 and slow bone loss in older people
- Make you feel good about yourself
- Reduce stress, anxiety and depression by shifting brain chemistry
- Reduce blood glucose and triglyceride levels
- Increase HDL – 'good' cholesterol
- Reduce blood pressure

- Reduce the risk of cardiovascular disease, Type II
  diabetes and early ageing
- Maintain aerobic fitness and overall energy
- Clear depression.

Lounge Lizards Beware

Because your body is genetically programmed to move, not getting enough physical activity carries a heavy price tag in terms of health, energy, emotional balance and looks. And if you have avoided physical activity as much as possible for many years, the good news is it's never too late to reap its benefits. A study carried out at Yale University showed quite clearly what the age-reversing and beneficial effects of taking up regular physical activity can be, even for people in their seventies who have been almost completely sedentary. A group of men and woman began an aerobics programme consisting of 40 to 60 minutes of mini-trampolining each week. The control group did only a gentle programme of stretching and yoga. Four months later, the researchers found that the aerobic group showed significant improvements in glucose tolerance, while the control group showed no such changes.

Use It Or Lose It

Break your arm and it will shed half its muscle and a third of its bone mass within a few weeks, simply because you stop using it. When the cast is taken off it will have shrunk to as little as half its size. If you are forced for any reason to stay in bed for a few months, the loss of minerals from your bones and the ageing of your muscle tissue can speed up by 10 years. But your body responds amazingly to exercise – and it doesn't have to be circuit training. Start now to make demands upon your muscles by doing both aerobic and weight-bearing exercise – nice and easy, even if you are not used to it. Not only will your muscles grow stronger and smoother, your bone tissue will become denser. Stop exercising again, and your body will turn to flab, your energy levels will drop, your muscle mass will shrink along with your ability to burn calories, and your overall sense of well-being will drain away.

What kind of exercise do you need for permanent weight control? Not the kind that goes all out to burn as many calories as possible. Far from it. That only *depletes* your energy, *slows* fat burning and can leave you feeling exhausted and looking haggard. Exercise for fat loss needs to be slow, sustained and regular and it needs to do three things: boost your metabolism, increase your supply of oxygen to the mitochondria of muscle cells for fat burning, and shift your LBM-to-fat ratio in favour of muscle. For this you need two kinds of exercise – *aerobic*, such as brisk walking, to stimulate oxygen supply; and *strength training* or *resistance work*. Together they will help your natural form emerge, burn fat and keep it off forever.

Fat Is Dead

Because your body's fat tissues have very low metabolic activity, they don't burn calories. Only mitochondria in your muscle cells do this. The more muscle tissue you have, the better your body burns calories, sheds fat, and keeps it off. A higher muscle mass also means you can eat more without gaining weight. But you need a lot of oxygen to do this. In fact, the more oxygen your muscles are supplied with via the bloodstream, the more calories and fat your body can burn. When we eat a high-carb/high-fat diet as we do in the West, the rate at which your blood transports oxygen to the cells is greatly slowed down. Fat in the blood makes red blood cells – the oxygen carriers – clump together. This happens very quickly after eating a meal rich in fat. It is the main reason why, after Christmas dinner, your brain doesn't function properly and all you want to do is go to sleep – the oxygen just isn't getting to your brain very efficiently.

Aerobic exercise enhances your body's ability to transport oxygen. Run, walk, swim, cycle or do any other activity that uses the large muscle groups, and where your heart beats steadily and your lungs breathe deeply, for 20 to 45 minute periods at least three, but preferably four, times a week. Aerobic exercise enhances overall fitness and well-being in other ways too. It improves the functioning of the heart, lowers cholesterol and affects your brain chemistry so that you produce natural opiates which make you feel good. It also increases noradrenaline – a brain chemical which carries an enormous feelgood quality – improving your self-image and confidence so you feel better about yourself and your life all round. Noradrenaline and its sister hormone adrenaline, which also increases with regular exercise, both stimulate the fat-burning ability of the mitochondria. Aerobic exercise enhances fat burning too, not only while you are working out but also for many hours afterwards. Interesting studies show that in many cases, aerobic exercise alone can bring about weight loss. Shedding weight while exercising regularly means that you lose fat instead of water or vital lean tissue. Once you get into it, you come to love it – while I have never met anyone who enjoys dieting!

AEROBIC EXERCISE PREVENTS
RAPID AGEING BY:

- Reducing blood pressure, triglycerides and body fat percentages
- Improving insulin sensitivity
- Maintaining lean muscle mass
- Maintaining aerobic fitness
- Increasing HDL – 'good' cholesterol
- Reducing blood glucose levels.

What Works For You

The most important things to consider when planning programmes of physical activity for yourself are the following. Do something that you enjoy. Explore new forms of exercise that you may never have experienced before, to find out what they can do for you. For many years exercise psychologists believed that the only form of exercise any of us ever needed was aerobic exercise. When you go aerobic, exercise for a period lasting 15 minutes to an hour or more.

WHAT WORKS FOR YOU:

- Aerobics
- Cycling
- Dancing
- Mini-trampolining
- Skiing
- Swimming
- Running
- Walking.

Of all of these activities, the one that fits best into most people's lives is simple walking. It doesn't cost anything. Anyone can walk anywhere without any special equipment. You can walk at whatever speed suits you – from a gentle stroll to a moderate pace. You can even try power walking. This is one form of aerobic exercise that has never appealed to me personally. I've tried it and found it very stress-producing. But everyone has their own tastes, so you never know – it might work for you.

Another important thing about walking is that you have little chance of getting injured while doing it. This makes it the safest exercise of all. Begin by taking a 20-minute walk each day. After a week or two, most people find they want to increase this to 45 minutes or even an hour. I was surprised at first by this phenomenon. When I questioned people as to why they increased it, each had a different story to tell. One man found he enjoyed walking in the evening with his partner, sometimes quite late at night. It renewed their relationship and gave them an opportunity to speak to each other he said. Another man told me he just found he felt so good that after the 20 minutes were over he just kept on doing it. This is a common experience with physical activity. Even if you are resistant to getting started, once you do, your body seems to lap it up and ask for more.

Easy Does It

You might begin by simply taking a walk around the block of even 10 minutes before going to work. There are all sorts of ways of fitting in a walk while hardly noticing that you are doing it. Park your car further away from the office, and walk to work. Climb stairs instead of taking a lift. A walk is a great way to spend time with a friend in a relaxed atmosphere. Take your children to the zoo. Take your baby for a stroll. Walk your dog. Don't limit yourself to walking in the same areas all the time. If you become bored with one area, drive to somewhere else and walk there – in a reserve or a park. Walk downtown in a city. Explore areas that you have not seen before. Most people who get into walking claim that even their holiday patterns change. Instead of choosing to go some place where they lie comatose on a beach, they become increasingly attracted to places that offer the possibility of hikes and activities.

To make good use of aerobic exercise as part of your Ketogenics or Insulin Balance programme, it must *not* be high-intensity. When you exercise too hard or become breathless while working out, the energy which feeds your movement is drawn not from your fat stores but from glycogen in your liver and your muscles. Aerobic exercise that works best is *moderate*, and of *long duration* since this kind burns both glycogen *and* fat. After 30 minutes of brisk, sustained walking, your body makes an important shift so that only 50 per cent of its energy comes from glycogen and the rest comes from your fat stores. Studies in exercise physiology suggest that the minimal threshold of exercise training to shed fat demands continuous movement of at least 20 to 30 minutes at least three times a week. Less than that and you are really wasting your time. The important thing to remember about fat burning is to exercise not *hard* but *long*. Most important of all...enjoy!

FAT BURNING BODY

Did you ever find yourself resenting the ability of young people to eat whatever they want, apparently lounge around all the time and never gain weight? This is because their lean-body-mass-to-fat-ratio is much higher than it is with older, sedentary people.

Loss of Power

Why is this so? It's all down to an incredible substance called human growth hormone (HGH). People under 25 have lots of it, and are far more sensitive to the chemicals in the body which stimulate its release. As we get older, our production of HGH decreases dramatically, along with our sensitivity to the chemicals that trigger it. This is caused by a number of things, not only the passage of time.

As we've seen, if we have lived on the standard Western diet, which emphasises carbohydrate and junk fats, our blood glucose levels tend to increase, which inhibits the normal flow of growth hormone released in the body. And we tend to get heavier – between the ages of 19 and 50, in fact, the average women gains 15lb. This further inhibits release of growth hormone. That's the bad news. The good news is that the body has a tremendous capacity for regeneration and transformation. The X Factor Diet, coupled with resistance training – working out with weights – can help you do this.

HGH is an anabolic, or tissue-building, hormone. Produced in the pituitary, a tiny gland at the base of the skull, it is secreted on and off through the day. It boosts growth in children, and also aids in tissue repair and helps direct the metabolism to burn fat instead of storing it, and to mobilise fat stores. In recent years there has been an enormous amount of research into the effects of introducing growth hormone by injection. Doctors use it with patients who have suffered severe burns or massive injuries to soft tissue and for people recovering from major surgery. They also give it to children that lack it and, as a result, are destined to a life of dwarfism. By injecting small amounts of growth hormone under the skin, doctors promote healing and ensure growth even in children that do not have the capacity to produce enough HGH themselves. It's extremely expensive stuff.

From Fat To Muscle

Recently, researchers have been exploring the use of HGH to prevent ageing. In one study reported in the *New England Journal of Medicine*, Dr Daniel

Rudman of the Medical College of Wisconsin discovered that very small amounts of growth hormone, injected just under the skin of men aged 61 to 81, increased their lean body mass by 8.8 per cent and decreased their body fat by 14.4 per cent. Bone density was increased in the spine, and the men's skin thickened by an amazing 7.1 per cent. The men did not exercise or change their diet during the study. In Dr Rudman's opinion, so powerful were the transformative and rejuvenating changes that they were 'equivalent in magnitude to the changes incurred during 10-20 years of [reversing] ageing.'

A number of studies show that injecting athletes with HGH even for only four to six weeks decreases their body fat dramatically and increases their lean body mass. In a very real sense, growth hormone is an elixir of youth. No wonder it is currently touted as the be-all and end-all for rejuvenation, and is being offered at enormous expense at clinics in Mexico and Eastern Europe.

Do It Naturally

But before you jump on the growth hormone bandwagon and rush off to have injections at your nearest clinic, you should know that by far the most powerful rejuvenating effects from increased levels of human growth hormone are brought about by changes in the way you eat and live.

Most of what stimulates the production of growth hormone are things over which we have total control:

■ A carbohydrate-restricted diet
■ A truly adequate protein diet
■ Deep sleep
■ Strength training
■ Decreasing blood glucose levels
■ Increasing blood protein levels
■ Increasing the levels of the prostaglandin E1.

And we can achieve all this through Insulin Balance and Ketogenics.

Build Lean Mass

That vital benefit of HGH – building lean body mass – holds the second secret to permanent weight control. Your lean body mass is always in flux – increasing or decreasing. When it changes, this is not because of alterations in your organs or bones, but rather because of alterations in your muscle. Under-muscled people have low levels of energy. Studies show they are at as great a risk from degeneration and early ageing as people who have too much body fat. When your muscles are strong, dense and alive, aches and pains vanish and posture is good too – for posture depends upon muscle alone. So does the proper elimination of waste from your cells. The lymphatic system, which carries these waste products away, is not powered by the heart but by muscle movement. So the more muscle movement you get, the better it works. This is particularly important for women – even slim ones. For unless your lymphatic system is working properly, you can end up with deposits of water, wastes and fat on localised areas of your body, better known as cellulite.

Total Effects

How your body performs both biochemically as well as physiologically is to a great extent determined by its ratio of LBM to fat. When for any reason, such as being inactive or going off and on slimming diets, you shed lean muscle tissue, your energy and the way your body performs is undermined. In most of us this is a slow decrease – often so slow that you don't notice it – over many years, only to awaken in midlife to find that your body is flabby even if you have remained thin, and that you suffer from chronic fatigue. There are other things too that can decrease muscle mass, such as illness, or too much exercise, or the wrong kind of exercise. Then, even if you appear to have stayed the same weight on the scales, the fat on your body will have increased and your body will have a lost great deal of its tone. The important thing to remember about weight control is this: stop worrying about how to whittle away just a bit more flab from your hips, thighs or tummy, and concentrate instead on improving your muscle mass.

So to shed fat and keep it off, you need to increase your lean body mass. For energy, beauty, health and weight control, most physiologists would say that 90 per cent LBM to 10 per cent fat is ideal for men. For women, 80 to 85 per cent LBM is just about perfect, which means carrying no more than 15 to 20 per cent of your weight in fat.

Check It Out

There are a number of methods for measuring your body composition. They are most often used by physiologists concerned with improving the performance of athletes. The procedure is sometimes done in sports clinics by hydrostatic weighing. With this method, the person sits on a chair in a tank of water to be weighed. The technique relies on Archimedes's principle that when a body is submerged, the buoyancy equals the weight of displaced water. Bone and muscle are denser than water, so a person who's got a higher LBM will weigh more in the water, and a person with a higher percentage of body fat will weigh less. Some physiologists do the measurements using what is called an impedance unit, where a very small current is sent through pads placed on your wrist or ankle to determine LBM-to-fat ratios, or sound or light waves are sent through the body. These can give a ballpark reading, but only hydrostatic weighing is truly accurate. The most common way of measuring – although not by any means the most accurate – is done with skin callipers, where you pinch your skin at various parts of the body and then measure the thickness of the pinch. Some complex calculations later, you'll have determined your body mass ratio. Easiest of all is to reach down and pinch your own flesh with your fingers at the bottom of the ribs, on your thighs, upper arms, belly, bottom and hips. If your pinch is thicker than half an inch to one inch, your LBM-to-fat ratio is not as good as it could be.

Here is a simple method which you can use as a quick rule of thumb both in Ketogenics or Insulin Balance.

PERCENTAGE BODY FAT CHART FOR WOMEN

If you are a woman – use this chart.

Use a ruler to line up your hip measurement with your height.
For example: If your hips measure 36.5 inches and you are
5 feet 2 inches tall, then your body fat is about 26 per cent.

Your relative body-fat measurement is at the point where the ruler crosses the percentage fat line.

From Sensible Fitness *(p.31) by J. H. Wilmore, Champaign, Illinois. Human Kinetics Publishers. Copyright © 1996 by Jack H. Wilmore. Reprinted by permission.*

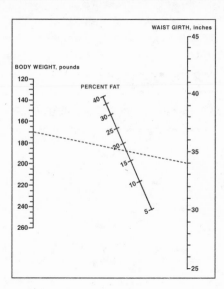

From Sensible
Fitness *(p.31) by J.
H. Wilmore,
Champaign, Illinois.
Human Kinetics
Publishers. Copyright
© 1996 by Jack H.
Wilmore. Reprinted
by permission.*

Forget Your Age

There is a widespread belief that as you get older, your body metabolism
naturally slows down and therefore you are less and less able to prevent
yourself from becoming fat. Actually, age has little to do with it. It doesn't
matter how old you are or how much you weigh now. What limits your ability
to burn fat and stay lean is how long you have been inactive. It is long-term
inactivity which wastes lean body mass and results in an inability at cellular
level to burn the calories you take in from wholesome food as energy. Start now
to improve your LBM by increasing the amount of muscle on your body, and
you can forget calorie counting forever. Once your LBM becomes prominent

enough, you will become one of those people you have always envied, who can eat whatever they like without ever gaining an ounce. But you have got to exercise to keep it that way.

That is where exercise designed specifically for building muscle comes in. Don't worry, this does not mean that you will end up musclebound. Quite the contrary. It's only women with hormonal disorders, or who take steroids, who sport those bulging arms and legs. Exercise to build muscle, such as weight training, using very light weights but many repetitions, is the most effective way of building LBM and uncovering your true body form. It increases your levels of growth hormone, and chisels and defines arms, legs, torso, hips and bottom, even if they have been neglected for many years and have lost their natural tone and shape. So good is this kind of body building at improving LBM that until recently no one considered that it might be an excellent form of protection against degenerative diseases such as coronary heart disease as well. There was a time when aerobic exercise was considered king for health fitness and longevity. Now, thanks to new research into the effects of weight training at prestigious centres such as McMasters University in Ontario, we know that aerobic exercise, in combination with weight training, is the very best you can get for health, fitness and longevity as well as good looks, stamina and energy. As a result, the much-respected American College of Sports Medicine have recently revised their long-standing assertion that aerobic exercise was the healthiest kind.

Weights Have It

Where aerobic exercise strengthens the heart and lungs, weight training goes far beyond. In the past five years an enormous number of studies have been carried out where the health of people in all age groups has been assessed before and after weight training. The results are amazing. They show that working out with dumbbells and barbells, or using the weight-training equipment you find in gyms, not only strengthens joints and increases muscle mass. It also raises the levels of growth hormone, as well as preventing and reversing osteoporosis. And it increases your bone density no matter what your age. Weight training improves just about everything in your life.

As long as you leave enough recovery time between sessions, the more weight training you do on the same body parts, the more you increase your lean-body-mass-to-fat-ratio. Far from making you musclebound, it will make you leaner. Many people who begin to do weight training find that they gain weight, although they have lost size. When they get dressed they discover their clothes have become loose, and that they have got rid of all the bulges that they have never been able to tackle. It often clears cellulite – provided, of course, that you cut out the high-carbohydrate junk foods in your diet. The more muscle mass you build, the more energy-burning factories you create in your cells, which in turn increases your metabolic rate. You are able to burn fuel for energy and lay down less fat, until eventually you can eat more than you are eating now, and never get fat.

Sleek Smooth Body

With time, your muscles will become become denser and more compact. Don't be worried if from time to time you step on the scales to find you weigh a pound or two more, instead of less. As your muscles become more dense, they also become heavier and the more muscle you create in your body the less fat there is. It is important to measure your fat loss progress by the size of clothes that you are wearing as well as the scales.

How long does it take to transform your body into a fat-burning organism? The process of building muscle is a slow one. It takes place over months. Having said this, people who are on a carbohydrate-restricted diet, and getting optimal quantities of high biological value proteins (see page 62-3) gain muscle far quicker than anything else. So Ketogenics and Insulin Balance can only speed up the process.

The Science Of Weight Training

I was introduced to the powers and the pleasures of weight training 10 years ago and began working with a young Welsh champion weightlifter who lived and breathed weights. My experience was so very different from the clichéd image that people have of doing weights. I learnt that it is a precise art and science. It is also incredibly stilling to the mind. When you are working with dumbbells or barbells you are fully present with the experience. You work a specific muscle group, while the rest of your body is still – a state very much like meditation.

To promote fat loss, weight training should always be done on an empty stomach. This way you use up the glycogen in your body quickly, and then turn to fat burning for energy.

Equipment Options

There are a number of different ways to do strength training. They include:

Free Weights
▨ For general strength and fitness, these are the best. Even top weightlifters depend heavily on free weights to develop their strength and skill. They consist of hand weights and ankle weights and they are great for use at home. Buy three pairs of weights in say, 3lb, 5lb and 8lb dumbbells

(although when choosing dumbbells make sure you pick them up and try the exercises you are going to do with them first). The heaviest weight should leave your muscle fatigued at the end of six to eight repetitions, but not be so heavy that you cannot lift it.

Weight Machines

▦ This is the kind of equipment you find in gyms. They're very popular, and it's easy to become dazzled by the technology. Some of equipment is particularly useful when doing exercises such as leg extensions or leg curls. It's easier to do these on weight machines than in any other way. Mostly, however, free weights are better than weight machines. For weight machines tend to limit your range of motion and in doing so negate the benefits gained by the balance itself that is established when you are actually moving free weights up and down.

Rubber Bands Or Tubing

▦ These can be good for travel. The rubber bands are huge versions of the office type, in different colours. The tubes, again in different colours, have lightweight plastic or nylon bars attached to them. Using either, you can mimic the effect of using weights and carry out a range of exercises for both upper and lower body. I prefer the giant rubber bands to the rubber tubing and plastic bars, for I find that the rubber tubing can very easily cause injury if you happen to slip or let go of it while you are exercising.

Gravity Resistance

▦ There are lots of exercises that use resistance to gravity to build strength, without the need for any special equipment. Push-ups, lunges, squats and sit-ups use your own body weight against gravity to increase strength. Even top athletes who use weight machines and free weights tend often to do many of their exercises through simple resistance, especially the abdominal or 'abs' exercises.

Water Works

▦ Exercising in water, and using its natural resistance, is enormously valuable for anyone with arthritis or other muscular or skeletal difficulties. It is gentle on the joints and makes it possible for you to gain strength without putting strain where it shouldn't be put. Many gyms and pools offer water-resistant work outs.

How To Get Started

First, check out your overall fitness. This you can do at a gym or with your doctor. The key to exercising well is to remember that it doesn't matter where you begin, for exercising at the right level for you will slowly and yet inexorably build strength and power. Remember that when you are lifting weights they need to be heavy enough to challenge you without causing injury. Don't be worried if you feel a bit sore after your first few workouts. What you should not feel, however, is serious pain.

Every time you lift and lower a weight, you form a repetition or 'rep'. Most reps take you 6 to 7 seconds to complete, 2 or 3 seconds to lift the weight, 1 second to hold it, and 3 to 4 seconds to lower it. You always want to pick up a weight that you can lift at least 8 times. The last rep should be difficult. As you work out and gain more strength, you will find that you will probably need to increase the weight of some of your dumbbells. If you can perform more than 12 reps in a row with no difficulty, this is an indication that your strength has increased so much you need a slightly heavier weight. A workout usually takes between 20 to 30 minutes to complete. The American College of Sports Medicine suggest 12 reps for each exercise, while people over 50 use somewhat lighter weights, light enough to allow 10 to 15 reps. The number of times you carry out each rep is called a set. For instance, 8 leg extensions followed by a couple of minutes' rest is considered one set. It's a good idea always to begin any resistance training by doing a 5- to 6-minute warm-up, such as marching, dancing to music or some other form of aerobic activity. This warms up cold muscles and helps to protect from injuries. Similarly, after doing your strength training, you will want to do a stretch and cool down which lengthens the muscles and helps prevent the build-up of lactic acid, which can cause aches.

Break Down To Build Up

Strength training works in a unique way. Many people believe that it is while you are doing the exercises that you are building lean body mass – increasing muscle density. This is not the case. Working out with a set of weights actually breaks down muscle tissue, causing very small tears in it. It is between 24 and 48 hours later, in response to these minor tears, that the body reacts and rebuilds new muscle. This makes it important to give yourself plenty of time between each exercise session for new muscle to be built. If you choose to carry out four sessions of strength training or weight training each week, you will need to exercise a different muscle group each of the four days. Say, shoulders Monday, legs Tuesday, skip a day for recovery, then do chest and back on Thursday, and then arms on Friday, then skip two days and begin the programme all over again.

I have looked at many different possibilities for people doing resistance work at home, and the very best that I have found are a series of four videos based on the work of Dr Michael Colgan, whom we met earlier. I think that Colgan probably knows more than anyone else in the world about exercise physiology and weight training, and all from a very practical point of view. Colgan has been advisor on nutrition to the American Olympics Committee, and has written a number of excellent books for top athletes. This programme is distributed through the American nutritional company Usana and is called *The Get Lean Video Programme.* While Usana's nutritional products are by no means what you would use in Ketogenics, I can't recommend the exercise programme highly enough for beginners.

There are also three books on strength training that I recommend highly. Wayne Westcott and Thomas Baechel's *Strength Training Past Fifty* (Human Kenetics, Leeds, 1998), Miriam Nelson's *Strong Women Stay Young* (Bantam, New York, 2000), and *The Wharton's Strength Book* by Jim and Phil Wharton (Random House, New York, 1999).

Wait For It

Not only is strength training the most powerful physical action you can take to make Ketogenics work better, faster and deeper in transforming the shape and vitality of your body – it is also something that you'll never want to give up once you've begun it. For you will notice that it improves your activities all day long, day after day. Carrying groceries is easier, clothes fit better, and you won't get back pains from gardening once your abs exercises have strengthened those stomach muscles that support the back.

Back On Your Bike

If for any reason you stop weight training for a period, you never seem to lose the knack. Once your muscles know the ropes, the moment you pick up your weights, your body seems to breathe a sigh of relief. It's a real pleasure to get back into training again. You never lose what you have learned and you can very rapidly rebuild the strength that may have been lost from being without exercise. Finally, resistance training, more than any form of exercise, brings you a sense of radiance. It's as though the whole of your body and your spirit sings. And because resistance training works so profoundly with the most important *real* force that any of us on the earth have to deal with – gravity – it seems to bring people an ability not only to dream their dreams but to make them happen.

PART THREE:

PATH TO POWER

DYNAMIC DUO

Both programmes in the X Factor Diet have the same goal: to help you shed excess fat permanently while enhancing your health. They accomplish this because of the way they are put together. Both help prevent and reverse insulin resistance and Syndrome X.

THE X FACTOR DIET

Ketogenics: a kickstart to fat loss
For women: more than 35 per cent body fat
For men: more than 22 per cent body fat

Insulin Balance: a diet for life
For women: less than 35 per cent body fat
For men: less than 22 per cent body fat

Both Ketogenics and Insulin Balance are based on the same principles:

- Eliminate both refined and high glycaemic index carbohydrates, including flour, starchy vegetables like potatoes, white rice, sugar and other sweeteners.
- Choose natural, fresh, organic, unprocessed foods.
- Eat many of your vegetables and fruits raw if you can, to get the benefits of the sunlight quanta they carry.
- Make non-starchy vegetables your primary source of carbohydrates.
- Steer clear of soft drinks, fruit juices, alcohol, and other highly processed drinks.
- Eliminate vegetable oils rich in omega-6 fatty acids from your diet. Use cold-pressed, extra-virgin olive oil instead.
- Enrich your diet with omega-3 fatty acids from fish and flaxseed oils.
- Refuse all trans fats, which are found in deep-fried foods, margarine, and foods that contain partially hydrogenated oils.
- Eat protein foods at every meal and snack.
- Eliminate coffee – especially on Ketogenics.

- Stay away from commercial foods.
- Gradually determine your own best level of carbohydrate for weight loss and maintenance and stick to it.
- Take a multiple vitamin plus plant factor antioxidant such as flavonoids, pygnogenal and alpha-lipoic acid regularly.
- Do some form of strength training four days a week for 30 minutes to strengthen your lean body mass.
- Walk briskly for 15 to 30 minutes each day to counter insulin resistance, enhance energy, improve your body's uptake of glycogen and maintain good emotional balance.

Gentle Transformation

Choosing the programme that's right for you depends on a number of factors. Insulin Balance is designed to help *moderately* overweight people reduce their fat levels and stave off premature ageing. It increases the lean-body-mass-to-fat-ratio, detoxifies the body, and heightens overall energy. The diet you follow on Insulin Balance reduces your intake of grains, improves the kind of fats you will be eating and introduces a calorific ratio of 35:35:30 for proteins, carbohydrates and fats at each meal. That mean 35 per cent of the foods you are eating will be chosen from top-quality proteins, 35 per cent from low glycaemic index carbohydrates and 30 per cent from health-enhancing fats.

INSULIN BALANCE IS THE RIGHT PROGRAMME IF:

- You are a woman with less than 35 per cent fat on your body or a man with less than 22 per cent.
- You want to improve your blood sugar control and enhance your energy levels so that you don't feel tired after a meal.
- You are only a few pounds overweight.
- You are generally healthy, and want to prevent the development of insulin resistance, or Syndrome X.
- You have only one or two symptoms of Syndrome X, such as high blood pressure or distorted cholesterol balance.
- You want to live longer and look better.
- You want to protect yourself from degenerative disease and hormonal imbalances from chronic fatigue, arthritis and weight gain.

On Insulin Balance you will eat three meals and two snacks each day. Each meal will be made up of one part protein to two parts low glycaemic carbohydrates, or one part protein to one part medium glycaemic carbohydrates. Your snacks will be in the same ratios.

Deep Revolution

Ketogenics is an ultra-low carbohydrate programme specifically designed for men who carry more than 22 per cent fat on their body and woman who carry more than 35 per cent. It is also for any healthy individual who prefers a more dynamic method of fat loss. People whose body fat is below these percentages lose weight on Insulin Balance, but above these percentages, the human body generally tends to maintain levels of free fatty acids in the blood which interfere with the fat-burning effects of the Insulin Balance programme. That is why they need Ketogenics. Once your percentage of body fat goes below the figures above, you should be able to switch to Insulin Balance. Many people who begin Ketogenics, however, like the diet so much that they prefer to remain on it until all excess weight is shed. Then they switch over to Insulin Balance as a permanent way of living and eating.

KETOGENICS IS THE RIGHT PROGRAMME IF:

- You are a woman with more than 35 per cent fat on your body or a man with more than 22 per cent fat.
- You have been unable to lose weight and need a swift reversal of insulin resistance.
- You have a number of the symptoms of Syndrome X or are borderline Type II diabetic.
- Because of all of the above, you need to kickstart your system to prepare yourself for the life plan, Insulin Balance.

Goodbye Grain

Compared to Insulin Balance, Ketogenics dramatically reduces the number of calories you consume. It is based on a maximum of 20 per cent of your calories coming from carbohydrates, 30 per cent from fats and a minimum of 50 per cent from protein. Unlike Insulin Balance, Ketogenics does not include grain foods. It uses only carbohydrates with a low glycaemic index and low carbohydrate density, such as fresh non-starchy vegetables. It uses protein foods which are reasonably low in saturated fats, and fats which consist of omega-3 fatty acids from flaxseed and fish oils, as well as mono-unsaturated extra virgin olive oil and coconut oil – a stable saturated fat which encourages fat burning. On either programme you will naturally get enough omega-6 fats through the foods you are eating. During Ketogenics you will be eating three meals and two snacks per day. Each meal will be made up of two parts protein to one part of low glycaemic vegetables. The snacks are protein only.

PROGRAMMES' BENEFITS

Insulin Balance	Ketogenics
Increases vitality and energy	Greatly reduces body fat
Balances hormones	Reduces insulin levels
Reduces 'brain fatigue'	Reduces sugar cravings
Increases longevity	Increases basal metabolism
Helps in fat reduction	Improves energy
Great for athletes	Improves moderate to severe
Increases basal metabolism	insulin resistance
Increases muscle mass	Increases muscle mass
Balances blood sugar levels	Eliminates constant hunger
Detoxifies the body	Detoxifies the body

Insulin Balance is designed both to prevent and reverse minor insulin resistance. Ketogenics stimulates quicker and more aggressive reversal of insulin resistance. It is the best plan for you if you have had difficulty or been unable to lose weight.

Regular physical activity features in both programmes, to increase your body's insulin sensitivity glucose tolerance and to lower your risk of getting degenerative illnesses. This is just simple weight training for half an hour four days a week (and easily done at home), combined with daily brisk walks of between 15 to 30 minutes. See the preceding chapter for the hows and whys of exercise, X-Factor style.

Key Differences
We've seen that the principles of Insulin Resistance and Ketogenics are the same, but that the diets diverge on a number of points. Here's a summary of the three key differences:

1 Both programmes use low-density carbohydrates, but Insulin Balance also uses medium glycaemic carbohydrates. On Insulin Balance you can eat freely of non-starchy low glycaemic carbohydrates, as well as the odd

starchy vegetable, legume, fruit and whole grain. On Ketogenics, even the amount of low glycaemic, low-density carbohydrates is limited.

2 With Ketogenics, you eat higher levels of protein foods and omega-3 fatty acids than you do with Insulin Balance. When you are hungry on Ketogenics you eat extra protein foods.

3 Insulin Balance is safe for just about everyone. Ketogenics should not be used by pregnant women, or anyone about to undergo surgery. It is also not suitable for someone with kidney or liver problems unless supervised by a doctor or other health professional, trained in functional medicine and aware of Syndrome X and its implications.

As the more dynamic of the two, Ketogenics brings about more rapid improvements in blood pressure, cholesterol and triglycerides as well as more rapid weight loss. Insulin Balance works more slowly and gently but, provided you are not carrying a large percentage of body fat, it gets the job done.

It's important to note that neither of these programmes are quick fixes. Both are designed to transform your body into a fat-burning, radiantly healthy organism at a physiologically sound pace so that you preserve precious lean muscle and enhance your health every step of the way. It may take from six months to a year to bring about a total reversal of symptoms and lose the fat from your body. But this time it is for keeps.

The Changeover

Let's say you've started on Ketogenics. Once you have been on it for some time and lost whatever weight you needed to lose, you can gradually change over to Insulin Balance. The best way to do this is by adding one daily serving of a medium glycaemic carbohydrate food, such as fruit, a grain or a legume. If you do not notice any weight gain or any sensations of bloating in your stomach from this, it is time to try a serving of another food. You can continue to do this for a month, always monitoring your progress, until you discover the level and kinds of carbohydrates which are ideal for you in order to maintain your weight permanently at its new level.

Whether you want to lose a little weight or a lot, these principles apply. Both programmes return you as much a possible to the paleolithic, genetically compatible way of eating and physical activity that I've been exploring with you.

▓ To lose weight it is essential that you avoid carbohydrate-dense high glycaemic foods, no matter how 'natural' they may be. In both cases your main source of carbohydrates should be non-starchy vegetables.

▓ After you've lost the weight, to prevent regaining it or getting Syndrome X, eat no more than moderate quantities of natural carbohydrate-dense foods, and then only occasionally. Such foods include high glycaemic fruits, legumes, grains and starchy vegetables. If you ever do eat these foods on Insulin Balance, always have them together with protein, fat and plenty of fibre at the same meal to minimise their insulin-raising tendencies.

Insulin Balance is an excellent way of eating to control blood glucose and insulin levels and protect yourself from Syndrome X and the early ageing and degeneration it brings.

Very overweight people cannot benefit from Insulin Balance because their body fat maintains circulating levels of fatty acids to feed insulin resistance. They need to lose fat tissue from their bodies below critical percentages (see Table) before Insulin Balance can take effect. This loss of fat can be achieved with Ketogenics.

Insulin Balance 35:35:30 carbs:proteins:fats	**Ketogenics** 20:50:30 carbs:proteins:fats
Longevity	Obesity
Fat loss/muscle gain for Women with less than 35% fat Men with less than 22% fat	Fat loss: Women with more than 35% fat
Hormonal Control	Men with more than
Blood sugar control	22% fat
Prevention of Syndrome X	Diabetes (Type II)
	Syndrome X

Whichever programme you follow, keep track of your progress by keeping a private personal journal. Record what you are eating each day and how you feel, as well as the amount of exercise you get and your experience of the whole process of transforming your life.

Riding The Waves
At times you will be filled with excitement and gratitude to have at last discovered a way to live at the high levels of energy and joy with which you may have been out of touch for some time. At other times, it could seem difficult. At the beginning you'll probably be excited over the change, but

remember that down the road, when your body is detoxifying, you'll need to give yourself a chance to rest. And your body will reward you with new vitality and swifter fat loss. Don't forget to write down what you feel in your journal. Human beings don't just detoxify on a physical level. We also cleanse ourselves on a psychological or spiritual one.

Each of us walks around with false ideas, often unconscious, which limit our lives and undermine our capacity for joy and creativity. And each of us carries emotional wounds that need healing. When you're busy healing the body with Ketogenics or Insulin Balance, these things tend to rise to conscious awareness to be experienced and dealt with. So the weight loss is really only part of the process – in a sense, it's not a goal in itself. Permanent fat loss becomes a wonderful gift that comes with restoring your body's metabolic functioning and physiological well-being. It often brings an exhilarating sense of freedom and that wonderful sense that you are becoming more fully yourself. Enjoy it. Meanwhile, let's look more specifically at Ketogenics and Insulin Balance and how to put them into practice.

INSULIN BALANCE STARTS HERE

If you've just started reading here, this is your introduction to Insulin Balance – the moderate-carbohydrate, adequate-protein programme in the X Factor Diet that's designed for people who are slightly overweight. Insulin Balance helps prevent both symptoms of mild insulin resistance and the cluster of degenerative diseases that make up Syndrome X. It's an excellent life-long programme that helps you shed fat and protects you from high cholesterol, hypertension and elevated triglycerides, and it's suitable for women carrying less than 35 per cent of their body weight as fat, and men carrying less than 22 per cent.

INSULIN BALANCE EATING

■ Promotes balanced ratios of carbohydrates, fats and proteins for high level health and vitality

■ Prevents hyperinsulinaemia and insulin resistance, which can contribute to heart disease, cancer, hormonal imbalance, diabetes, arthritis, chronic low energy, weight gain, high blood pressure and high cholesterol

■ Enhances your energy, prevents chronic disease and protects from premature ageing

■ May lengthen your lifespan.

Carbs Control

As you'll probably know – to your cost – most weight-loss diets are calorie controlled, low in fat and protein, and high in carbohydrates. The very fact that the protein content of these diets is low means that by following them you lose precious muscle tissue from your body – ageing it, undermining your health and making it virtually impossible to keep off any weight you've lost. Most slimming diets also raise insulin levels, which in turn encourages an increase in body fat.

In the last 50 years, all over the world, we have eaten more and more carbohydrates and junk fats. For the last 20 years we have been urged to increase our intake of complex carbohydrates and reduce fat and protein. Yet clinical experience shows that the commonly eaten high-carb/low-fat diet that is also low in protein raises serum insulin levels, lowers metabolic rate and fosters weight gain. Insulin resistance appears to be the underlying source of most of these ills, as well as a highly stressed immune system and accelerated biological ageing. Coupled with a sedentary lifestyle, this diet can leave you feeling fat, fatigued and futile.

Insulin Balance is specifically designed to reverse these problems. For a moderately overweight person, it promotes significant changes in the ratio of lean body mass to fat, improves overall vitality and reduces toxicity in the body. The Insulin Balance diet includes a balanced intake of macronutrients – 35:35:30 at each meal (35 per cent low to medium glycaemic index carbohydrates, 35 per cent top-quality protein and 30 per cent beneficial fats).

INSULIN BALANCE EATING YOUR CALORIES

35 per cent should come from carbohydrates

35 per cent from protein

30 per cent from 'good' fats

NORMALISED BLOOD SUGAR

↓

BALANCED INSULIN LEVELS

↓

A HEALTHIER YOU

↓

Emotional stability	Vitality	Enthusiasm
Normal blood pressure	Energy	Good vital signs
Mental activity	Restful sleep	Creativity	Ideal body size
Good lean body mass	Balanced hormones

HOW MUCH PROTEIN

To calculate your daily protein requirement for Insulin Balance, it is important to calculate your lean body mass. This is an easy thing to do once you have calculated the percentage of body fat that you carry (see page 92-3).

Multiply your weight in kilos times your percentage of body fat. This gives your total body fat weight.

_____	_____	_____
Weight x	**% of body fat** =	**Total body fat weight**

Once you know the weight of your total body fat, subtract this from your total weight. What you get is your lean body mass. Your lean body mass measurement is the total weight of all of the non-fat tissues in your body. You'll need this measurement to work out your ideal level of protein each day. This in turn will enable you, by comparison, to work out how much carbohydrate foods to balance with it.

Total weight   _____

(minus) Total body fat   _____

= _____   **Your Lean Body Mass**

Now we have to take into account how much physical activity you get, because the more you exercise, the higher your need for protein will be. Here is a chart to help you make that calculation.

Activity	Protein Requirements	Adjustments (If any apply, add to your Physical Activity Factor)
Sedentary	0.5	Pregnancy increase by 0.2
Light (i.e. walking)	0.6	Lactation increase by 0.1
Moderate (30 mins daily, 3 times per week)	0.7	Children increase by 0.2
Active (1 hour daily, 5 times per week)	0.8	Body building increase by 0.1
Very active (2 hours daily, 5 times per week)	0.9	Significantly overweight increase by 0.1
Heavy weight training or twice-a-day exercise (5 days per week)	1.0	(30 per cent for men) (40 per cent for women)

Let's calculate your daily protein requirement:
Here's how to:

Your Lean Body Mass x 2.2 x Physical Activity Factor = Your Total Daily
Protein Requirement

Example: An 82-kilo man has 21 per cent body fat and is sedentary
Weight of Body Fat 82 x 0.21   = 17.2 kilos body fat
Lean Body Mass   82 – 17.2 kilos body fat = 64.8 kilos lean
body mass
Physical Activity Factor (sedentary) is 0.5
Daily Protein Requirement 64.8 x 2.2 x 0.5 = 71.3g of protein
per day

Example: A 59-kilo woman has 34 per cent body fat and is active
Weight of Body Fat   59 kilos x 0.34 = 20 kilos
Lean Body Mass   59 kilos – 20 kilos = 39 kilos
Physical Activity Factor (active) = 0.8
Daily Protein Requirement 39 x 2.2 x 0.8 = 68.6g of protein
per day

It's vital to note that this is NOT the weight of meat or fish, but the weight, in
grams, of the *protein* it contains. Most meats and fish, for instance, are only 20
to 30 per cent protein.

How do you figure out the protein content of food, on a practical, day-by-day
basis? Of course, you could always spend hours mulling over long lists of the
protein, fat and carbohydrate contents of every food that you eat. In my
opinion, this does little more than make people neurotic. It could even turn you
into one of those obsessive 'health foodies', who think of little beyond the
amount of nutrients they are getting. Happily, there is another way. You may
recall the *palm method* I described in an earlier chapter. It's a technique
frequently used by doctors, nutritionists and other practitioners trained in
functional medicine. Once you grasp the general idea, the answer to how much
protein you have to eat literally lies in the palm of your hand. And the method
can be used for both Insulin Balance and Ketogenics.

How The Palm Method Works
The size of the palm of your hand, including its thickness and excluding your
fingers and thumb, is about the same as the volume of protein food you will
need to eat at each Insulin Balance meal. It may be a little more or a little less,

depending on your lean body mass. In any case, the ratio of how many palms of protein to carbohydrate you should eat remains constant. For snacks, you will want a third of a palm of protein food. If you get a great deal of exercise, or are pregnant, you will need to add an extra third of a palm to each meal.

The only way in which the palm method breaks down in measuring protein is when you are having a meal or a snack based on microfiltered whey protein. This doesn't matter too much since the exact protein content of a specific amount of whey protein – a scoop or a tablespoon, for example – is invariably given on the package. So you will need to judge your whey protein by grams of protein content rather than the palm method. Most micro-filtered whey protein snacks should contain between 10 and 15g of pure protein. As a meal replacement, you are looking at 15 to 30g.

How Many Carbs

Use the same method to find out how much carbohydrate to eat – except that here things become slightly more complicated. On Insulin Balance you will need two palms of good carbohydrates – that is, low glycaemic carbohydrates such as steamed broccoli, spinach, cauliflower, green beans and salad vegetables. Alternatively, you can have one palm of medium to high glycaemic carbohydrates. You can even, if you want to get fancy and combine best-choice carbohydrates and higher glycaemic carbohydrates, have one palm of the best choice and half a palm of the higher glycaemics.

Gauging The Fats

The amount of fat that you need at each meal is about one tablespoon of the best: extra-virgin olive oil, flaxseed oil, coconut oil, or the fats in foods such as avocados, olives, fish or game, macadamia nuts, almonds or tahini. The amount of fat you eat usually doesn't cause deficiency. From the point of view of the palm method, you will need to eat fat equivalent to the size of your smallest finger at each meal.

Great Protein Meal Choices

Fish, shellfish, chicken, organic beef, organic lamb, low fat cheese (occasionally), turkey, venison, eggs, wild duck, rabbit, and game, micro-filtered whey protein.

= 1 palm full as thick as your palm

Good Carbohydrate Meal Choices

Celery, sprouted seeds and grains, lettuce, spinach, radicchio, cauliflower, broccoli, snow peas, cabbage, dandelion greens, fresh fennel, mustard greens, bok choy, Swiss chard, asparagus spears, cucumber, leeks, marrow, mushrooms, parsley.

= 2 palms full as thick as your palm

Poor Carbohydrate Meal Choices

Baked potato, carrots, parsnips, bananas, chopped dates.
½ palm full as thick as your palm

Great and Poor Carbohydrate Meal Choices

Steamed green beans, broccoli, spinach, cauliflower, sautéed mushroom/onion. Salad: lettuce, snow peas, radish, onion, endive, celery.
= 1½ palms full as thick as your palm
Fresh banana and chopped dates
= ½ palm full as thick as

The palm method is an easy way to go about getting the right balance between top-quality proteins, good carbohydrates and good fats on Insulin Balance.

GREAT CHOICE PROTEINS	POOR CHOICE PROTEINS
Meat and Poultry	
Beef (organic, lean)	Bacon
Beef, minced – organic (less than 15 per cent fat)	Beef, fatty cuts
Micro-filtered whey protein	Liver, chicken
Chicken breast (free range, organic, skinless)	Pepperoni
Liver, lamb (organic)	Salami
Turkey breast	Sausage: pork, beef, turkey, or chicken
Eggs	
Egg whites	

Fish and Seafood

Bass
BluefishCalamari
Clams
Cod *
Crab
Grouper
Haddock
Halibut
Lobster
Mackerel *
Prawns
Salmon *
Sardines*
Scallops
Snapper
Swordfish
Taraki
Trout*
Tuna, canned in water
Tuna, steak*

* rich in Omega-3 essential fatty acids

Protein-Rich Dairy Foods	
(only occasionally)	
Cheese, fat free	Parmesan
Cottage cheese, low fat 1%	
Cottage cheese, no fat	

CARBOHYDRATES GOOD CHOICES

Raw Vegetables	Cooked Vegetables	Fresh Fruit
Alfalfa Sprouts	Artichoke	Apple
Bamboo shoots	Asparagus	Apricots
Broccoli	Aubergine	Blackberries
Cabbage	Beans, green	Blueberries
Capsicum	Bok choy	Boysenberries
Cauliflower	Broccoli	Cantaloupe melon
Celery	Brussels sprouts	Cherries
Cucumber	Cabbage	Grapefruit
Endive	Cauliflower	Honeydew melon
Escarole	Chick peas	Kiwi fruit
Fennel	Collard greens	Lemon
Lambs' Lettuce	Courgette	Lime
Lettuce	Hommus	Mandarin
Mushrooms	Kale	Nectarine
Onions	Leeks	Orange
Radishes	Lentils	Peach
Rocket	Mushrooms, boiled	Pear
Salsa	Okra	Pineapple
Snow peas	Onions, boiled	Plum
Spinach	Sauerkraut	Raspberries
Tomato	Silverbeet	Strawberries
	Spinach	Tangerine
	Turnip	Watermelon
	Yellow squash	

Grains
Barley
Steel-cut oatmeal

CARBOHYDRATES POOR CHOICES

Vegetables Cooked
Acorn squash
Baked beans
Beetroot
Butternut pumpkin
Carrot
Chips, potato
Corn
Lima beans
Parsnips
Peas
Pinto beans
Potato, baked
Potato, boiled
Potato, mashed
Re-fried beans
Sweet potato, baked

Condiments and Treats
Barbecue sauce
Cocktail sauce
Honey
Ice-cream
Jam or jelly
Molasses
Plum sauce
Relish, pickle
Sugar
Sugar, icing
Sweets
Syrup, 'Golden'
Syrup, 'Maple'
Teriyaki sauce
Tomato sauce

Grains, Cereals and Breads
Bagel
Biscuits
Bread crumbs
Bread, whole-grain or white
Bread sticks
Buckwheat
Bulgar wheat
Cereal
Cornflour
Couscous, dry
Crackers
Croissant
Croûtons
Doughnut
English muffin
Granola
Grits, cooked
Melba toast
MilletCake

Alcohol
Beer
Spirits
Wine

FATS

Good Choices	Poor Choices
Almond butter	Bacon bits
Almonds	Butter
Avocado	Cream
Coconut oil	Cream cheese
Guacamole	Lard
Macadamia butter	Margarine
Macadamia nuts	Sour cream
Olive oil	
Olive oil and vinegar dressing	
Olives	
Peanut butter, natural	
Tahini	

Drink Up

What you drink is important, too. You may be in the habit of drinking fruit juice, but it doesn't fit well into an insulin-balanced way of life. If you feel you must have a glass of apple juice or orange juice every now and then, try diluting it – one-third juice to two-thirds water – and treat it as a serving of fruit when calculating your carbohydrates for meals and snacks. Fruit juices are very high on the glycaemic index. Your body soaks them up like pure sugar and absorbs them very rapidly.

Coffee also has a tendency to raise blood glucose levels, especially if you drink a lot of it. People on Ketogenics need to steer clear of coffee altogether, but on Insulin Balance, most people can get away with a cup or two a day – no more. Tea is a better choice. Both green tea and black tea contain some caffeine, but can lower glucose and triglyceride levels. Coffees, teas and anything else containing caffeine, however, tend to have a diuretic effect on the body, which you don't need.

If you drink sugar-free colas and soft drinks, this is another thing you will want to avoid (see 'Sweet Nothings' – page 207). Fruit-flavoured mineral waters are fine provided they contain no carbohydrates and no artificial sweeteners (check the labels) .

Although alcohol – that is, hard liquor like whiskey, gin and vodka – raises insulin levels and is best avoided, a glass of dry white or red wine with one of your meals is okay. It may even have a beneficial effect. A number of recent studies indicate red wine in particular increases the body's sensitivity to insulin.

This is one of the main goals of Insulin Balance, so adding a glass of wine to your lunch or dinner may further enhance the process. Wine does have some carbohydrate in it – dry white and red wines usually contain from 1 to 1.5g of carbohydrate per ounce. So if you do choose to drink a glass or two of wine with one of your meals – no more than one or two small glasses – be sure to take this carbohydrate into account when calculating your daily allotment.

By far the best drink of all is water. To calculate optimum quantities for your body, see page 159. Drink this much every day even if you have to carry a bottle of water around with you to remind you to get your quota.

Now let's look at some typical meals for breakfast, lunch and dinner and some good Insulin Balance snacks.

Insulin Balance Breakfasts

Breakfast is the most important meal of the day. Here are some suggestions for Insulin Balance breakfasts that will help keep your energy high all through the morning.

Three scrambled eggs in olive oil with two cloves of garlic, chopped tomatoes, onions and homemade salsa.
i.e. The eggs = 1 palm protein
1 tsp olive oil = 1 little finger of fat
Tomatoes, onions, homemade salsa = 1 palm of carbohydrate

A slice of melon and naturally smoked kippered herring.
i.e. Kippers = 1 palm of protein (contain omega-3)
Melon = 1 palm of carbohydrate

A large bowl of yoghurt and strawberries, sprinkled with almonds and sweetened with stevia (see page 209-11).
i.e. Low-fat yoghurt = mixture of protein and carbohydrate
Strawberries = a good source of carbohydrate
Almonds = good source of essential fatty acids

A small breakfast steak quick-seared in coconut oil with sliced onions, mushrooms, and green beans.
i.e. The breakfast steak = the protein
The mushroom, onions and green beans = good-quality carbohydrate
Olive oil = the fat

Three poached eggs on a slice of 100 per cent rye toast drizzled with low-carb jam.

A quick shake made with 20-30g of microfiltered whey protein, a teaspoon of flaxeed oil, an apple and 2 heaped teaspoons of psyllium husk sweetened with stevia (see page 209-11).

Insulin Balance Lunches

Caesar salad with hard-boiled egg, croutons and carrot sticks.

Chef's salad with turkey slices, grated cheese, olives, artichoke hearts and a creamy dressing.

Big Greek salad with 28g of left over lamb or chicken made with sliced red onions, romaine lettuce, cucumber, tomato wedges, sprinkled with a teaspoon of sesame seeds and a teaspoon of pumpkin seeds, Greek olives and 2 teaspoons of crumbled feta cheese with an oil and lemon dressing.

Chicken kebabs skewered with onion pieces, red and geen pepper chunks and mushrooms dipped in olive oil and seasoned with herbs and a dash of lemon.

Bun-free hamburger – organic beef, turkey or chicken burger with sliced lettuce, tomatoes and cucumbers.

Tuna or rye sandwich with tomatoes, fresh garlic, homemade mayonnaise, sprouted seeds and grains, mixed sprouts and fresh tomatoes.

Fennel, orange and grape salad with snow peas and leftover slices of turkey or lamb

Crudités with three dips – aubergine, tapenade and curried guacamole.

Insulin Balance Dinners

Sautéed sea bass with garlic, steamed broccoli and courgettes with almonds.

Three small grilled lamb chops with garlic, oregano and lemon juice, grilled sliced aubergine and tomatoes, brushed with olive oil and seasoned with fresh herbs.

Grilled tiger prawns and rocket salad served with aeoli.

Grilled salmon, baked asparagus with butter, lambs' lettuce salad with blue cheese dressing.

Stir-fried chicken with bok choy, bean sprouts, ginger, green onions, garlic, water chestnuts cooked in coconut oil with a coconut cream sauce and sprinkled with toasted sesame seeds.

How Quick Can You Tell?

How long will it take to begin to experience the benefits of Insulin Balance? The time varies greatly from one person to another. Most people start to see changes very quickly. Within a week or two they find they have more energy, and fewer cravings for food. Their digestion works better, their tummy is flatter. By all accounts it should take three months or longer before you experience a fall in blood pressure and a shift in cholesterol levels. What has surprised me is that many people experience measurable positive change in these areas in as little as four or five weeks.

On a personal level, you will feel more alert and have more energy to keep you going – signs that your insulin sensitivity is enhanced and your blood sugar stabilised. You are likely to be less moody. In the beginning, you will lose a few pounds immediately because of water loss when you cut out high-carbohydrate eating. It will then turn into a slow, steady loss of, say, a pound or a pound and half a week. But again, people are highly individual. If within the first three weeks you don't notice your clothes becoming a great deal looser and your tummy a great deal flatter, it might be wise to shift to the more dynamic Ketogenics to jump-start your body's ability to burn fat.

Life Plan

Once Insulin Balance has bought you to the place where you have got the results you were looking for, it will start working for you long term. Experiment with modifying your diet enough so that it becomes slightly more flexible – say, to accommodate the odd bowl of ice cream or a cocktail without it affecting how you look and feel. Everyone has to find their own way as to what works for them: a flexible eating plan that you can follow for the rest of your life. When they begin Insulin Balance, many people do so feeling they can hardly wait until it has worked its wonders so they can go back to eating chocolate ice cream again. The irony is that after six months of Insulin Balance, 85 per cent of them come to the point where chocolate ice cream no longer has much allure. Some people report that they find the desserts they used to long for taste too sweet. Then you know for sure that Insulin Balance has done its work, and done it well.

KETOGENICS – MIRACLE OF NATURE

You are about to enter a whole new world of health, good looks, energy and fat loss. It's called Ketogenics, and we'll spend the next few chapters exploring it.

In the last chapter we looked at how the Insulin Balance plan worked. But it's not suitable for everyone at the beginning. If you're a woman with over 35 per cent body fat, or a man with over 22 per cent body fat, you'll need to begin with the more radical programme in the X Factor Diet, Ketogenics, to kickstart your system.

Within the first two weeks on Ketogenics, you are likely to lose a remarkable amount of weight, usually between 4 to 12 pounds if you are a woman, and 8 to 16 pounds if you are a man. From then on, you can steadily shed from ½ to 2 pounds of stored fat a week, while you marvel at your body reshaping itself to a new sleek firmness without hunger. More importantly, during the next few weeks you can discover just how wonderful it is possible to feel following a high-nutrient/low-carbohydrate diet.

But Ketogenics is not in any real sense a diet at all. It's a scientifically based method for shifting your body out of a static vegetative state into a dynamic – and completely natural – fat-burning mode. At the same time it helps re-establish healthy blood sugar and insulin levels, and helps to eliminate insulin resistance or Syndrome X, which is undermining the health of vast numbers of people throughout the world. It does this by eliminating the *wrong kind* of carbohydrate foods from your diet, and shifting the balance between the *right kind* of carbs/fats and protein.

KETOGENICS:

- Reduces the levels of insulin in the blood, making sure your stored body fat can be metabolised for energy
- Protects valuable muscle tissue and keeps metabolism high so that you never get any diet rebound after weight is lost

---

- Lowers the amount of glucose that can be stored as fat and creates a state in the body of dietary ketosis, which not only enables your body to burn fat as energy but also has a remarkable rejuvenating effect on it
- Is the safest and fastest way to normalise blood sugar and hyperinsulinaemia while shedding excess body fat
- When your carbohydrate intake is low enough your metabolism shifts from a glucose-based method of burning energy to one that uses its own fat stores
- Once ketosis is established, your body goes on burning fat stores while you eat, while you sleep, while you work – even while you meditate on how much better you are going to look and feel in a few weeks' time
- Ketogenics helps restore insulin balance and glucose balance in your body.

Dramatic Cut

Right at the very beginning, you'll reduce your carbohydrate intake dramatically to help your body enter fat-burning mode quickly and effectively. Don't worry, you are not going to be doing this for long – just until your metabolism gets used to turning its attention away from using glucose as a source of energy, towards burning fat stores. Based on a maximum of 20 per cent of calories from carbohydrates, 30 per cent from fat and a minimum of 50 per cent from protein, Ketogenics uses only carbohydrates with both low density and a low glycaemic rating in its salads and cooked vegetable dishes. The beneficial fats we've been reading about – omega-3 fatty acids from fish oils in particular, monounsaturated omega-9 oils like extra-virgin olive and grapeseed oils, and tropical coconut oil for cooking – are all vital to the plan.

Even during the first three weeks of Ketogenics you will by no means be eliminating *all* carbohydrates. You will only be lowering the level of your carbs to 20g a day and increasing your protein to 150g a day for the same period. After that, you yourself will be able to monitor how and when to increase carbs, and by how much.

The carbohydrates you eat on Ketogenics will come mostly from vegetables rich in phyto-nutrients, either served raw in gorgeous, well-dressed salads, or lightly steamed, wok-fried, baked or puréed. You can even have a little of the right kind of fruit if you wish. What this first three-week period will do for you is force your body to enter fat-burning mode by using up all of the stored energy that came from previously eaten carbohydrate foods.

KETOGENICS

- Changes the balance of protein, fat and carbohydrate in your diet
- Is based on a maximum of 20 per cent of calories from carbohydrates, 30 per cent of calories from fat, and a minimum of 50 per cent of calories from protein
- Uses only carbohydrates with a low glycaemic index – which release glucose slowly – in salads, steamed and wok-fried vegetables
- Uses fats mostly from omega-3 (fish oil) and monounsaturated (olive, canola, grapeseed) oils
- Uses protein foods low in most saturated fats.

An End To Hunger

And – great news – as soon as you enter ketosis, usually within a few days, you will not feel hungry. (We'll be looking at ketosis in detail in the following chapter.) Nor will you ever need to count calories. There is no limit to the amount of protein foods you can eat in the first three weeks, but you need to ensure that you get at least 150g per day. Nor is there any limit to the amount of fat that you eat, so long as it is *healthy fat*. What you won't be eating are all of the cereals, breads, pastas and sweets you may be used to. For it is these carbohydrate-based foods, especially refined sugars, that caused you to lay fat down on your body in the first place.

WHAT WILL KETOGENICS DO FOR YOU?

- Lower your body fat in a safe and effective way usually at a rate of ½ to 2 lb fat loss per week
- Lower blood insulin levels, which will help control your appetite
- Drastically decrease the amount of glycogen in your system which can be stored as body fat
- Protect valuable muscle tissue
- Encourage body fat to be burnt for energy

- Release small quantities of ketones in the urine – chemicals that indicate fat is being used for energy
- Banish cravings for sugar and carbs
- Enhance your energy
- Detoxify your body.

Forget Slimming Diets

Calorie-restricted diets don't work. First, they leave you hungry, so there is always an internal battle going on as to whether you stay on the diet or not. Secondly, they don't correct the underlying metabolic imbalances in your body that have caused you to store fat in your tissues. These stores have probably developed over a lifetime of eating a high-carbohydrate diet – especially the wrong kind of dense, refined carbohydrates. It is the imbalances and the biochemical distortions which our modern diet brings about that caused you to gain weight in the first place. They are also responsible for food cravings, chronic fatigue and much of the depression that can accompany being overweight. Ketogenics helps correct these things forever, and Insulin Balance keeps them away forever, while providing you with the leaner, stronger, healthier body that is your birthright.

Lean And Ageless

Ketogenics also protects your muscle tissue, so your body only becomes firmer and sleeker as you lose weight. Muscle mass – that part of your body that's good, strong muscle – is the single most important indicator of biological ageing. The higher your ratio of lean body mass to fat, the better your body is going to function. Ketogenics preserves muscle mass while encouraging fat burning. This is essential for long-term weight control. For it is within the cells of muscle tissue that the fat in your body gets burnt to make energy. The better the quality of muscle tissues you have, the better your body can produce energy and the less it lays down fat stores. Low-calorie slimming diets, high in carbohydrates, low in fat and often lacking enough protein, bring about a significant loss of muscle tissue. This lowers your metabolic rate so that you burn fewer calories for energy, and also contributes to "rebound" weight gain, where a reduced metabolism forces you to eat less and less in order not to regain the weight you have shed. After such dieting, weight gain is inevitable. But when you regain those pounds, you're not regaining the muscle you lost while dieting. They return in the form of more fat stores to undermine your health, strength and beauty and to make weight loss even tougher next time around.

Where Insulin Comes In

I gave you the lowdown on insulin and insulin resistance in the first part of this book – but as a huge part of Ketogenics is overcoming insulin resistance and its attendant ills, I've included the essential points again here.

If you are someone who has tried again and again to lose weight unsuccessfully despite exercise programmes and diets, you are likely to be one of the hundreds of thousands of people who are producing too much insulin and whose cells have therefore become insensitive to it so it can't do its job. This, as we've seen, is a condition called *insulin resistance.*

We've seen how insulin works in the body and makes it possible for your cells to absorb glucose, derived from carbohydrates, from your blood (see page 18-19). All carbohydrates, whether potatoes, wholegrain breads, sweets or breakfast cereals, are broken down into glucose in the body. It's insulin's job to deliver this sugar all over the body, to muscle cells, brain cells and other tissues so it can be used as energy. Trouble looms, however, if you eat too much sugar or too many carbohydrates – especially the *wrong* kind of carbohydrates – in proportion to the amount of protein that you are eating. Eventually insulin can't do its job properly, your cells can't make use of all the available sugar you have consumed as energy, and the excess glucose gets shuttled into your fat cells, where it is stored. You gradually get fatter and fatter, after having to wrestle with a chronic lack of stamina and energy. For your body is able to do little more than store the energy you take in from carbohydrate foods.

BEWARE SLIMMING DIETS

■ Low-calorie weight loss sheds both fat and muscle mass.
■ Loss of muscle mass and the slowed down metabolic rate that comes with them explain why 95 per cent of people cannot maintain their lowered body weight after the slimming diet is finished.

How Fat Gets Stored

Even if you restrict the fat intake in your diet – as much of the Western world has been doing for the last 15 years – you will still lay down more body fat. For it is the glucose from carbohydrates, not fat, that causes your body to get fat. And if insulin resistance sets in, yet more insulin will be secreted in an attempt to make use of all those carbohydrates and nourish energy-starved cells. The excess insulin further suppresses your blood sugar level, lowering your overall sense of vitality and creating those intolerable carbohydrate cravings where you want to eat more and more chocolate and sticky buns just to keep going. For instead of your body being able to use energy from the foods you are eating, most of it is now being delivered to fat cells. This can leave you depressed, low in energy, bad-tempered and wanting yet more carbohydrate. Here's how it works:

TOO MUCH INSULIN MEANS TROUBLE

Pumping out too much insulin exhausts the pancreas so that it is no longer be able to produce enough insulin. In some people this can lead to late-onset, or Type II, diabetes.

High levels of insulin in the body result in insulin resistance where there is so much insulin in the blood that the insulin receptors in the cells either become immune to its presence or are no longer produced in a great enough number. In either case, they no longer respond to the presence of insulin and their ability to burn glucose as energy gets depleted.

Insulin resistance spurs your pancreas to produce yet more insulin leading to overproduction, or *hyperinsulinaemia*, which in turn produces more insulin resistance.

Insulin forces your body to store glucose from carbohydrate foods as fat and prevents stored body fat from being used as energy.

Ongoing high levels of insulin not only make you fatter, they also keep you fat.

Breaking Through

It's a vicious circle. And it needs to be broken once and for all if you are to shed the excess fat on your body and keep it off without ever having to diet again. The vicious circle looks something like this:

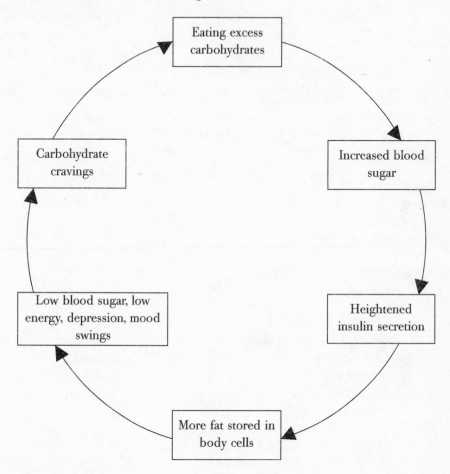

Ketogenics breaks this circle once and for all. In the next chapters we'll find out how.

LET IT BURN

Is Ketogenics safe? This is the usually the first question asked by anyone unfamiliar with the expanding research into the powers of low-carbohydrate eating. These include a majority of doctors for whom the word 'ketosis' sets alarms bells ringing. The reason? In medical school, all trainee doctors learn about ketosis, which develops in Type I diabetes. More accurately called ketoacidosis, this condition is very dangerous indeed and can endanger a diabetic's life. But the pathological condition associated with ketoacidosis bears little resemblance to the benign dietary ketosis generated through a state of fasting or a low-carbohydrate diet.

Benign Dietary Ketosis

This natural form of ketosis is far from dangerous. It is a powerful and positive metabolic process which takes place when your body switches from using glucose as its primary fuel for energy to burning stored fat. It even promotes natural detoxification. Ketones, which are found in the body when ketosis is happening, are simply by-products of the breakdown of free fatty acids that takes place when glucose is not available. They are then used as fuel. Dr Lubret Stryer, professor of biochemistry at Stanford University in California and the author of the standard biochemistry textbooks used in most American medical schools, says that ketones are 'normal funnels of respiration and are quantitatively important as sources of energy…indeed heart muscle, and the kidneys use ketones in preference to glucose'. Meanwhile, Drs Donald and Judith Voet, authors of another widely used biochemistry textbook, report that ketones 'serve as important metabolic fuels for many peripheral tissues, particularly heart and skeletal muscles'.

Sadly, diets based on ketosis continue to get a bad rap from uninformed journalists – and even from a few doctors themselves. You still hear ketones commonly referred to as 'waste products of fat which pollute the blood' or 'toxic compounds which cause damage to the brain, fatigue, nausea and apathy'. All of these statements are false. Anyone who wants to take the trouble to dig a little will discover what the experts above have stated – that ketones are a perfectly normal fuel used by many tissues of the body to meet its energy needs. In fact, there is a great deal of scientific evidence to indicate that certain tissues in the body, including the brain, actually prefer using ketone bodies for energy, even over glucose.

Define It

Any way of eating which results in the formation of ketones, or ketone bodies, can be called ketogenic. Fasting will do this. So will restricting carbohydrate consumption below a certain level – usually somewhere between 20 and 70g a day. The level varies greatly from one person to another.

In the West, the normal diet generally consists of proteins, carbohydrates and fats. When you remove or dramatically decrease the amount of carbohydrates you are taking in, the body's stores of glycogen produced from them is quickly used up. Your body then has to find other ways of providing energy. Free fatty acids help. They can be used by most of your tissues for energy, but not by all. The nervous system and the brain, for instance, cannot use them. What they can use are ketone bodies. In a glucose-deprived state, your body quickly makes ketone bodies, which go on to produce ketosis and make it possible for Ketogenics to work its healing.

How It Works

As we've seen, the Ketogenics way of eating is low-carbohydrate but adequate in protein foods and essential fatty acids. Within a day or two of starting the diet, a good quantity of ketone bodies are present in your body. Now some interesting things start to happen. Your production and utilisation of glucose decreases. There is less breakdown of muscle tissue or protein for energy – a phenomenon know as *protein sparing*, which is essential for long-term weight control. This is because the protein it spares in the muscle tissue in your body together with adequate protein enables you to shed excess body fat while, at the same time, maintaining your lean body mass. In addition, your energy levels and immune system are given a boost. The condition of your skin and look of your body improves. All of these things bring you a real sense of power as well as lasting good looks, plus the ability to keep fat from accumulating once you have lost whatever weight you need to lose. Unlike low-calorie slimming diets, ketogenic fat loss doesn't lower your metabolic functions, so that you end up with weight-gain rebound once you have lost weight. Instead, it actually enhances your metabolism. Eventually, you will be able to eat more and still maintain your lean body – forever.

Hormone Keys

Ketogenics, together with regular weight-bearing exercise, brings about weight loss without loss of lean body mass because it alters the relationship of those two big-time hormones, insulin and glucagon. Insulin, as we've seen, is the hormone of holding, of storing, of keeping, of building up. It's responsible for moving nutrients and energy out of your bloodstream and into your cells. It is insulin which takes glucose into the muscle cells, where it's stored as glycogen. And it is insulin that moves free fatty acids into fat cells to be stored as triglycerides, or body fat. Glucagon works in the opposite way from insulin. It is a fuel-mobilising hormone, triggering the breakdown of stored glycogen in your tissues, especially in the liver, to provide energy as glucose for your body to use.

The moment you drastically reduce the level of carbohydrates you are eating, the level of insulin being secreted by the pancreas decreases, while glucagon levels rise. When this happens, more free fatty acids are released from the fat cells where they have been stored and the burning of free fatty acids for energy increases. As the burning of free fatty acid in the liver accelerates, ketone bodies are formed and ketosis begins.

Of course, insulin and glucagon are not the only hormones in your body which are affected positively by a low-carbohydrate diet. Others also help shift your body's fuel source away from burning glucose towards burning fat. Exercise plays a powerful metabolic part in the success of Ketogenics, too. For exercise increases ketosis and lowers raised insulin levels, countering insulin resistance.

The Ketogenic Fast

Ketogenic diets are not newcomers. They have been used for healing throughout the ages. In no small part this is because when well-designed, they bring about many of the same detoxifying and rebalancing metabolic changes in the body that fasting – that is, complete abstinence from food – does. So similar are the two metabolic states that a true fast, used through history for healing and spiritual clarity, is referred to as *starvation ketosis*, while a ketogenic diet supplying adequate protein and essential fatty acids is known as *benign dietary ketosis*.

The main difference between them is that during a total fast, your body wastes. That is, it feeds upon its own muscle tissues, eating away precious lean body mass which in time leaves you weaker and highly susceptible to rebound weight gain. Ketogenics spares muscle. From the point of view of weight loss, this is particularly important. When people have been put on a complete fast or very low-calorie diets and given only vitamins and minerals for months at a time, they do indeed lose weight. However, a large part of this comes from body protein – muscle tissue. As much as half the total weight lost during a complete fast or very low-calorie diet consists of muscle and water loss. This weakens the body, decreasing the number of its energy-burning 'factories' – mitochondria – within the muscle cells which, in turn, decreases the metabolic rate and makes your body highly susceptible to rebound weight gain. What's worse, the weight that is regained later comes in the form of fat, not muscle. This is why it becomes harder and harder to lose weight with each low-calorie diet you try.

Ketogenic Treatments For Illness

As far back as the Middle Ages, ketogenic diets were used to treat many illnesses, including childhood epilepsy. The ketogenic treatment came out of the discovery that a complete fast would prevent epileptic seizures in children. However, since there was no way of sustaining a fast indefinitely, most especially in growing kids, a ketogenic diet offered a viable alternative.

It still does. In the 1920s, researchers discovered that when they fed children on a diet that was low in carbohydrates, high in fat and provided enough protein for growth, they were able to maintain ketosis for long periods of time and by doing so, control paediatric epilepsy – even where drugs and other treatments failed. Then, from the 1930s to the 1950s, new drug treatments were developed for epilepsy, and the use of the ketogenic diet dwindled for a time. In the United States it was 'rediscovered', thanks to a two-year-old boy named Charlie.

Charlie suffered from uncontrollable epileptic seizures which no drug treatments, not even brain surgery, were able to control. In a desperate search to help his son, Charlie's father found references to a ketogenic diet used for epilepsy which had been developed back in the 1920s by an American doctor named Wilder. Charlie's father put the diet into practice, and so successful was it in banishing the boy's seizures that it spurred his father to set up the Charlie Foundation. This organisation trains doctors and dieticians from all over the world on how to use the diet, and produces videos as well as a book, *The Epilepsy Diet Treatment: An Introduction to the Ketogenic Diet*, to help people learn how to use it. In recent years a very large project in treating childhood epilepsy has been carried out at Stanford University. The ketogenic diet used for controlling epilepsy is quite different from Ketogenics, however. It is much higher in fat, for instance, to provide energy for growth in children, as it is used for many years. Other medical uses of the ketogenic diet in the past include the treatment of childhood trauma, as well as respiratory failure.

Ketones Crack The Fat Code

Aside from its medical uses, the ketogenic diet has mainly been used for weight loss over the last century. Various diets – some good, most poor, a few even dangerous from a nutritional point of view – have made use of the ketogenic metabolism to initiate fat loss. Some have recommended fasting for up to a year on nothing more than water, vitamins and minerals. Others, developed in the 1970s, were fasts designed to spare proteins, but the recommended proteins were very low quality, and nowhere near enough of it was allowed. Because some of the diets were badly formulated in relation to the quality and quantity of the basic nutrients the body needs to thrive, they may have brought about weight loss, but muscle tissue was also lost and certain deficiency diseases took hold. Luckily, they were quickly abandoned.

But what came out of the clinical experience of that period was an awareness that low-carbohydrate diets do indeed help clear obesity. They do this not because they initiate any extraordinary peculiarity of metabolism. Instead, it's because the moment you remove a lot of carbohydrate from the diet, food cravings end, as does false hunger – which causes people to eat more than their bodies need. People quite naturally eat less and lose weight. Researchers and clinicians have discovered that this occurs in most people whenever carbohydrates are restricted to 75g a day or less. Unfortunately, in the early days of ketogenic weight loss, there was too often too little concern with making the ketogenic diet truly healthy. For in addition to restricting carbohydrates, good ketogenic weight loss needs to provide high-quality proteins and optimal levels of vitamins, minerals and essential fatty acids.

Enter Dr Atkins

In the early 1970s the book *Dr Atkins' Diet Revolution* (now *Dr Atkins' New Diet Revolution*) appeared, sold millions of copies and stirred up the whole ketogenic question once more. Instead of going the semi-starvation route or opting for the 'very low-calorie' diet that experimenters had dipped into in previous decades, New York physician Robert Atkins put together a weight loss diet based on unlimited protein and fat. The only limits made were placed on carbohydrates. He insisted that the Atkins Diet was a diet for a lifetime, and would provide quick and easy weight loss with no hunger, and would allow dieters to eat as much as they wanted. Unfortunately, some of the research that Atkins originally cited to support his claims suffered from methodological flaws. He and his diet were severely criticized by the American Medical Association for what they deemed unsupported claims. Before long, the low-fat-high-carbs dogma raised its commercial head, with all of the health claims being made for such a way of eating – a hullabaloo widely promoted by powerful food manufacturers. For a few years, talk of the ketogenic diet was silenced.

Recently, thanks to revolutionary research into the growing incidence and health implications of insulin resistance, including mounting rates of obesity and degenerative conditions which have come in the wake of high-carbs/low-fat diets, many new books advocating a ketogenic approach have appeared, such as *Protein Power* by Michael and Mary Dan Eades. The ketogenic diet is at last beginning to come into its own. It has matured and in the process become more balanced and nutritionally sound. As a result, clinics and hospitals in many countries are beginning to use it as a therapeutic approach, not only to manage obesity in both children and adults, but also as a way of treating certain kinds of cancer. Researchers report that a ketogenic diet can be used to shrink tumours while maintaining a patient's nutritional status, and recently an Australian team discovered that the presence of ketone bodies inhibits malignant cell growth as well as reducing melanoma deposits in the lungs of mice by two-thirds.

Ignorance Is Not Bliss

Most of the critics of a ketogenic diet base their judgments on the notion that it can cause kidney or liver damage. Yet many of the most vocal critics of ketosis itself appear completely uninformed as to what ketosis even is, and often speak of ketones as if they were made from protein. In truth, ketone bodies are fragments of carbon-based fuels created by the burning of fat. Then there's the evidence of some children with epilepsy, who are routinely fed on a diet which keeps them in deep ketosis for years with few side effects. Awareness of the benefits of a ketogenic diet grows slowly. Mention at a dinner party or to your GP that you are using a ketogenic diet, and you are still likely to get all sorts of warnings – reflections of ignorance about the physiology of ketosis, and how powerful a healing agent a ketogenic diet can be.

If you suffer from a liver or kidney complaint or some other metabolic abnormality, however, it is vital that you get your doctor's permission before embarking on Ketogenics. It is not wise for anyone to undertake dietary change without doing so under the guidance of a physician or health practitioner knowledgeable about functional medicine and metabolic nutrition. For you want to get the very best out of the experience as well as respect your own biochemical individuality. No diet is right for everyone.

Only The Best

As with any other way of eating, a ketogenic diet, to be healthy, needs to consist of the best you can get. It needs to contain optimal quantities not only of vitamins and minerals, but also of top-quality – preferably organic – vegetables. It needs to be rich in the phytonutrients which enhance immunity and act as free radical scavengers. It needs to provide essential fatty acids in good balance. After all, you could live on nothing but Brie cheese on a ketogenic diet. You would lose weight, but healthy? Most certainly not. Both programmes in the X Factor Diet make use of the finest natural foods on the planet – foods as close as possible to those our paleolithic ancestors thrived on. Their goal is not just fat loss, but the transformation of your body and your life to a higher level of energy, good looks and well-being.

KETOGENIC KICKOFF

So how do we harness the power of ketosis, in which body fat alone is burnt as energy? In this chapter we'll be looking in detail at how to get started.

The Power of Ketosis

The calorie ratios in Ketogenics – 50 per cent protein, 20 per cent low glycaemic index carbohydrates, and 30 per cent therapeutic fats – force your body to burn fat instead of glucose by switching it into benign dietary ketosis – a natural, healthy response to the drastic cutting of carbohydrates. In the process it will:

- End addictive eating habits and banish cravings for foods such as sugar, wheat and corn derivatives, milk products, caffeine, gluten, grains and sugar.
- Stabilise your blood sugar, evening out the peaks and troughs that put you on a rollercoaster of fatigue, mood swings, weak spells and brain fog, and bring you a sense of personal power in their place.
- Effectively switch your body from glucose burning to fat burning, eliminating your own body fat.
- Dazzle you with a demonstration of just how much fat can be burnt from your body while eating delicious, health-enhancing foods.

Within the first 48 hours on Ketogenics, your body should switch its metabolic functioning and begin using fat as fuel instead of sugar. As this happens, ketone bodies – the by products of fat breakdown from your cells – will be released into your bloodstream. They will then be eliminated from your body through your breath and your urine. Ketones are biochemical proof that you are consuming your own stored fat. Ketosis suppresses your appetite – so much so that after the first 48 hours you will probably no longer think about food obsessively.

Measure It

Ketosis can be monitored by measuring the levels of ketones in your urine. This is a good indicator of the balance of carbohydrate and insulin in your body. To make sure that you are not eating too many carbohydrate-rich foods, it is important that you test your urine for ketones twice a day – before breakfast and again before your evening meal.

For successful ketogenic fat loss, your ketone levels must be maintained between 'trace' and 'small' (0.5–1.5mmol-l). You will be able to test these levels using urinary test strips which you can buy at any pharmacy. They are called Ketosticks®.

Because the presence of ketones in the urine indicates that fat burning is taking place, you might be tempted to believe that the higher the level of ketones the more quickly your body is burning fat. This is not the case. Ketone levels above 'trace' and 'small' – in excess of 'moderate' (4-6mmol) – can actually stimulate insulin secretion. This in turn would lead to a reduction in free fatty acid release from fat tissues and a consequent slowing of fat loss. So it is essential that you maintain ketone levels at 'trace' or 'small'. If your ketone levels are greater than 4mmol, you may need to increase the number of low glycaemic index carbohydrates you are eating slightly or reduce the amount of exercise you are doing. If you are not producing ketones, chances are that you are eating too many carbohydrate foods or you may need to do more exercise.

Caution – if ketone bodies reach levels above 'moderate' (4mmol-l) this may indicate that you are not eating enough and may be wasting muscle tissue. This can cause electrolyte imbalances and alterations in the pH so that your body becomes to acid. Always drink plenty of water (see page 159) and increase your carbohydrates until the ketones are reduced to (0.5–1.5mmol-l) i.e. trace' and 'small'.

If you do not appear to be in ketosis within the first three or four days, or if later on in your Ketogenics programme you go out of ketosis for 24 hours or more, check back to your diary and find out if there are any of the Ketogenics rules that you may not be following. For instance, are you still drinking coffee? Caffeine inhibits Ketogenics by causing the liver to release extra glucose into the bloodstream. Don't drink it. If you continue not to show ketones in your urine you may need to reduce even further the number of carbohydrates you are eating or increase your level of exercise.

There are also some insulin-sensitising nutrients which may be added as supplements to encourage fat burning: chromium, magnesium, omega-3 fatty acids, lipoic acid and n-acetyl carnitine, for instance (see page 154-7).

In most people, the metabolic changeover from burning glucose to burning fat takes about two days, during which you may feel hungry. If you break your programme and have a starchy meal, it will take you another two to three days to get back into ketosis. This is the only time when you are likely to be hungry on Ketogenics.

KETOGENIC RULES

■ Drink 8 to 10 glasses of water daily (see page 159 to calculate your own water needs). You can also drink herb teas and organic vegetable broths (provided you check carbohydrate content). A high water intake is essential for ketones to be effectively processed via the kidneys. It prevents any negative effects of them accumulating. Avoid alcohol and soft drinks of all kinds, including fruit juice and cordials. Mineral waters and flavoured mineral waters are fine provided they contain no artificial sweeteners and no calories (i.e. carbohydrates). You can prepare an excellent alkaline broth which serves the double purpose of providing you with a delicious warm drink and helping to balance any acidity caused by the release of stored fats from your tissues into your blood stream.

Here's How:
Chop half a cup to a cup of several kinds of low glycaemic vegetables and toss them into a large pot (for example, broccoli, cabbage, cauliflower, bean sprouts, asparagus, mustard greens, spinach, watercress, ginger). Add three or four cloves of garlic and a litre and half of water. Bring to a boil and simmer for 15 minutes. Season with some herbs and a little sea salt. Strain and store in the refrigerator. Reheat when needed.

■ **Avoid all sweeteners except stevia and Splenda.** (see pages 209-11 and 208-9) This includes honey, raw sugar, fruit juice concentrates, molasses and malt extracts, as well as artificial sweeteners such as saccharine and aciculae-K. Avoid the use of aspartame (Equal or NutraSweet), which may stimulate insulin secretion and prevent weight loss. Also beware of sweeteners such as mannitol, sorbitol, and other hexitols. When using Splenda be aware that each teaspoon contains about 1g of carbohydrate, so monitor your intake. Too much can slow down weight loss.

■ **Make good use of snack drinks and meal replacements based on microfiltered whey protein.** Unfiltered undenatured whey protein has the highest biological value of any protein source in the world. Rich in immune-enhancing glycomacroproteins, immunoglobulins and other health enhancing factors, whey protein isolates promote healthy intestinal flora and help you build a firm, sleek, shapely body, better and faster than any other foods.

Eat plenty of raw food to ensure you keep your sunlight quanta intake high. This means at least one salad per day, made with delicious high-fibre, low-glycaemic vegetables.

Eat enough. Ketogenics is not a low-calorie programme. It is essential that you eat enough of the recommended foods and that you continue to produce ketones in order for fat burning to take place without loss of muscle tissue. You do not need to overeat. Most people find that they naturally take in approximately 20 per cent less calories per day than 'normal'. This is not something that usually needs to be measured. Just be aware that if your calorie intake drops below this, you will need to make sure that you eat more in order to spur fat burning.

Do not eat starchy food such as bread, flour, pasta, pastry, potatoes or rice. If a food is not part of the Ketogenic programme it is vital to have absolutely none of it. The idea that 'just one taste won't make any difference' is a kiss of death to Ketogenics. This is a *qualitative* diet not a *quantitative* one. During Ketogenic Kickoff your daily carbohydrate levels should be kept below 20g per day. If your ketone levels rise above 'small' (1.5mmol-l) then you can increase gradually your intake of low glycaemic carbohydrates until levels come down to 'trace' to 'small'. Use the charts on the page 141-2 to familiarise yourself with great carbohydrate choices – fewer than 3g of usable carbohydrate per serving. Good carbohydrate choices – fewer than 5g of usable carbohydrate per serving, and super carbohydrate choices – less than 1g of usable carbohydrate per serving.

Eat three low carbohydrate meals plus 2 protein snacks each day.
Do not assume that any food is low in carbohydrates unless you absolutely know its carbohydrate content. Read labels. Make good use of the usable carbohydrate tables in the Appendix (page 303-21).

■ **Spend your carbohydrate allowance wisely.** Choose healthful low glycaemic carbohydrate foods. Not only could one cream-filled donut halt ketosis and therefore fat loss for several days, it will only feed your carbohydrate addiction. Ketogenics puts you on the road to permanent leanness and radiant health. An important part of that process is clearing all of the food addictions that helped make you fat in the first place – the sugars and starches which cause Syndrome X.

■ **Steer clear of diet products unless they are specifically labelled 'no carbohydrates'.**
Most 'low' diet products are low in fat but not low in carbohydrates. Many products contain the word 'sugar-free'. This does not mean that there is no carbohydrate in them, and indeed it is no guarantee that they don't contain some form of sugar. Many products you would not think twice about are full of carbohydrates – cough syrups, chewing gum (even sugar-free chewing gum) and cough drops are filled with sweeteners, for instance.

■ **Beware of hidden carbs in sauces, gravies and dressings.** In restaurants, always ask that your foods be cooked without sugar or flour.

■ **Keep motivated.** Build a good support team of friends around you and make sure your kitchen is ketogenic. Clear out biscuits, pastas and restricted breads from your cupboards and change your shopping habits. While the rest of your family may not need Ketogenics, virtually all of them will thrive on a lower carbohydrate diet such as Insulin Balance. You will find that most people are fascinated by the transformation taking place in you. Give them a chance to benefit from what you have learned.

What Do I Eat?

Your menus will be made up exclusively of foods and drinks chosen from good-quality protein sources and low glycaemic index, low-density carbohydrates, plus the very best fats. Let's look at protein first.

Eat Freely Of These Foods

Fish – all kinds of fresh and canned fish including bass, trout, sole, sardines, herring, mackerel, salmon, tuna, terakihi, dory.

Shellfish – mussels (the green-lipped variety are best), calamari, oysters, clams, crayfish, lobster, crabs.

Game and Poultry – wild duck, pheasant, quail, venison, turkey, organic or free-range chicken, rabbit, wild boar.

Meat – organic bacon, organic beef, organic pork, organic lamb, organic ham.

Eggs – soft-boiled, in omelettes, poached, hard-boiled, scrambled, fried and in any other no-carbohydrate egg dishes.

Cheese – only occasionally, and limit intake to 4oz. Many cheeses contain carbohydrates, so check the content. Use parmesan, camembert, feta, cottage cheese, tofu cheese, ricotta.

Carbohydrate Foods

Eat three cups a day of loosely packed salad or two cups of cooked vegetables chosen from the following lists:

SUPER CARBOHYDRATES
(LESS THAN 1G OF USABLE
CARBOHYDRATE PER SERVING)

1 cup alfalfa sprouts (0.4g)
1 cup sliced bok choy (0.8g)
1 stick celery (0.9g)
½ cup sliced endive (0.8g)
1 cup shredded lettuce (0.4g)
½ cup sliced raw radicchio (0.9g)
5 radishes (0.8g)
½ cup rocket (0.4g)
1 tablespoon minced spring onions (0.1g)

GREAT CARBOHYDRATES
LESS THAN 3G OF USABLE
CARBOHYDRATE PER SERVING

6 fresh asparagus spears (2.4g)
½ cup raw beetroot tops or 1 cup cooked (1.8g)
¼ cup blackberries (2.9g)
1 cup chopped raw broccoli (2.2g)
½ cup chopped capsicum (2.4g)
1 cup cauliflower florets (2.6g)
½ medium cucumber (3g)
¼ cup chopped leeks (2g)
½ cup boiled sliced marrow (2.6g)
½ cup sliced raw mushrooms (1.1g)
½ cup cooked mushrooms (2.3g)
5 whole enoki mushrooms (2g)
½ cup chopped raw spring onions (2.5g)
½ cup chopped parsley (1.9g)
1 tablespoon chopped raw shallot (1.7g)

GOOD CARBOHYDRATES
FEWER THAN 5G OF USABLE
CARBOHYDRATE PER SERVING

½ cup diced aubergine (3.2g)
½ medium avocado (3.7g)
¼ cup blueberries (4.3g)
4 brussels sprouts (3.4g)
2 cup red or green cabbage (3.6g)
½ cup chopped dandelion greens (3.3g)
½ cup chopped fresh fennel (3.1g)
½ cup sliced French beans (3.8g)
1 cup mustard greens (4g)
1 whole hot chilli pepper (4.3g)
½ cup strawberries (3.3g)
½ cup chopped Swiss chard (3.6g)
1 medium tomato (4.3g)
½ cup canned, sliced water chestnuts (4.5g)

Salad Dressings And Sauces

Extra-virgin olive oil with vinegar, lemon or lime juice (watch carbs – see chart below), home-made mayonnaise, low-carb bottled dressing (not diet dressings, as these almost invariably have sugar in them – read labels). Be sure to count as part of your carbohydrate intake whatever kind of vinegar or lemon juice you are using to make your salad dressing. Here is a useful chart to help you calculate carbs.

CARB GUIDE FOR DRESSING INGREDIENTS	
1 tablespoon of:	No. of grams carb
fresh lemon juice	1.3
fresh lime juice	1.4
apple cider vinegar	2.0
balsamic vinegar	2.0
rice wine vinegar	6.0
champagne vinegar	0.0
red wine vinegar	0.0
white wine vinegar	0.0

Herbs And Spices

Use all fresh herbs and spices freely. When it comes to dry herbs, check labels for sugar or other carbohydrates. The ones you buy in the supermarkets are notorious for having additives in them.

Drinks

Filtered or distilled water, sparkling water, flavoured sparkling water (must have no calories and contain no artificial sweeteners). Clear broth – bouillon (read labels).

Fats And Oils

Extra-virgin olive oil, walnut oil, grapeseed oil, coconut oil, home-made mayonnaise made with extra-virgin olive oil, small amounts of butter, flaxseed oil, omega-3 fish oils, heavy cream (very occasionally), sour cream (very occasionally). Olives (check carbohydrate levels).

Alcohol

Not allowed, with a few exceptions as below. Your body uses alcohol immediately as fuel, even before it uses carbohydrate and fat. Alcohol can interfere with ketosis but once the calories from it are used up you get right back into ketosis metabolism. Once you get through the first three weeks of Ketogenics, you can experiment with adding a glass of red wine every now and then and see if this interferes with fat burning. It varies tremendously from one person to another. Any wine that you drink further down the road on Ketogenics needs to be only in small quantities, only infrequently, and must be dry. Sweet wines are far too high in carbohydrates. You can use wine in small quantities when cooking, for as soon as the alcohol is heated to simmering it will be lost or reduced in whatever sauce you are preparing.

GLYCAEMIC INDEX FOR FRUITS AND VEGETABLES

VEGETABLES

Low Glycaemic Index		High Glycaemic Index		
3 Per cent	**6 Per cent**	**15 Per cent**	**20 Per cent**	**25 Per cent**
Asparagus	Beans, string	Artichokes	Beans, dried	Potato, sweet
Bean Sprouts	Beets	Oyster Plant	Beans, lima	Yams
Beet Greens	Brussels Sprouts	Parsnips	Corn	
Broccoli	Chives	Peas, green	Potato, white	
Cabbage	Collards	Squash		
Cauliflower	Dandelion Greens	Carrots		
Celery	Aubergine			
Chard, Swiss	Kale			
Cucumber	Kohlrabi			
Endive	Leeks			
Lettuce	Okra			
Mustard Greens	Onions			
Radishes	Parsley			
Spinach	Peppers, red			
Watercress	Pimento			
	Pumpkin			
	Rutabagas			
	Turnips			

FRUITS

Low Glycaemic Index		High Glycaemic Index	
3 Per cent	**6 Per cent**	**15 Per cent**	**20 Per cent**
Cantaloupe	Apricots(fresh)	Apples	Bananas
Rhubarb	Blackberries	Blueberries	Figs
Strawberries	Cranberries	Cherries	Prunes
Tomatoes	Grapefruit	Grapes	Any dried nuts
Watermelon	Guava melons	Kumquats	
	Kiwifruits	Loganberries	
	Lemons	Mangoes	
	Limes,	Mulberries	
	Oranges	Pears	
	Papayas	Pineapple (fresh)	
	Peaches	Pomegranates	
	Plums		
	Raspberries		
	Tangerines		

Getting Started

As you enter the Ketogenics programme, stop taking any over-the-counter medications which are not absolutely necessary. It is important that you never stop taking prescription medications without first consulting your doctor. Naturally if you have any medical condition that requires you to take prescription medication it is essential that you get your doctor's permission and support for entering the Ketogenics programme. Ketogenics makes significant dietary changes, and there are some drugs which can interfere with weight loss, such as oestrogens and steroids, for instance. There are other drugs, including anti-diabetic medications and diuretics, that could prove problematic during Ketogenics simply because your body becomes much more susceptible to their effects as it detoxifies. Therefore, your doctor will want to reduce the amounts you are taking so that you do not end up with overdoses.

Check-Up

If possible, get a check-up from your doctor before starting the diet. A thorough check, including blood tests which determine cholesterol levels, the relationship of HDL ('good' cholesterol) and LDL ('bad' cholesterol), triglycerides, insulin and glucose levels and uric acid, will give you a benchmark against which to measure progress. It is likely that both you and your doctor will be delighted with the dynamic health-enhancing changes that will have taken place as measured by these conventional medical parameters, three months down the road.

Clear the Deck

During the first few days of Ketogenics, clean out your cupboards. Get rid of all the flour, sugar and other high-carb stuff which forms an important part of most people's daily food intake. Lay in a good supply of all of the foods you are planning to enjoy. (See 21st-century Hunter Gatherer, page 200, for details on all this.)

Don't be surprised if in the first two or three days of Ketogenics you feel tired, hungry or even have a headache. This may be particularly true if you have been drinking a lot of coffee. Ketogenics puts you into a profoundly detoxifying metabolic mode very much like fasting. Your body is throwing off stored wastes at a rate of knots. This can temporarily create minor symptoms. If possible, start Ketogenics on a Friday so you have the weekend to get some extra rest. By Monday you should be feeling remarkably fit and much better. Should your symptoms last more than two or three days – and this only happens in a very few people – try eating more low glycaemic index vegetables (see page 144) until they subside. Then lower your carb intake back down to 20g per day. Be sensible. If after three days you feel genuinely unwell it is important that you see your doctor.

Never skip a meal and always have a protein snack between meals. If you experience any constipation add one to three teaspoons of fibre (see page 157) three times a day and increase your water intake. Try drinking a herbal tea with mild laxative effects. Should you feel weak or find that you are losing weight very rapidly make sure that you getting *enough* protein. Try increasing your intake of microfiltered whey protein. Make yourself some alkaline broth (see above) full of potassium-rich foods (avocados, spinach, broccoli) seasoned with sea salt.

Get Into Exercise

Exercise is almost as important on Ketogenics as what you eat. Begin with a 20-minute walk per day. After the first three or four days add to that a weight-training programme. This will increase muscle mass and help in the vital task of building a fat-burning body for life (see page 98). Weight-training need take no more than half an hour four times a week. Remember, it is within the mitochondria of muscle cells that fat is burnt, so the better your muscle, the more efficiently you will burn fat.

How Much Protein?

For the first three weeks of Ketogenics, it is essential that you take in 150g of protein a day, unless you are a man weighing 285 to 300lb (129 to 136kg), in which case you should eat 157g and 164g of protein, respectively. Remember that this is not 150g of a protein food such as fish; this will only contain between 20 and 30 per cent protein. What I mean by 150g of protein is 150g of biologically available protein. After three weeks, reduce the level of protein down to whatever is most appropriate for your weight. Here is a table to give you some guidelines for amounts of protein to eat *after* the first three weeks.

MEN		WOMEN	
Weight (lb/kg)	Minimum Daily Protein (g)	Weight (lb/kg)	Minimum Daily Protein (g)
175/79	118	150/68	85
200/91	126	175/79	88
220/100	134	200/91	90
240/109	142	220/100	92
260/118	150	240/109	94
285/129	157	260/118	96
300/136	164	285/129	98

Remember, as your weight decreases you will gradually need to decrease the amount of protein that you consume.

Factor In Activity
Now it is important to factor into your protein requirements the amount of exercise you get. If your exercise is only light – say you walk for 20 to 30 minutes a day three times a week – multiply your protein requirement by 1.1. If your exercise is moderate – you go walking or swimming for 20 to 30 minutes a day five times a week – then multiply your protein requirement by 1.2. If you take part in heavy exercise where you are doing weight training three or four times a week together with aerobic exercise, such as walking 20 minutes or more a day, multiply your protein requirement by 1.3.

How Many Carbs?
You will need a daily carbohydrate intake of 20g for the first two weeks until you are well established in ketosis. Then increase your intake of low glycaemic index carbohydrates gradually, keeping track of the level of ketones in your urine (they must remain 'trace' or 'small') until you establish the right carbohydrate intake for you. Look at the carb charts on pages 141-142, or check out the at-a-glance chart below.

Carbs At a Glance

Eat up to three cups of good (low glycaemic) carbohydrate foods each day. These carbohydrate foods are high in fibre, vitamins, minerals and phytonutrients and low in simple carbohydrates. Make them the focus of your salads and stirfries.

Vegetables

Alfalfa	Garlic
Asparagus	Green beans
Bok Choy	Kale
Broccoli	Lettuce
Cabbage	Mushrooms
Capsicum	Onions
Cauliflower	Parsley
Celery	Radish
Coleslaw	Silverbeet
Courgette	Sprouts
Cucumber	Turnip

Fruits

If you want to eat fruits, half a cup a day is OK. But then you will need to cut one cup from the 'carbohydrate foods' list above for every half cup of fruit you eat. These low glycaemic index fruits are the best for reducing blood glucose and insulin responses:

Apricots	Raspberries
Blackberries	Melons
Grapefruit	Strawberries

How Much Fat?

In addition to fats that come with your foods, take two teaspoons of flaxseed oil and/or 1000 to 3000mg of omega-3 fish oils per day.

How Much Should I Eat?

Use the palm method (see page 111-2) on a day-to-day basis to become familiar with the size of servings which are appropriate. For Ketogenics, each palm and a half of protein foods you eat you will complement with one palm of low glycaemic index carbohydrates (see list on page 141). If ketones don't appear in your urine, you will know that you need to decrease your carbohydrate levels until they do appear and/or to increase the intensity and duration of the exercise you are doing. This forces your body to use fat stores instead of glucose as fuel. Always maintain your carbohydrates and exercise at levels which produce 'trace' to 'small' levels of ketones as indicated by Ketosticks®.

The Palm Method Revisited

While the palm method is not as accurate as weighing your foods, it works pretty well. Here are the guidelines for using it for Ketogenics:

▓ For each palm and a half of protein foods you eat, add one palm of low glycaemic index carbohydrates.

▓ Each snack will be entirely protein and will equal one-third to one-half of a palm. If you get hungry, eat more protein.

Putting It All Together

You will find masses of wonderful Ketogenics recipes in 'Sheer Pleasures', starting on page 231. By checking the carbohydrate and protein content of a recipe you will able to identify those that are suitable both for Ketogenic kickoff and for later on, once ketosis is well established, as well as for Insulin Balance. Do make good use of them. I think you will be surprised at just how delicious these foods can be. Meanwhile, here are some simple suggestions for breakfast, lunch and dinner.

Ketogenic Breakfasts

Scrambled tofu with mushrooms and green onions, herb tea.

Spinach omelette, two crisp strips of organic bacon, herb tea.

Poached eggs on tomato slices sprinkled with spring onions, sautéed grated fresh ginger and a clove of garlic.

A breakfast shake or smoothie made with microfiltered whey protein concentrate, water, one to three teaspoons of ground psyllium husks, or other suitable fibre (see page 162) a few drops of stevia (see page 209-11), and a quarter of a cup of low glycaemic fruit such as blueberries, raspberries or strawberries.

Low-carb pancakes sprinkled with a dab of butter and sprinkled with cinnamon.

Crunchy rocket leaves topped with cucumber slices and organic, naturally smoked salmon, with a wedge of lemon.

Ketogenic Lunches

Spinach salad with sliced chicken, dressed with olive oil and champagne vinegar. Lemon flavoured sparkling spring water.

Chef's salad with chicken slices, 28g (1oz) of slivered fresh Parmesan, avocado dressing.

Egg salad with chopped onions and homemade mayonnaise wrapped within crunchy lettuce leaves. Peppermint tea.

Roast lamb sandwich with homemade garlic mayonnaise served on a bed of shredded rocket and sliced tomatoes. Decaffeinated green tea.

Egg, tuna, chicken or tepanyaki tofu, mesclun salad with minced chives and olives (read labels for carbs). Homemade lemonade sweetened with stevia (see page 209-11).

Ketogenic Dinners

Lobster served with garlic butter, steamed spinach spiked with Cajun seasoning, side salad of lambs' lettuce and thin slices of red onion.

Sole almandine served with steamed broccoli, slivered almonds and sliced mushrooms.

Free range or organic charbroiled steak with fresh asparagus spears and melted butter. Side salad of sprouts, enoki mushrooms and celery.

Grilled chicken breast with stir-fried courgettes, watercress side salad dressed in olive oil, lemon juice and garlic, sprinkled with a grated hard-boiled egg.

Grilled lamb chops garnished with mint leaves and served with cauliflower 'mashed potatoes', side salad of cucumber, endive and walnuts, dressed in walnut oil and champagne vinegar.

Grilled salmon with fresh dill and lemon slices, served with green beans and Brussels sprouts.

Stir-fried scallops with garlic and snow peas. Lambs' lettuce salad with rich avocado dressing and fresh strawberries.

KETOGENIC SUPER SNACKS

Snack	Portion	Protein	Carbs
Microfiltered whey protein smoothie	1 cup	10-15	0
Cottage cheese	¼ cup	7	2
Hard-boiled egg	1 large	6	0.6
Lean meat slices	1oz	7	0.1
Macadamia nuts	1oz	3	4
Sunflower seeds	1oz	5	4
Walnuts	1oz	4	5

HELP WHEN YOU NEED IT

Popping vitamin pills has become a way of life for some, but apart from a good multiple vitamin and mineral supplement and perhaps some extra vitamin C – which in my opinion all of us in the Western world need – there are no special supplements required for the X Factor Diet. Some, however, can be enormously helpful for specific purposes. Except for magnesium and alpha-lipoic acid, which benefit everybody, my attitude towards these supplements is to use them when you need them, not long term. The body tends to grow accustomed to whatever you are giving it and likes to have a break every now and then.

Step By Step

It's also a good idea, if you are going to add extra supplements, that you do so one at a time. Leave a couple of weeks in between and before adding another so you can see how your body is responding. For if you start taking more than one thing at a time, you won't know what is doing what. Always remember that each of us has an absolutely individual biochemical make-up. Our response to various foods and nutritional supplements is also individual. Just because something may work well for someone else, don't expect that it will automatically do a lot for you.

Here are some of the most useful supplements to take when following Ketogenics and Insulin Balance. And by the way, when choosing a multiple vitamin and mineral supplement, as a general rule, you get what you pay for (see Resources).

THESE NUTRIENTS PROMOTE INSULIN SENSITIVITY

- Antioxidants
- Magnesium
- Omega-3 essential fatty acids
- Chromium
- Soluble dietary fibres.

Antioxidant Help From Nature

Wherever you find high levels of insulin and blood sugar as well as insulin resistance, that person's metabolism naturally generates higher levels of free radicals. An excess – that is, when more free radicals are present than your body's antioxidant enzymes can quench – of these unpaired electrons damage healthy cells and play a significant role in the development of obesity, early ageing, heart disease and other degenerative conditions. Supplements of antioxidants help neutralise them.

Antioxidants are found in vitamins A, C and E and the minerals selenium and zinc, as well as in phyto-nutrients – carotenoids, flavonoids and many other beneficial plant chemicals. Brightly coloured vegetables such as broccoli, red capsicum and pumpkins are very rich in phytonutrients. They can play a very important part in your success. Fresh vegetables are also rich in important minerals and trace elements to help the metabolic pathways of your body to run smoothly.

Colour Your World

Many studies show that a diet high in the flavonoids and carotenoids contained in certain vegetables and fruit puts people into a relatively low-risk category for cancer, stroke and heart disease and other diseases related to glucose problems (see page 19-21). In plants, flavonoids act as the principal defence against free radical damage, much as they do in our bodies when we eat foods rich in these plant factors. As well as making sure that your meals rely heavily on colourful vegetables and low glycaemic fruits (see suggestions, page 145), there are a number of other flavonoids which may be helpful to take as nutritional supplements – especially on Ketogenics, where carbohydrate foods are highly restricted.

- **Pycnogenol** – This is a complex of more than 40 flavonoids taken from the bark of the French maritime pine. An oligomeric proanthocyanidin – OPC for short – pycnogenol has anti-inflammatory properties as well as being a superb herbal antioxidant which reinforces the protective effects of other antioxidants. It is 50 times more potent as an antioxidant than equivalent amounts of vitamins C and E. You'll need to take 100-200mg of it daily, measured as 95 per cent OPCs.
- **Green tea** – This tea is rich in polyphenols – potent antioxidant compounds made up of some 30 flavonoids by dry weight. It has been shown to lower cholesterol levels and is useful for strengthening the walls of the capillaries as well as the collagen in the skin. It increases the activity of other antioxidants in the body. One cup can contain 300–400mg of polyphenols. You can buy it decaffeinated. You'll need 1 to 3 cups a day.

■ **Citrus bioflavonoids** – These are found in lemons, grapefruit and oranges as rutin and hesperidin. These plant factors are also excellent for improving the strength of collagen in the skin as well as the health of blood vessels and capillaries. Take 2000–6000mg daily.

■ **Grapeseed extract** – This is much like pycnogenol, but more intense in its free radical scavenging properties. Grapeseed extract is also rich in antioxidants. It is less expensive but probably just as potent. Take 150–300mg daily.

■ **Quercetin** – A flavonoid found in apples and onions, quercetin has potent anti-inflammatory properties. It also helps to control high insulin levels. Recent studies show that a typical Western diet contains from 23–170mg of flavonoids a day, whereas it is likely that the figure for our paleolithic ancestors was 1000mg. Take 200–400mg three times a day before meals.

Taking all these plant factors together in one or several supplements is an excellent plan.

Class Of Its Own

Alpha-lipoic acid (ALA) is unique. An antioxidant also found in foods like liver and yeast, it is now increasingly taken in therapeutic doses ranging from 100-600mg a day. It is a sulphur-containing, vitamin-like substance needed in the body's production of energy at a cellular level. It has a proven ability to lower chronically high levels of insulin and glucose. Researchers using it increasingly believe that it may be possible to use ALA to prevent or reverse damage caused by high levels of insulin and glucose in the body. Generally speaking, people with hyperinsulinaemia or diabetes have inadequate levels of this substance in their bodies. ALA is especially important in restoring and preventing nerve damage. It is also an excellent anti-ageing supplement, and appears to be capable of recycling vitamin E and vitamin A in the body after they have been used up in free radical reactions. Many experts in functional medicine believe not only that it helps improve glucose metabolism, restore liver and brain health and prevent nerve disorders, but that it can also reduce the incidence of glaucoma and protect the body against heavy metals and radiation damage.

If you are considering taking ALA as a supplement, there is one thing to be cautious about, however. This is the fact that, in the body, it works very closely together with the B complex vitamin thiamine. If someone is deficient in thiamine this could cause a further deficiency resulting in skin conditions or other symptoms. This is relatively rare, however, and certainly not a problem for people taking a multiple vitamin containing thiamine.

> ## ALPHA LIPOIC ACID – HOW IT HELPS
>
> - Reduces insulin resistance
> - Improves insulin sensitivity, so insulin functions more effectively
> - Lowers glucose levels
> - Reduces the formation of AGEs
> - Neutralises free radicals.

Magnesium Is A Must

The daily diet of our paleolithic ancestor is estimated to have contained between 800 and 1500mg of the mineral magnesium. By contrast, the average Western diet provides us with a mere 200-300mg of this important mineral. Food processing, non-organic agricultural methods, and long-term food storage have vastly depleted the magnesium available to us. As a result, magnesium deficiencies are widespread. They contribute hugely to sudden death, to cot deaths in infants, diabetes, heart disease, high blood pressure, chronic bronchitis, chronic fatigue syndrome, migraine headaches, asthma, muscle cramps, PMS and depression, as well as many psychiatric disorders. Magnesium deficiency also creates a susceptibility in the body to the brain-damaging effects of food additives such as monosodium glutamate (MSG) and aspartame. If you don't have enough magnesium, you basically don't have enough energy for your body to carry out efficiently and gracefully the metabolic processes which support high-level health. Having lived on a poor-quality diet, many of us have (at least temporarily) impaired our ability to absorb what magnesium *is* present in the foods we are eating. These are some of the reasons why magnesium supplements can be useful in Ketogenics and Insulin Balance.

Measuring the exact levels of magnesium in your body and determining just how much supplemental magnesium may be useful to you is difficult. You cannot do a simple blood test. For this will only indicate the levels of *blood* magnesium, and blood magnesium levels shift continually. What is of real concern is levels of this element in your cells. These levels shift much more slowly. Indeed, if you are severely deficient in the mineral you need to take a magnesium supplement for three or four months to get enough magnesium back into your cells. And it needs to be in a bio-available form of the mineral – not elemental magnesium, but magnesium tartrate, magnesium citrate or chelated magnesium.

Magnesium helps to counter insulin resistance extraordinarily well. If you choose to take a magnesium supplement, you will probably want between 230 and 600mg of magnesium a day. But note: there are two groups of people who should not take magnesium without the express permission of their physicians. These are people with kidney failure – who should never be on a ketogenic diet anyway – and people with a high degree of AV heart block, a condition affecting the heart's natural pacemaker. For the rest of us, magnesium often holds an important key for weight loss while building overall energy and vitality.

The Marvellous Omega-3s

Omega-3 fats, as we've seen, help in weight reduction. Studies using them show, without question, that with the fat you eat, type is far more important than amount when you're shedding fat stores. When animals are fed with abundant omega-3 fatty acids, they gain less weight compared to those given omega-3 fats and saturated fats. Omega-3 fatty acids help to reduce the levels of triglycerides – one of the blood fat characteristics of Syndrome X – and improve both blood pressure and overall heart function. The way to get more omega-3s is to cut out vegetable oils from your diet, except for extra-virgin olive oil, which is rich in omega-9 fats. And to eat more fish – particularly oily fish rich in the omega-3 fatty acids DHA and EPA. If you can't manage eating the fish itself, you might consider taking between 1000 and 3000mg of omega-3 fish oils daily in capsule form.

Flaxseed oil is also rich in omega-3 fatty acids. However, many people who have lived for a long time on a convenience food diet with a high ratio of omega-6 oils to omega-3 fats cannot efficiently convert the oil into a usable form. In this case you are better off taking fish oils as a supplement and/or eating plenty of fatty fish in your diet, to add up to 3000 to 6000mg of omega-3s daily.

How About Chromium?

An essential trace element, chromium is vital for good carbohydrate metabolism and the maintenance of insulin sensitivity. Chromium sits right at the core of a molecule called the glucose tolerance factor. It regulates blood sugar and works with insulin to encourage your body to take glucose into its cells to be burnt as energy. Where there is a deficiency of this element, you often find insulin resistance, hyperinsulinaemia and high blood sugar.

The results of chromium supplementation have been well studied in many clinical trials. So effective is its action on blood sugar that in one double-blind study of both Type I and Type II diabetics, researchers discovered that supplements of chromium picolinate made it possible for almost three-quarters of the patients taking part in the study to reduce their medications – some by as much as 30 per cent.

In recent years chromium has become a popular weight-loss supplement. It appears to help the body decrease its fat stores and at the same time protects against loss of muscle tissue. In one 90-day double-blind clinical trial, researchers found that giving participants on a slimming diet 400mcg of chromium daily encouraged an average loss of 17lb of body fat, without loss of muscle tissue. The control group, who were not given the chromium, lost only 3lb of fat and over half a pound of muscle. A good daily dose is generally considered to be between 400 to 600mcg (note that these are micrograms, not milligrams) of chromium picolinate or chromium polynicotinate a day, in divided doses, taken with meals.

Carnitine Burns Fat

Carnitine is a very special nutrient when it comes to building lean body mass and shedding fat. Sometimes classified as an amino acid, it is intimately involved both in the formation of ketone bodies and the burning of fat in muscle cells. Carnitine is frequently used as a weight-loss supplement. There is much controversy over whether or not it actually works in this way. What is known for sure is that it helps promote maximum endurance and peak performance in aerobic sports, and that it is useful to anyone who needs more energy. Carnitine does this by acting as a gate-keeper for fat burning. In effect, it picks up stored fats and carries them to mitochondria in the cells, where it can be burnt off as energy. The usual dose of carnitine is between 1000 and 3000mg a day, always in the form of L-carnitine or acetyl-L-carnitine. Acetyl-L-carnitine is increasingly used for brain health and longevity, but it is a great deal more expensive than L-carnitine. The L-carnitine form is fine for use in weight loss. Take 1000–3000mg a day.

Fibre Matters

Sugar-free fibre supplements can be useful too, especially with Ketogenics, where your levels are greatly reduced. They can be very helpful when beginning the programme. Some people find that with Ketogenics, the number of bowel movements is reduced, and some people can even suffer constipation. This is the result of eating less fibre, and boosting the capacity of your gastrointestinal system to absorb nutrients from the foods you are eating. In most people, a big salad full of lovely, fibrous vegetables rich in phyto-nutrients is enough to counter any tendency to constipation. If you feel you need more help, you can add some psyllium husks to your protein drinks or mix it with soups and sauces, or you can simply take it in a glass of water (although it tastes like straw). Start with one to two teaspoons and gently increase the dose until your bowel movements are normal. You can also find more expensive fibre supplements which are even better, such as combinations of insoluble and soluble fibres (see page 162).

Water Is Best

Believe it or not, the best supplement you can take on Ketogenics and Insulin Balance is pure, clean water. Next to oxygen, water is the most important factor keeping us alive. And it does a great deal more when it comes to weight loss. As your the body becomes ketogenic and fat molecules are burnt up as energy, whatever wastes and toxins have been stored in the fat tissue are let loose into the bloodstream. When you drink plenty of water, this helps your body clear these wastes from your system safely and quickly. Drinking plenty of water is also essential in order to take an accurate reading with Ketosticks®. For when the urine becomes too concentrated, the readings can go awry. Water also plays a part in successful Ketogenics by making sure the concentration of blood ketones doesn't become too high. Remember that the measurement should always remain in the 'trace' or 'small' range. When it gets higher than 'trace' (5mg/dl) or 'small' (15mg/dl), insulin levels can rise and fat release from your fat cells fall. Water helps dilute blood ketone levels and keep this from happening. Ketogenics tends to eliminate excess water stores, so drinking plenty of water helps to counter the dehydrating effect of ketosis – a couple of litres a day is good.

Get Energy

There are other reasons why water is so important, not the least of which is its effect on your energy levels and appetite. Not only does dehydration lead to your feeling weak and tired, it leads to overeating, since failing to drink enough water disturbs your perceptions, leading you to think you're hungry even when you are not. The appetite control centre in the hypothalamus in your brain does not distinguish well between hunger and thirst. Drinking lots of water helps make sure you are not eating more than your body actually wants and needs. For it is easy for any of us to mistake thirst for hunger.

Another valuable characteristic of water – which science can still not explain – is that it acts like liquid energy. Research projects with athletes as well as anecdotal experience from mountain climbers show that when you drink more water than you think you need, your energy levels remain high. I don't know how many people I have told this to in the past who have greeted the information with a flat disbelief until they increase the amount of water they are drinking. Then they report back to me, usually still surprised by the experience, that drinking more water creates an abundance of energy throughout the day – vitality they have not often experienced before.

How Much H²o

Keep a large bottle or two of pure fresh mineral water or filtered water within easy reach and make sure you consume your quotas of this clear, delicious, health-giving drink. Here's how to work it out:

Divide your current weight in kilos by 8 – if you weigh 58 kilos, then 58 divided by 8 = 7.25 big glasses. Then round the figure upwards to the next glass and there you have it – 8 glasses a day. (A big glass of water is between 250 and 280ml).

Remember that this is only a base calculation on a cold day – you will need a lot more during exercise or on a hot day.

Whatever other supplements you decide to take or not to take, put water at the top of your list. Make sure, too, that it's good clean water. Most tap water is not in any way what you would want to put into a detoxified, ketogenic body.

THE LOW DOWN

Now we're ready for the FAQs on the X Factor Diet – those frequently asked questions that address any concerns or curiosity you may have about the programmes you're about to begin.

Q: How are Ketogenics and Insulin Balance going to change my body and my life?
A: Ketogenics and Insulin Balance can help restore your metabolic biochemistry, balance insulin and blood sugar and restore insulin sensitivity which has been lost. They not only reduce the fat stores in your body, gradually restoring it to its natural shape and size – they also help protect you from premature ageing and degenerative diseases and increase your overall energy. As your body restores itself, you will experience an increasing sense of power on a personal level. You can feel – in some people for the first time in their life – as though you can do whatever it is you really want to do. I am continually surprised when I see the changes take place in people when they shift to this way of eating and living – of how not only their physical imbalances and distortions disappear, but so do many of their psychological ones. I see people feeling good about themselves instead of feeling guilty or inadequate. For me, this is one of the most exciting aspects of the programme. On a merely practical level, both Ketogenics and Insulin Balance will make you look and feel younger, improve the quality of your skin, build sleek-curved arms, legs, torso and belly. And they also help eliminate that feeling of powerlessness and being out of control in relation to food and eating which many women experience. For when your body gets back in balance, you no longer feel hungry all the time. Gradually, all of those cravings for something sweet that lead to addictive eating disappear forever.

Q: Why do I always gain weight after losing it?
A: Many get caught between a rock and a hard place by going on and off slimming diets. They come to the point where they know if they lose weight they will gain it back again – usually more weight than they lost. Then they feel worse, so it all comes down to feeling hopeless and pointless. Many ask themselves why they should bother at all. If you want to grow lean for life, there is no worse way to do it than on a low-calorie diet. When you diet without getting sufficient protein or calories, this lowers your metabolic rate. In your body's attempt to conserve its energy reserves – fat in your fat cells – your

metabolism becomes incredibly efficient at wringing the last drop of energy from any food that you eat, and storing it. In addition to this, slimming diets remove not just fat but a great deal of muscle – protein tissue – from your body. This further lowers your metabolic rate, which means that you need to eat fewer and fewer calories in order to lose weight and keep it off. It also reduces the number of mitochondria – the little factories in muscle cells where fat can be burnt as energy. In effect, your whole metabolic chemistry goes into conservation mode, making it harder and harder to lose weight each time you try.

Once muscle tissue is lost from your body and weight is regained – as it is in at least 95 per cent of the people who go on slimming diets – your metabolism slows down even further. You have lost muscle tissue, so you have lost your body's ability to burn fat, along with a great deal of strength and stamina. There are many people walking around – especially women – who are 'thin' but who actually have a very high ratio of fat to muscle in their body as a result of years of slimming diets and depriving themselves. They have no vitality and are continually counting calories since they have to eat less and less to keep from gaining weight.

Ketogenics and Insulin Balance can change all of this forever. I can help you overcome the inertia of weight loss and shift your metabolic functioning into a dynamic mode where your body is burning stored fat and producing energy. You no longer have the big ups and downs which have you reaching for a cup of coffee or something sweet just to keep you going. On Ketogenics or Insulin Balance you are giving your body exactly what it needs to thrive. Your body rewards you by building beautiful lean tissue, enhancing metabolism and slowly but inevitably burning off all of those excess fat stores. It is such a different experience than what people get from dieting, and there is no way that you can know about it without experiencing it. It brings about nothing short of a dynamic revolution in your life. Many who experience it claim it is one of the most exciting things ever to happen to them.

Q: I've heard that eating excess protein can cause osteoporosis and damage my kidneys. Is this true?

A: First of all, you won't be eating excessive protein on these diets. With Ketogenics and Insulin Balance you'll eat adequate protein. Despite the old wives' tale that eating protein may harm the kidneys and cause osteoporosis, neither of these things is true. In 1995, a study in Germany showed unquestionably that kidney function actually improves when the protein content of one's diet is increased. As far as osteoporosis is concerned, there is no evidence whatsoever that diets adequate in protein – which humans have consumed for hundreds of thousands of years – contribute to osteoporosis. The traditional diet of the Inuit in the Arctic Circle and of the Masai in Africa consists primarily of protein. Osteoporosis was completely unheard of among both groups until they added Western convenience foods high in refined carbohydrates to their daily fare.

Q: *Will using Ketogenics and Insulin Balance not only make me lean but also healthy?*
A: Absolutely. That is how Ketogenics and Insulin Balance bring about what many consider miracle changes in their body and their life. This way of eating and living – including exercise which helps build lean tissue in the body and shifts brain chemistry into a 'feelgood' state – works its wonders entirely because it enables the body to detoxify itself as well as to restore normal functioning to organs and systems. Ketogenics and Insulin Balance are truly holistic approaches not only to fat loss but also to high-level health, good looks and energy. You may be surprised by just how far-reaching their beneficial effects are.

Q: *I am worried about constipation. If I am not eating my bran-filled breakfast cereals, rice and sandwiches, will I not get constipated?*
A: It is not likely. For the nutrient-rich carbohydrates you'll eat, which are full of phyto-nutrients and antioxidants, also contain a lot of excellent-quality fibre – broccoli, cauliflower, asparagus, spinach, kiwi fruits, berries and the other low-density carbohydrates all have plenty. They help prevent constipation even better than the so-called fibre supplements that we are continually being sold. Also, as you reduce your insulin levels, your body begins to make more of the helpful prostaglandins such as PGE1, which increase the water content of the colon and help prevent constipation. Finally, the omega-3 fatty acids, which you will be getting either through flaxseed or fish oil, also help prevent constipation.

If, right in the beginning, you do find yourself a bit constipated, you can use a good fibre supplement temporarily. The cheapest and most widely available are ground psyllium husks. Start with 1 teaspoon and gradually increase up to 2½ to 3 teaspoons a day. You can mix these with microfiltered whey protein drinks or take them in water. Even better are the blends of soluble and insoluble fibres that have a low-allergy potential, such as oat fibre, beet fibre, rice bran cellulose and apple fibre. But be sure you read labels of any product you want to buy. Lots of fibre supplements are full of sugar. Be sure also to subtract the amount of fibre in grams any supplement contains from the amount of total carbohydrate that these supplements show on the label. For you are only concerned with *usable* carbohydrate – not with the fibre itself, which, although counted as carbs on the label, passes right through you.

In any case, during the first few days it's far more likely that you will experience loose stools while your body is adjusting to the new diet. In part, I believe, this is the result of the detoxification that takes place when you make the metabolic shifts that Ketogenics and Insulin Balance depend upon. If this is the case, consider reducing your intake of fish oil capsules, and check out the possibility of any allergy or food sensitivity to some food you have been eating. Gradually, as your body adjusts to this new way of living, you will find that the diarrhoea will disappear. If it does not disappear within a couple of days, it's important that you consult a doctor to check out the possibility of any infection.

Q: Why does my doctor not know about the effect carbohydrate foods have on the body and what it can do for us?
A: Sadly, throughout most of the world, medical schools give budding doctors virtually no training in nutrition or functional medicine. During his medical training, my son Jesse received only two hours of nutritional training in some six years of study. That consisted of telling him what kind of 'special diets' were available in hospitals for diabetics and people going into surgery. Hopefully in the next few years this will change. Meanwhile, the rising cost of medical care in every country in the world is forcing governments to look seriously at nutrition as a tool for prevention. Often government advisors themselves are out of touch with recent discoveries in metabolic nutrition and functional medicine. As a result, changes in advice take place only slowly. Doctors are very busy people. Few make time to go to special seminars that would train them in these areas. I suggest that if your doctor does not know about the benefits of a low-carbohydrate, adequate-protein diet, give him some of the references in this book so that he can check them out for himself. I think it's a question of leading the horse to water. Whether or not a particular horse is ready to drink is not something any of us have any control over, but certainly the information is there in terms of clinical experience and scientific studies, if anyone wants to put in the time to research it.

Q: I've just started on Ketogenics and find that I'm totally exhausted. My legs feel heavy when I go upstairs and my energy levels are even worse than before. Why?
A: Some people feel great right from the start of Ketogenics. Others take a few days to make that shift. I know personally that the first two or three days on it, I experienced this enormous heaviness in my legs when I went upstairs. I also wanted to rest a great deal. Partly this is a result of your body making a shift over from the kind of enzymes that have been processing lots of carbohydrate food to those that are needed for breaking down proteins. Partly I believe it is also a result of the detoxification process it is experiencing.

This is a powerful cleansing programme very much like the experience of a fast or a juice fast, with the exception that what you are doing now is not only cleansing your system but rebuilding strength at the same time. It takes your body a few days to produce the new enzymes you need as you make that shift. And remember that the detoxifying process itself takes energy. Ideally you should begin Ketogenics on a Friday so that you can spend the weekend getting some extra rest should you need it. By Monday – the third day – most people are already in ketosis and finding that their energy is beginning to build. Remember, too, that if you have just given up caffeine or alcohol and have been more or less dependent on them, you may even get the odd headache or exhausted feeling until your body begins to restore its balance. This usually happens within two or three days. Should this occur, get plenty of rest, take long baths and do pleasant things so long as fatigue is present – just as you would if you were on a juice fast. You will be surprised at how quickly this builds into high levels of vitality.

If you have been on the diet for two or three weeks, feeling great, and then find yourself with a sense of lightheadedness, muscle aches or great fatigue, it may be that you need to increase the potassium in your body. The easiest way of doing this gently and safely is to go and buy one of the potassium salts from a health food store and use that on your food. These are designed to be substitutes for ordinary table salt. If you are taking any medicines to control blood pressure or any diuretics, however, it is important that you check with your doctor before taking any potassium supplement, since a few of these medicines can interfere with the body's release of potassium and cause problems. Finally, if right at the beginning you are still hungry and low in energy, eat more protein and fat in the form of microfiltered whey drinks including fibre, a handful of almonds or macadamia nuts, hardboiled devilled eggs, chicken or fish.

Q: I am still worried about ketosis. Will it not be dangerous for my body?
A: The answer is no. Ketosis is not dangerous unless you happen to be a Type I diabetic. If you are a woman with more than 35 per cent of your body weight as fat or a man with over 22 per cent as fat, then you will most definitely go into ketosis when you have spent a couple of days on Ketogenics. But that's good news, not bad. If you are not that overweight, you will probably opt for Insulin Balance with its more liberal carbs and end up right on the edge of ketosis.

Ketosis is still a much-maligned and little-understood phenomenon. The name comes from ketone bodies which are produced when fat stores break down. Everybody produces ketones all the time. However, unless you are on a ketogenic diet or have been fasting, you will not be in a state of ketosis. This is a metabolic state in which one is able to measure a level of ketones in your blood. So they are far from being 'poison' or dangerous as they are still described by a few who remain unaware of the natural role they play in the body's metabolism. Some organs, such as the heart, actually prefer ketones to any other kind of fuel. This is probably true of the brain as well. A ketogenic way of eating brings about the breakdown of stored fats, creating a significant quantity of ketones – especially if you are very overweight. The level of carbohydrate you are eating is kept low so your body does not burn them all. This means that the extra ketones circulating in your blood are then eliminated through urine, bowels and breath. Ketone bodies are fats which are not completely burned, so if you eliminate some without using them for energy, you are getting rid of unwanted fat and not even having to burn it off. Ketones are an absolutely normal source of energy. There is no evidence, except with people who have Type I diabetes or severe alcoholism, that ketones are dangerous.

Q: How do I know what level of ketosis in best for fat burning?
A: Use Ketosticks® to determine changes in your own level from day to day. These are simple plastic strips which you pass through a stream of urine once or twice a day, usually in the morning on awakening and then late in the afternoon or just before going to bed. They will tell you just how much overspill of ketone bodies is taking place. As I've said elsewhere, the ideal level for fat burning is 'trace' or 'small'. You do not want to go above that. If you find that you are not showing 'trace' or 'small' on the ketone strips, then it is time either to look seriously at your carbohydrate intake and reduce it further until you can pick up these measurements, or to increase your level of exercise. If you go above 'trace' or 'small', it is time to increase your intake of low glycaemic, low-density carbs like green vegetables until the levels of ketones come down to 'trace' or 'small'. Many people think that since ketosis burns fat, more fat will be burned the higher the level of ketosis. This is not the case. In fact, there is some anecdotal evidence to indicate that people with levels of ketones in their urine above 'trace' or 'small' are actually *inhibiting* fat burning in their body. So it is very important to keep the levels of ketone in your urine down.

Q: What about coffee?
A: Coffee increases insulin in the body and therefore does not belong in Insulin Balance or Ketogenics. I have known people plateau on Ketogenics who were drinking coffee. On giving it up, they begin to shed weight again. Coffee, of course, is highly polluting to the system in general. I would certainly avoid it altogether for the first couple of months, then maybe try drinking a cup of coffee a day, monitor your fat loss, and see what happens.

Q: My breath smells bad. Why is this?
A: Ketones are not only released through the urine and the bowels, but also through the lungs. This can create a kind of 'acetone breath' as well as a funny taste in the mouth. See page 224 in 'Troubleshooting' for ways to combat this problem.

Q: How closely do I need to follow the programme to get results?
A: If you are above that key percentage of body fat – 35 per cent for a woman or 22 per cent for a man – you will need to be extremely exact about how you follow the programme. For simply reducing your carbohydrate intake, as happens on Insulin Balance, won't help you lose weight. If you are below that level of fat in your body, then simply following Insulin Balance with its more liberal carb allowance will slowly and gradually bring about any weight loss that needs to be accomplished to restore your body to its perfect form. If you are going the Ketogenic route, it is important to cut carbohydrate way down at the beginning – in some people as low as 20g per day – in order to restore damaged insulin receptors and normalise levels of insulin in the blood. Until this is accomplished, you may find that any carbohydrate and sugar cravings you tend to have will continue. Once you are continuously in ketosis and the rebalancing process is taking place, all of your false hunger will simply disappear.

For in the same way that your insulin receptors get resistant to the presence of insulin over a long time, and demand more and more insulin in order to work at all, the 'sweet' receptors in your tastebuds also become resistant, and you need to eat more and more sugary foods to satisfy your cravings. Restore normal sensitivity and you find that the gentle sweetness of a piece of melon is enough to satisfy you. After a few weeks of Ketogenics or Insulin Balance, most people discover that anything that's really sweet, such as the kind of chocolate they used to absolutely adore, no longer appeals to them. Sometimes the mere taste of it makes them feel quite queasy. For their body's sweet receptors have returned to normal sensitivity. Your craving for sweets inevitably diminishes over time.

Q: On Ketogenics can I eat as much I want and still lose weight?
A: For most people, the answer is yes, simply because the protein and essential fats you're eating on Ketogenics have a natural appetite-suppressing effect. Most people following Ketogenics find that they can be guided entirely by their appetite. This does not mean, however, that calories don't count. If someone were determined to gorge themselves on protein-rich and fat-rich foods, they could well find that they don't lose weight, even though they have reduced their carbohydrate down to below, say, 50g per day.

There are three components that determine how many calories a human being needs to maintain weight. 1. How much energy they expend while resting. 2. The thermal effect of activity – that is, how many calories they burn while exercising and after exercising. 3. The thermal effect of eating – that is, the slight increase in metabolic rate that occurs when you eat food. Take the example of a woman weighing 10 stone 10 pounds who is on Ketogenics. She is likely to burn 1500 calories a day simply from the energy she expends while resting. Say she has a moderately active life and exercises four to five times a week at a moderate intensity. This would increase the number of calories she needs to take in to maintain her weight by a factor of 1.5, or 2250 calories a day. Add to that the thermal effect of eating, which is roughly 10 per cent per day or 225 calories in her case, and you come up with a total of 2475 calories a day. This is the number of calories that she would need to maintain her body weight at a stable level. As long as she is eating less than 2250 calories a day, given her current weight and level of activity, she will gradually lose weight. A rough way of estimating the calories needed for daily maintenance is to multiply a woman's body weight in pounds by 15 to 15.5 calories per pound. In practice, this seldom becomes an issue with Ketogenics because appetite itself is diminished and the high quality of nutrition, rich in fresh vegetables plus top-quality proteins and essential fatty acids, brings most people a level of satiation that makes any considerations of counting calories unnecessary.

Q: I've heard that low-carb diets only work because they cause water loss. Is this true?
A: No. In the first few days of Ketogenics or Insulin Balance, you will find that you lose three to four pounds in weight – sometimes even more – which is water loss. Once you eliminate all of the excessive carbohydrates from your body, however, there is no longer a need for your system to produce more water in order to dilute the negative effects they can have. After this, all weight loss comes from your body slowly, steadily and progressively burning its fat stores – not protein tissue. This makes Ketogenics and Insulin Balance very different from slimming diets. The important thing to remember (and please don't get neurotic about weighing yourself all the time – once a week is plenty) is that it is *fat loss*, not weight loss, that you are after. You may even find there are days when you see yourself temporarily gaining weight instead of losing it. This is because muscle tissue is much heavier than fat tissue. As you build more fat-burning muscle, restoring normal body form, you may go up a pound or two in weight temporarily. However, what you will find, too, is that your clothes will have become looser. For muscle tissue is very heavy, while fat tissue is light. (This is why fat people float so easily in swimming pools while muscular people tend to sink.) Don't only rely on your scales as a way of measuring progress.

Use your tape measure and the way your clothes fit.

Q: I've heard of other people who have written about low-carb diets, such as Robert Atkins, Barry Sears and Michael and Mary Eades. How do they differ from one another?
A: The average Western diet contains at least 300g of carbohydrate, and the food pyramids recommended by most governments these days call for even more. On any low-carbohydrate diet, calories become far less important, simply because the proteins and fats that you eat on a low-carb diet are satisfying and most people find that they automatically eat less food, although the food is far more nutritionally dense.

Dr Robert Atkins, the author of *Dr Atkins' New Diet Revolution,* is the most famous of all the low-carb gurus. His diet has two phases. 'Induction' is the first, and during it carbohydrates are restricted drastically down to 15g for two weeks. This phase of his diet is followed by an increase of carbohydrate of approximately 5g a week until you return to what he calls your maintenance level of weight, ie your ideal level. For most people, an ideal carb intake on any ketogenic diet is considered to be between 25 and 90g a day. This is less than one-third of what people on the average Western diet get. Atkins allows you to eat all the protein and fat you want but never allows starches like potatoes and pasta, nor sugar. The Atkins diet can be very high in saturated fat, which concerns many experts in functional medicine, since our paleolithic ancestors had very little saturated fat in their diet, while today's meats and dairy products are full of it. The Atkins diet is certainly not for anyone with an allergy to milk products as it also uses a considerable amount of cream and cheeses. I have much respect for Dr Atkins and his work. My major concern about his diet is that instead of helping us rediscover a truly natural diet high in fresh vegetables and simple clean protein, it recommends too many ersatz foods – for instance, muffins and sweets, which are made to look like the foods that most people eat on a Western diet. I personally would rather get away from them altogether. I find that people feel better once they make a switch more towards a paleolithic way of eating.

Barry Sears, author of *The Zone* and *Mastering the Zone,* has a passion for biochemistry. His books are fascinating to read if your share his passion. They can, however, become difficult to understand and many people claim they are very complex to use. Sears is not concerned with a ketogenic diet, nor is he particularly concerned with weight loss. He is using foods to shift the hormonal system into producing optimal performance, both mentally and physically. This is a state that he calls 'the zone'. Elite athletes like his programme very much. It does reduce weight in some people – usually those with relatively low levels of excess fat on their bodies – since the protein level is higher and the fat and carbohydrate levels lower than those of the ordinary Western diet. Many people with cravings for carbs who have tried it claim it does not reduce their cravings. Sears maintains that each of us has an exact protein requirement and that we must eat no more and no less than that. He matches this with specific amounts of carbohydrate. He has created a complicated system of protein and carbohydrate blocks as a guide for people using it. His diet is 40 per cent carbohydrate and 30 per cent protein and fat. It's a diet that can work for many people whose body fat is less than 35 per cent for women and less than 22 per cent for men. But it takes a lot of measuring and discourages many.

Michael R. Eades and Mary Dan Eades are the authors of *Protein Power*. These two American doctors have created a programme which also tags an individual's protein needs to a complex formula. Their intensive weight-loss programme is ketogenic and restricted to 30g of carbohydrate a day. Eades and Eades calculate the grams of carbohydrate differently than Atkins does, subtracting the fibre – the metabolically inactive content of food – from the amount of total carbohydrate in a food to determine what they call 'significant carbohydrate count' (in other words, *usable* carbs). Like Atkins, the Eades are not too concerned with fats except that they warn you to stay away from trans fats and say that eating too much heavy cheese can restrict weight loss. Once a person reaches his or her ideal weight, the Eades suggest they add 5g carbohydrates a day each week until they reach a level at which they can maintain the weight. The Eades are not concerned about the glycaemic index in relation to fat loss. They tend to look at all carbohydrate as sugar. They too, to some extent, have created menus akin to the kind of foods people on an ordinary Western diet are used to eating, ie breakfast cereals, low-carb breads, artificial syrups, etc. I have tried the low-carb ready-made foods they sell and don't find them wonderful. But then I don't like manufactured foods with artificial sweeteners anyway. They have a good website: www.eatprotein.com.

Q: How do I break out of the prison of dieting forever?

A: This is an enormously important question. Many people spend all their time thinking about food, depriving themselves and being miserable. They feel there is no place to go. They feel they are stuck between four walls, have no choices or options and are well and truly trapped. The first thing to do is to remember that the power for bringing about the changes in your body you want lies entirely with you. What Ketogenics and Insulin Balance do is allow your body to begin re-establishing normality. In the beginning of either programme you may have trouble trusting this. As the days and weeks go on, you will gradually come to know that the path you are on will take you to where you want to go. At that point something wonderful happens. All of that fear and guilt and confusion and obsession with food simply and gently drifts away. This brings a sense of freedom which is impossible to describe unless you have experienced it. People give up worrying about how fast or how much weight they are losing, knowing that what's happening to their body is natural and truly wonderful and can only get better and better.

THE X FACTOR DIET
IDIOTS' GUIDE

Welcome to the Idiots' Guide to the X Factor Diet. Here you will find a 14-day plan for each of the X Factor programmes – Ketogenics and Insulin Balance.

If you are a veteran of countless high-carbohydrate, low-fat diets and you are still overweight – and/or exhausted, depressed and plagued by food cravings, yet unable to put your finger on why – it is very likely that one of the X Factor Diets can help you shed fat forever and build high-level health. You, like so many of us, are likely to be experiencing the negative effects of Syndrome X. This is exactly what the X Factor Diet is designed to counter. Syndrome X, also known as insulin resistance, is an umbrella term for a collection of metabolic disorders such as high blood pressure and overproduction of insulin – the hormone that helps ferry blood glucose into body cells to be burnt as energy. Left unchecked, Syndrome X predisposes you to disorders like obesity, Type II diabetes, heart disease, cancer and Alzheimer's, to mention only a few. Congratulations on making the decision to change your life. Let's dive right in.

How the X Factor Diet works
Both Ketogenics and Insulin Balance vanquish Syndrome X by:
- **Rebalancing levels of insulin**
- **Encouraging your body to burn fat instead of glucose**
- **Forging a lean, sleek body**
- **Boosting your vitality**
- **Slowing the process of ageing.**

Ketogenics and Insulin Balance work their magic in a simple, natural way – by turning the high-carb/low-fat rule on its head. Instead of eating all that pasta and bread, you will:
- **Eliminate refined and high glycaemic index carbohydrates, including flour, starchy vegetables like potatoes, white rice, sugar and other sweeteners**
- **Concentrate on natural, fresh, organic, unprocessed foods**
- **Eat many of your vegetables and fruits raw if you can**
- **Make non-starchy vegetables high in phyto-nutrients and antioxidants your primary source of carbohydrates**
- **Steer clear of soft drinks, fruit juices, alcohol and other highly processed drinks**

- Eliminate processed vegetable oils rich in omega-6 fatty acids from your diet – and all convenience foods containing them – and use cold-pressed, extra-virgin olive oil and flaxseed oil instead
- Enrich your diet with omega-3 fatty acids from fish and flaxseed oils
- Refuse all trans fats, which are found in deep-fried foods, margarine and foods that contain partially hydrogenated oils
- Eat good-quality protein like fresh fish, free-range chicken, eggs, game, organic meat and low-carb soya products at every meal and snack
- Eliminate coffee – especially on KETOGENICS
- Stay away from commercial foods
- Gradually determine your own best level of carbohydrate for weight loss and maintenance and stick to it
- Take a multiple vitamin plus plant factor antioxidant such as flavonoids, pygnogenal and alpha-lipoic acid daily
- Practise strength training four days a week for 30 minutes to enhance your lean body mass and create a fat-burning body
- Walk briskly for 20 to 30 minutes each day to counter insulin resistance, enhance energy, improve your body's uptake of glycogen and maintain good emotional balance.

Ketogenics Or Insulin Balance – Which Is Right For You?

Ketogenics and Insulin Balance use the same principles to work their wonders. But they differ in important ways. Ketogenics rapidly kickstarts your system into burning fat. INSULIN BALANCE is a gentler way of losing body fat, and can be adjusted to form a lifelong way of eating. Remember, these are not low-calorie slimming diets. They are eating programmes designed to help your body shed fat naturally.

Are you a KETOGENICS person or an INSULIN BALANCE person? Turn to page 92-3 and calculate what percentage of your body is fat. Then...

...go for KETOGENICS if as a woman you carry more than 35 per cent body fat, or as a man you carry more than 22 per cent – or if you're a healthy individual who wants a more dynamic method of fat loss.

*Do not use Ketogenics if you are pregnant, about to undergo surgery,
have kidney or liver problems or are a Type I diabetic.*

**...go for INSULIN BALANCE if as a woman you carry less than 35 per
cent body fat, or as a man you carry less than 22 per cent. INSULIN
BALANCE is safe for just about everyone.**

Ketogenics

Insulin Balance

**Turn to page 000
and follow the steps.**

**Turn to page 184
and follow the steps.**

Ketogenics Step By Step

Ketogenics is a programme of high-protein, ultra-low-carb eating and simple
exercise that will kickstart your system into burning the fat it has accumulated.
After your body fat levels fall below the key limit of 35 per cent for women,
and 22 per cent for men, you can move on to Insulin Balance, the permanent
eating and exercise plan that will keep insulin levels balanced and your body
lean and healthy (that plan starts on page 184). Or you can stay on
KETOGENICS until you've lost all your excess body fat, then switch. But note:
KETOGENICS is not a slimming diet. You've got to eat enough of the foods
recommended below for it to work.

Step One: Gen Up

Keeping levels of protein and carb in your diet at an optimum ratio helps your
body switch to burning stored fat instead of glucose. The metabolic process is
known as benign dietary ketosis. While it's happening, your body will start to
produce less glucose, so that fatty acids will be released from fat cells to burn
as fuel. Food cravings will go, detoxification will begin and your body fat will
start to disappear. Within the first two weeks you are likely to lose:

- 4 to 12lb if you're a woman, or
- 8 to 16lb if you're a man.

Afterwards, expect a steady permanent weight loss of approximately 2lb of fat
stores a week until your body fat levels are low enough for Insulin Balance.

Step Two: Make The Switch

Shift the ratios of carbohydrates, fats and proteins so that:

▒ 20 per cent of your calories will be low glycaemic carbohydrates
▒ 30 per cent of your calories will be good fats
▒ 50 per cent of your calories will be high-quality proteins.

Get to know the very best in all these categories (see lists below). After that, check out the 14-day suggested menus on page 179-83.

Your Ketogenics Carbs

The carbs you'll eat on KETOGENICS are all low glycaemic index. That means they release glucose slowly, which helps keep insulin levels balanced and Syndrome X at bay. Starchy, high glycaemic index carbohydrates such as bread, pasta, pastry, potatoes and rice are off the menu.

From the lists below make up three cups of loosely packed raw vegetables, or two cups of cooked, a day. This is essential so that you get adequate fibre plus vitamins, minerals and phytonutrients to create a fat-burning metabolism and build vitality. Eat at least half of them raw. This will give you the best boost from phyto-nutrients and sunlight quanta, or energy. In all, you'll be eating a maximum of 20g of carbs a day for the first two weeks. After that, you can gradually increase the amount of low glycaemic carbs you eat until you establish the right level for you while still remaining in ketosis. (See Step Five page 183 for how to monitor ketosis.)

SUPER CARBS (LESS THAN 1G USABLE CARBS/SERVING)

☐ 1 cup alfalfa sprouts
☐ 1 cup sliced bok choy
☐ 1 stick celery
☐ ½ cup sliced endive
☐ 1 cup shredded lettuce
☐ ½ cup sliced raw radicchio
☐ 5 radishes
☐ ½ cup rocket
☐ 1 tsp minced spring onions

GREAT CARBS (LESS THAN 3G USABLE CARB/SERVING)

- 6 fresh asparagus spears
- ½ cup raw beetroot tops or 1 cup cooked
- ¼ cup blackberries
- 1 cup chopped raw broccoli
- ⅟ chopped capsicum
- 1 cup cauliflower florets
- ½ medium cucumber
- ¼ cup chopped leeks
- ½ cup boiled sliced marrow
- ½ cup sliced raw mushrooms
- ½ cup cooked mushrooms
- 5 whole enoki mushrooms
- ½ cup chopped raw spring onions
- ½ cup chopped parsley
- 1 tsp chopped raw shallot

GOOD CARBS (LESS THAN 5G USABLE CARBS/SERVING)

- ½ cup diced aubergine
- ½ medium avocado
- ¼ cup blueberries
- 4 Brussels sprouts
- 2 cup red or green cabbage
- ½ cup chopped dandelion greens
- ½ cup chopped fresh fennel
- ½ cup sliced French beans
- 1 cup mustard greens
- 1 whole hot chilli pepper
- ½ cup strawberries
- ½ cup chopped Swiss chard
- 1 medium tomato
- ½ cup canned sliced water chestnuts

Your Ketogenic Fats

The fats you'll eat on KETOGENICS are the healthiest available. They can be used in salad dressings or for cooking. There is no official limit, but remember that 30 per cent of your calorific intake should come from fats. In addition to the fat you get from food, take two teaspoons of flaxseed oil every day, or consider using a good supplement of omega-3 EPA and DHA fish oils (see 'Nutritional Supplements' on page 178). Omega-3 fatty acids help your body burn fat.

- extra-virgin olive oil
- walnut oil
- grapeseed oil
- coconut oil
- homemade mayonnaise made with extra-virgin olive oil
- small amounts of butter
- very occasionally, small amounts of cream or sour cream.

Your Ketogenic Proteins

The proteins you'll eat on KETOGENICS are high quality, and low in most saturated fats – so you'll avoid fatty cuts of beef, most kinds of sausage, and chicken livers.

The easiest way of measuring proteins is by the palm method. All this means is that the protein food you're going to eat should cover your palm (excluding fingers and thumb) and also be about the same thickness as your palm. You will eat about a palm and a half of protein food per meal, balanced by a cup of carbohydrate from the recommended list on page 174-5. You will also have two all-protein snacks a day, each about a third of a palm's size. In all, you'll be eating 150g of protein a day – and that means protein content, not the weight of the meat, fish or other food itself.

You can't use the palm method to measure microfiltered whey protein. Instead, use the scoops provided with the powder to make up the required number of grams in the recipes supplied in recipe chapters.

PROTEINS

Meats
- organic beef
- organic pork, bacon and ham
- organic lamb

Game and Poultry
- organic or free-range chicken
- turkey
- wild duck
- pheasant
- quail
- rabbit
- venison
- wild boar

Fish and Shellfish
- bass
- trout*
- sole
- sardines*
- herring
- mackerel*
- salmon*
- tuna, fresh*
- tuna tinned in water
- terakihi
- dory
- cod*
- haddock
- halibut
- snapper
- swordfish
- green-lipped mussels
- calamari
- oysters
- clams
- crayfish
- lobster
- crab
- scallops

Eggs
Just ensure you cook them the no-carb way: soft- and hard-boiled, in omelettes, poached, scrambled or fried.

Cheese
An occasional treat, limited to 110g a time. Be sure to check any carb content.
- Parmesan
- Camembert
- feta
- cottage cheese
- ricotta

Vegetarian Options
- tofu, tempeh, miso and other soya products – but check carb content on label
- microfiltered whey protein – this is the highest value biological protein in the world. It's great for non-vegetarians too. Be sure to use plenty of it. (See Resources on page 339 for stockists.)

* rich in omega-3 essential fatty acids

Your Ketogenic Drinks and Extras

Drinks

▨ filtered or spring water – drink 8 to 10 glasses a day

▨ herb teas, flavoured mineral water (although only those with no sweeteners or calories) and organic vegetable bouillon or broth

▨ vegetable broth made with broccoli, cabbage, cauliflower, bean sprouts, asparagus, mustard greens, spinach, watercress, ginger, garlic or any combination thereof is good. Bring to the boil and simmer for 15 minutes. Season with herbs and sea salt and store in the fridge, reheating as needed. A good drink if you're feeling weak or headachy at the start of KETOGENICS.

BEWARE: avoid all alcohol, soft drinks, fruit juices and cordials. They will interfere with ketogenic fat burning.

Sweeteners

Avoid all sweeteners except for stevia and (if you must go artificial) Splenda (see pages 209-11 and 208-9).

Salad Dressings And Sauces

You can make these with recommended oils from the list on page 176. Just count as part of your carb intake any vinegars or juices you use. Champagne vinegar, red wine vinegar and white wine vinegar have no carbs, but each tablespoon of balsamic or apple cider vinegar has 2g and fresh lemon or lime juice approximately 1.3g.

Herbs And Spices

Use all spices and fresh herbs. Be sure to check carb content of dried herbs.

Fibre

If you become constipated on KETOGENICS, dried psyllium husks are an excellent source of fibre: they contain no carbs, and can be added to smoothies. For stockists, see 'Resources', page 339.

Nutritional Supplements

Take the following daily:

▨ a good multiple vitamin including phytonutrients (see Resources, page 339)

▨ 400-600mcg chromium picolinate or chromium polynicotinate

▨ 230-600mg magnesium tartrate or magnesium citrate or chelated magnesium

▨ 1000-3000mg omega-3 EPA and DHA fish oils in capsule form.

For information on other supplements, see 'Help When You Need It', page 223.

Step Three: Plan Your Menus
Here's a 14-day plan to help you ease your way into this wonderful new way of eating. You don't need to follow it by rote – simply use it as an inspiration for your own creativity. Have a microfiltered whey protein drink whenever you can – preferably once a day. Just carry a shaker full of it for instant snacks on the go. It's great for building your fat burning body. Don't hesitate to keep that leftover piece of chicken for tomorrow's snack. You might even carry a tin of tuna for emergencies. KETOGENICS foods can be absolutely delicious. Have fun planning your menu.

Be sure to remember to:
- Measure the protein using the palm method (see page 111-2), except for microfiltered whey protein – use the scoop that comes with the tub.
- Keep your vegetable carbs to three cups a day.
- Use the recommended fats in cooking or to make salad dressings. You can add your omega-3 fatty acids in the form of flaxseed oil to smoothies or salad dressings as you please.
- Drink 8 to 10 glasses of water a day – ringing the changes with herb teas, no-carb flavoured spring water or homemade lemonade sweetened with stevia (page 209-11).

Once you've got the hang of KETOGENICS eating, you can put together your own recipes. Use the 'Sheer Pleasures' section, starting on page 231, for more ideas. For advice on shopping to find the best available foods, see '21st-century Hunter Gatherer' on page 200. For stockists of organic meats and other ingredients, see 'Resources' on page 339.

Day 1
Breakfast: 1 or more patties Hand-made Sausage (page 241-2) with grilled tomato.
Snack: Smoothie made in the blender with 10-15g chocolate-flavoured microfiltered whey protein, 1 cup of spring or filtered water, and 3 ice cubes.
Lunch: Spinach salad with sliced chicken, dressed with olive oil and champagne vinegar.
Snack: ¼ cup cottage cheese.
Dinner: Grilled organic steak with Char Grilled Capsicums (page 272-3). Side salad of lettuce and minced spring onions with an olive oil and red wine vinegar dressing.

Day 2
Breakfast: Cottage cheese with snipped chives and slices of fennel bulb and cucumber.
Snack: 1 hard-boiled egg.
Lunch: Rocket and red onion salad with chunks of roast lamb, and olive oil and red wine vinegar dressing.
Snack: 28g macadamia nuts.
Dinner: Grilled swordfish with a scatter of pickled peppercorns. Stir fried bok choy with garlic.

Day 3
Breakfast: Poached egg on tomato slices sprinkled with spring onions, sauteed grated fresh ginger and a clove of garlic.
Snack: 28g walnuts.
Lunch: Fish Paté (page 258-9) with celery and radishes.
Snack: Slices lean lamb.
Dinner: Chicken Curry (page 265-6). Steamed green beans and cauliflower.

Day 4
Breakfast: Light as Air Pancakes (page 237-8) with a dab of butter and a sprinkle of cinnamon.
Snack: 28g sunflower seeds.
Lunch: Chef's salad with chicken slices, 1oz slivered fresh Parmesan and avocado dressing.
Snack: Smoothie made in the blender with 10-15g vanilla-flavoured microfiltered whey protein, 1 cup spring water, and 3 ice cubes, sweetened with stevia or Splenda, as desired (see page 208-11).
Dinner: Grilled salmon with fresh dill and lemon slices. Steamed or wok fried green beans and brussels sprouts.

Day 5
Breakfast: Scrambled Tofu (page 238-9).
Snack: Slices lean organic beef.
Lunch: Egg salad with chopped onions and homemade mayonnaise, wrapped in crunchy lettuce leaves.
Snack: 28g cottage cheese.
Dinner: Organic pork marinated in Japanese Teriyaki Marinade (page 253), then stir fried with garlic, snow peas and spring onions.

Day 6
Breakfast: Crunchy rocket leaves topped with cucumber slices and organic,

smoked, sugar-free salmon served with a wedge of lemon.

Snack: Smoothie made in the blender with 10-15g honey nut-flavoured or plain microfiltered whey protein, 1 cup spring water, and 3 ice cubes, sweetened with stevia or Splenda if needed (see page 208-11).

Lunch: Broccoli Soup with tofu (page 279-80).

Snack: 1 hard-boiled egg.

Dinner: Organic charbroiled steak. Fresh asparagus spears and melted butter. Side salad of alfalfa sprouts, enoki mushrooms and celery.

Day 7

Breakfast: Sweet Nothing Soufflé (page 235).

Snack: Slices organic chicken.

Lunch: Caesar Salad with Hard-boiled Croûtons (page 244-5).

Snack: 28g macadamia nuts.

Dinner: Lobster with garlic butter. Steamed spinach spiked with Cajun seasoning. Side salad of lambs' lettuce and thin slices of red onion, with an olive oil and red wine vinegar dressing.

Day 8

Breakfast: Smoothie made in the blender with 30g microfiltered whey protein, 200ml spring water, 3 ice cubes, 1-3 teaspoons psyllium husks, a few drops of stevia (see page 209-11) and a quarter-cup of blueberries.

Snack: 1 hard-boiled egg.

Lunch: Teppanyaki Tofu Strips (page 261-2) stir fried with green beans, chopped chilli and garlic.

Snack: 28g walnuts.

Dinner: Sole almandine served with slivered almonds. Steamed broccoli. Salad of radicchio with olive oil and balsamic vinegar dressing.

Day 9

Breakfast: Spinach omelette with crisp strips of organic bacon.

Snack: 28g sunflower seeds.

Lunch: Chunks of cooked turkey, minced spring onion and finely chopped raw broccoli tossed in homemade garlic mayonnaise.

Snack: 28g chunk of feta.

Dinner: Poached cod with Winning Pesto (page 253-4). Mesclun side salad with olive oil and white wine vinegar dressing.

Day 10

Breakfast: Phytonutrient Eggs (page 236-7).

Snack: 28g walnuts.

Lunch: Roast lamb with homemade parsley mayonnaise, served on a bed of shredded rocket and sliced tomatoes.
Snack: ¼ cup cottage cheese.
Dinner: Stir-fried scallops with garlic and snow peas. Lambs' lettuce side salad with mustard vinaigrette. Melon balls.

Day 11

Breakfast: Smoothie made in the blender with 30g microfiltered whey protein, 200ml spring water, 3 ice cubes, 1-3 teaspoons psyllium husks, a few drops of stevia (see page 209-11) and ¼ cup strawberries.
Snack: 28g macadamia nuts.
Lunch: Salad of celery, red onion, lettuce and shredded fresh ginger, topped with diced cooked free-range duck and drizzled with olive oil and lime juice dressing.
Snack: 1 hard-boiled egg.
Dinner: Broiled lamb chops garnished with mint leaves. Cauliflower Mash (see page 276). Side salad of cucumber, endive and walnuts dressed in walnut oil and champagne vinegar.

Day 12

Breakfast: 1 or more patties Hand-made Sausage (page 241-2) with grilled mushrooms.
Snack: 28g sunflower seeds.
Lunch: Salad of cos lettuce with chopped hard-boiled eggs and dressed with Basil and More Basil Dressing (page 257).
Snack: ¼ cup cottage cheese.
Dinner: Grilled chicken breast with stir-fried courgettes. Watercress side salad dressed with olive oil, lemon juice and garlic.

Day 13

Breakfast: Omelette on the Run (page 235-6).
Snack: Smoothie made in the blender with 10-15g honey nut-flavoured microfiltered whey protein, 1 cup spring water, and 3 ice cubes.
Lunch: Salad of romaine lettuce, green onions and radishes with masses of Tofu Cheese dressing (page 285-6).
Snack: 28g sunflower seeds.
Dinner: Sautéed Sea Bass with Garlic (page 263-4). Side salad of alfalfa sprouts and cucumber with olive oil and red wine vinegar dressing.

Day 14

Breakfast: Quick Shake (page 233).

Snack: 1 hard-boiled egg.

Lunch: Avocado, lettuce and tomato salad with grilled diced bacon and olive oil and balsamic vinegar dressing.

Snack: Slices organic turkey.

Dinner: Nut Crusted Tuna (page 264). Steamed broccoli and cauliflower.

Step Four: Get Moving

It's time to start walking 20 to 30 minutes a day. After the first three or four days, add in a weight training programme to increase your muscle mass and spur fat burning (see page 94). You'll be doing this for 30 minutes, four days a week.

Step Five: Do Your Twice-A-Day Checkup

Monitor whether you're staying in ketosis by measuring the levels of ketones – by-products of fat breakdown from your cells – in your urine. Do this before breakfast and again before dinner, using Ketosticks®, available at any pharmacy. For successful fat burning, your ketone levels must be maintained between 'trace' and 'small' – that is, 0.5 to 1.5mmol. If they go higher, add a little more low glycaemic vegetables to your diet until the Ketostick measurement returns to 'trace' or 'small'.

Step Six: Get Help When You Need It

Go to Troubleshooting on page 223.

You'll find ideas for negotiating menus in restaurants in Eat Out with Savvy (page 212), help for those moments of weakness in If You're Craving (page 219), and more information in Further Reading and Resources. (pages 323 and 339).

READY, SET, GO – LIFE CHANGES BEGIN HERE. HAVE FUN WITH THEM.

INSULIN BALANCE STEP BY STEP

You've chosen Insulin Balance. It's a wonderful way not only to shed fat but to regenerate and rejuvenate your body and to help keep it in great shape year after year. Insulin Balance combines a high-protein, low-carb way of eating with simple exercise. If your body fat level is below the key limit – 35 per cent for women, and 22 per cent for men – Insulin Balance is your X Factor Diet.

Step One: Gen Up
Like Ketogenics, Insulin Balance will spur fat burning and balance insulin levels, but it will do the job more gently. Your body will not need to go into ketosis, so you won't need to bother with monitoring it. More than that, Insulin Balance can be adjusted to become a permanent way of living, whichever programme you started with. It ensures you'll stay lean, healthy, younger-looking and full of vitality.

If you started on Ketogenics and are now ready to change over to Insulin Balance, you'll find you can do this bit by bit. Basically, you'll be eating more carbs and easing up a bit on the protein. Start by adding one serving a day of medium glycaemic index fruits or vegetables (see opposite) to your basic Ketogenics menu. Go on until you reach the level that seems right for you – that is, you're still in optimal health, and you're not gaining any weight.

Step Two: Make The Switch
Shift the ratio of carbohydrates, fats and proteins so that:
- 35 per cent of your calories will be carbohydrates
- 30 per cent of your calories will be fats
- 35 per cent of your calories will be proteins.

You'll need to fine-tune your protein needs a bit. The amount of lean body mass you have ultimately determines how much protein you'll eat. See page 109 for how to calculate your lean body mass.

Get to know the very best in all three food categories (see lists on pages 185-8). After that, check out the 14-day suggested menus on page 190.

Your Insulin Balance Carbs
A lot of the carbs you'll eat on INSULIN BALANCE are low glycaemic index. That means they release glucose slowly, which helps keep insulin levels balanced and Syndrome X at bay. You're also free to eat medium to moderately high glycaemic index carbs, but you'll have to eat correspondingly less of them. Starchy, high glycaemic index carbohydrates such as bread, pasta, pastry and rice are out, although barley (good in soup), steel-cut oatmeal,100 per cent rye bread or Ryvita can be eaten on occasion.

The palm method is a handy way of measuring carbs. An amount of carbohydrate food about as big as your palm minus thumb and fingers, and the same thickness, equals one palm of food.

From the lists below, make up **2 palms of low glycaemic carbs per meal – or 1 palm of medium to high glycaemic carbs**. Eating them raw will give you the best boost from phytonutrients and sunlight quanta, or energy.

LOW GLYCAEMIC INDEX CARBS

Vegetables

- asparagus
- bean sprouts
- beet greens
- broccoli
- cabbage
- cauliflower
- celery
- cucumber
- endive
- lettuce
- mustard greens
- radishes
- spinach
- Swiss chard
- watercress

Fruits

- cantaloupe
- rhubarb
- strawberries
- watermelon
- tomatoes

MEDIUM GLYCAEMIC INDEX CARBS

Vegetables

- aubergine
- beets
- Brussels sprouts
- chives
- collards
- dandelion greens

Fruits

- apricots (fresh)
- blackberries
- cranberries
- grapefruit
- lemons
- limes

French beans
kale
kohlrabi
leeks
okra
onions
parsley
pimento
pumpkin
red pepper
swede
turnip

oranges
plums
raspberries
papaya
tangerines
peaches
kiwi fruits

HIGH GLYCAEMIC INDEX CARBS

Vegetables
artichokes
carrots
green peas
oyster plant
parsnips
squash

Fruits
apples
blueberries
cherries
grapes
kumquats
loganberries

mangoes
mulberries
pears
pineapple (fresh)
pomegranates

Your Insulin Balance Fats

The fats you'll eat on Insulin Balance are the healthiest available. They can be used in salad dressings or for cooking. Eat about a tablespoon or so per meal from the list below. In addition to the fat you get from food, take **2 teaspoons of flaxseed oil every day, or consider using a good supplement of omega-3 EPA and DHA fish oils** (see 'Nutritional supplements', page 178). Omega-3 fatty acids help your body burn fat.

almonds and almond butter
avocados (and guacamole)
coconut oil

■ extra-virgin olive oil

■ macadamia nuts and macadamia butter

■ olives

■ peanut butter, unsweetened

■ tahini

Your Insulin Balance Proteins

The proteins you'll eat on INSULIN BALANCE are high quality, and low in most saturated fats – so you'll avoid fatty cuts of beef, most kinds of sausage, and chicken livers.

The easiest way to measure proteins is by the palm method – see under the carbs section, above. You will eat about a palm of protein food per meal, depending on your lean body mass. You can't use the palm method to measure microfiltered whey protein. Instead, use the scoops provided with the powder to make up the required number of grams in the recipes found in the recipe sections.

PROTEINS AND FATS

Meats
- organic beef
- organic pork, bacon and ham
- organic lamb

Game and Poultry
- organic chicken
- turkey
- wild duck
- pheasant
- quail
- rabbit
- venison
- wild boar

Fish and Shellfish
- bass
- trout*

- sole
- sardines*
- herring
- mackerel*
- salmon*
- tuna, fresh*
- tuna tinned in water
- terakihi
- dory
- cod*
- haddock
- halibut
- snapper
- swordfish
- green-lipped mussels
- calamari
- oysters
- clams
- crayfish   *continued over*

☐ lobster
☐ crab
☐ scallops

Eggs

Just ensure you cook them the no-carb way: soft- and hard-boiled, in omelettes, poached, scrambled or fried.

Cheese

An occasional treat, limited to 110g a time. Be sure to check any carb content.

☐ Parmesan
☐ Camembert
☐ feta
☐ cottage cheese
☐ ricotta

Vegetarian Options

☐ tofu, tempeh, miso and other soya products – but check carb content on label
☐ microfiltered whey protein – this is the highest value biological protein in the world. It's great for nonvegetarians too. Be sure to use plenty of it. (See Resources on page 339 for stockists.)

* rich in omega-3 essential fatty acids

Your Insulin Balance Drinks and Extras

Drinks

▨ filtered or spring water – 8 to 10 glasses a day
▨ herb teas and no-carb flavoured mineral water
▨ fruit juice diluted with spring water as an occasional treat (treat it as a serving of fruit)
▨ vegetarian bouillon
▨ coffee – up to 2 cups a day
▨ green or black tea in moderation
▨ dry white or red wine – up to 2 small glasses a day.

Sweeteners

Avoid all sweeteners except for stevia and (if you must go artificial) Splenda (see pages 209-11 and 208-9).

Salad Dressings And Sauces

You can make these with recommended oils from the list above.

Herbs And Spices

Use all spices and fresh herbs freely.

Fibre

If you need it, dried psyllium husks are excellent, as they contain no carbs and can be added to smoothies. For stockists, see Resources, page 339.

Nutritional Supplements

Take the following daily:

- a good multiple vitamin including phytonutrients (see Resources, page 339)
- 400-600mcg chromium picolinate or chromium polynicotinate
- 230-600mg magnesium tartrate or magnesium citrate or chelated magnesium
- 1000-3000mg omega-3 EPA and DHA fish oils in capsule form.

If you feel the need for others, see Help When You Need It on page 194.

Step Three: Plan Your Menus

Here's a 14-day plan to help you ease your way into this wonderful new way of eating. On Insulin Balance you have more freedom than you did on Ketogenics. And you certainly don't need to follow the suggested menu by rote – simply use it as an inspiration for your own creativity. Have a microfiltered whey protein drink whenever you can – preferably once a day. Just carry a shaker full of it for snacks on the go. It's great for building your fat burning body. Don't hesitate to keep that leftover piece of chicken for tomorrow's snack. You might even carry a tin of water pack tuna for emergencies. Insulin Balance foods can be absolutely delicious. Have fun planning your menu – including all those mouthwatering desserts.

With the menus and recipes that follow, remember to:

- Measure carbs and protein using the palm method (see page 111-2), except for microfiltered whey protein – use the scoop that comes with the tub.
- Use the recommended fats in cooking or to make salad dressings. You can add your omega-3 fatty acids in the form of flaxseed oil to smoothies or salad dressings.
- Drink 8 to 10 glasses of water a day – ringing the changes with herb teas, no-carb flavoured spring water or homemade lemonade sweetened with stevia (page 209-11).

Once you've got the hang of Insulin Balance eating, you can put together your own recipes. Use the Sheer Pleasures section, starting on page 23, for more ideas. For advice on shopping to find the best available foods, see 21st-century Hunter Gatherer on page 200. For stockists of organic meats and other ingredients, see Resources on page 339.

Day 1
Breakfast: Three scrambled eggs in olive oil with two cloves of garlic, chopped tomatoes, onions and homemade Energy Salsa (page 259).
Snack: 28g cottage cheese with a sprinkle of Cajun spice.
Lunch: Herb salad with flaked tuna, sliced red onions, sunflower seeds, and olive oil and balsamic vinegar dressing.
Snack: 28g Spicy Nuts (page 286).
Dinner: Organic pork stir fried with garlic, grated ginger, cauliflower and spring onions. Strawberries topped with vanilla-flavoured Protein Whip (page 291-2).

Day 2
Breakfast: Vanilla Nutmeg Smoothie (page 233-4).
Snack: 1 hard-boiled egg.
Lunch: Chicken kebabs skewered with onion pieces, red pepper chunks and mushrooms dipped in olive oil and seasoned with herbs and a flash of lemon.
Snack: 28g pork rinds.
Dinner: Courgette spaghetti tossed with grated Parmesan and a sautée of garlic, crumbled Hand-made Sausage (page 241), minced chilli and fresh herbs. Sliced peach served with Almond Macaroons (page 290).

Day 3
Breakfast: A slice of melon and naturally smoked kipper herring.
Snack: 28g pumpkin and sunflower seeds.
Lunch: Caesar Salad with Hard-boiled Croûtons (page 244-5) and carrot sticks. Protein Fudge Treats (page 291).
Snack: 28g cottage cheese with a sprinkle of Mexican spice.
Dinner: Chargrilled steak. Spinach and sprout salad with a scatter of avocado chunks and olive oil and red wine vinegar dressing. Crunchy Potato Skins (page 283).

Day 4
Breakfast: Omelette on the Run (page 235-6) made with chopped organic ham.
Snack: Slices of wild salmon.
Lunch: Greek Salad (page 246-7), adding 4oz cubed cooked lamb and a

tablespoon of mixed sesame, sunflower and pumpkin seeds to the basic recipe.
Snack: 3 Parmesan Wafers (page 286).
Dinner: Roast cod with Coco-almond Broccoli (page 280). Cucumber and
radish crudités. Raspberry Chocolate Mousse (page 293).

Day 5
Breakfast: Large bowl of yoghurt and strawberries, sprinkled with almonds
and sweetened with stevia (see page 209-11).
Snack: 28g walnuts.
Lunch: Crunchy Broccoli Salad (page 248-9) sprinkled with slivers of organic
ham.
Snack: Flaked water-pack tuna.
Dinner: Three small grilled lamb chops with garlic, oregano and lemon juice.
Grilled sliced aubergine and tomatoes, brushed with olive oil and seasoned
with fresh herbs. Ambrosia (thinly sliced navel oranges thickly sprinkled with
grated fresh coconut and drizzled with Grand Marnier).

Day 6
Breakfast: Scrambled Tofu (page 238) made with turmeric and chopped red
pepper.
Snack: Smoothie made in the blender with 10-15g chocolate-flavoured
microfiltered whey protein, 1 cup spring water, 1 tablespoon of psyllium husks
and 3 ice cubes.
Lunch: Crudités with three dips – aubergine, tapenade and Curried Avocado
(page 257-8).
Snack: 1 hard-boiled egg sprinkled with Cajun seasoning.
Dinner: Grilled tuna steak. Baked asparagus with butter. Romaine lettuce salad
with blue cheese dressing. Lemon Cream Pie (page 295) made with Easy Going
Piecrust (page 294-5).

Day 7
Breakfast: A small breakfast steak seared in coconut oil with sliced onions,
mushrooms and green beans.
Snack: 28g Camembert.
Lunch: Fennel, orange and grape salad with snow peas and slices of organic
turkey.
Snack: 28g sunflower seeds.
Dinner: Chunks of tofu stir fried in soy oil with shredded ginger, bok choy,
cashews and tamari. Slices of melon served with Protein Whip (page 291-2).

Day 8
Breakfast: Omelette on the Run (page 235-6) made with ham and served with chopped fresh tomatoes and basil.
Snack: 28g cottage cheese.
Lunch: Mock Potato Salad (page 250-1) served with a salad of walnuts, chicken and romaine lettuce with olive oil and white wine vinegar dressing.
Snack: 28g pork rinds.
Dinner: Sautéed Halibut with Garlic (page 236). Steamed broccoli and courgettes with almonds. Protein Icecream (page 296) sprinkled with extra coconut and drizzled with Raspberry Syrup (page 240).

Day 9
Breakfast: Three poached eggs and a slice of 100 per cent rye toast drizzled with low-carb Blueberry Jam (page 240-1).
Snack: Smoothie made in the blender with 10-15g vanilla-flavoured microfiltered whey protein, 1 cup spring water, 1 tablespoon of psyllium husks and 3 ice cubes.
Lunch: Chef's salad with turkey slices, grated cheese, olives, artichoke hearts and a creamy dressing.
Snack: 28g Tofu Cheese (page 285-6).
Dinner: Perfect Peppers (page 273-4). Roasted pumpkin. Mesclun salad with olive oil and champagne vinegar dressing. Lemon Posset (page 293-4).

Day 10
Breakfast: Rocket salad with chunks of marinated tofu, alfalfa sprouts and an olive oil and lemon juice dressing.
Snack: Slices lean organic lamb.
Lunch: Salmon Salad (page 250).
Snack: 28g cottage cheese with a sprinkle of Mexican spice mix.
Dinner: Chicken stir fried with carrots, bean sprouts, ginger, green onions, garlic and water chestnuts cooked in coconut oil with a coconut cream sauce. Toasted sesame seeds. Blueberries, strawberries and melon balls served with Almond Macaroons (page 290).

Day 11
Breakfast: Blueberry Curds and Whey (page 239).
Snack: 28g macadamia nuts.
Lunch: Organic beef hamburger without the bun, served with sliced lettuce, tomatoes and cucumbers. Protein Icecream (page 296) topped with crushed almonds and a sprinkle of organic unsweetened cocoa.
Snack: 1 Devilled Egg (page 284).

Dinner: Grilled tiger prawns with a slice of lemon. Rocket salad with slices of red pepper. Garlic mayonnaise.

Day 12

Breakfast: Light as Air Pancakes (page 237-8) with butter and Raspberry Syrup (page 240).

Snack: Smoothie made in the blender with 10-15g honey nut-flavoured microfiltered whey protein, 1 cup spring water, 1 tablespoon of psyllium husks and 3 ice cubes.

Lunch: Flying Soup (page 275) served with a RyVita 100 per cent rye cracker and cottage cheese.

Snack: 28g sunflower seeds.

Dinner: Baked almond-crusted swordfish steak (page 264). Cauliflower Mash (page 276). Salad of lettuce and red cabbage with a mustard vinaigrette. Blueberry cream pie (page 000) made with Easy Going Piecrust (page 294-5).

Day 13

Breakfast: Scrambled egg with organic sausage and a grilled tomato.

Snack: 28g walnuts.

Lunch: California Sprouted Salad (page 249-50) with organic chicken chunks tossed in curried mayonnaise. Protein Fudge Treats (page 291).

Snack: Flaked water-pack tuna.

Dinner: Strips of organic beef marinated in Japanese Teriyaki Marinade (page 253) and stir fried with sliced onions, bok choy, green beans and water chestnuts.

Day 14

Breakfast: Berry Bliss Smoothie (page 234) made with blackberries and strawberries.

Snack: Slices of organic lamb.

Lunch: Tuna on 100 per cent rye sandwich, with tomatoes, homemade garlic mayonnaise and sprouted seeds and grains.

Snack: 28g macadamia nuts.

Dinner: Sautéed chicken breasts seasoned with cracked pepper. Steamed spinach with Hollandaise Sauce (page 254). Raspberries and crushed Almond Macaroons (page 290) folded into vanilla-flavoured Protein Whip (page 291-2).

Step Four: Get Moving

If you started on Ketogenics, you'll already be well into your daily exercise routine. If not – it's time to start walking 20 to 30 minutes a day. After the first three or four days, add in a weight training programme to increase your muscle mass and spur fat burning (see page 94). You'll be doing this for 30 minutes, four days a week.

Step Five: Get Help When You Need It

If you experience any problems with INSULIN BALANCE, go to Troubleshooting on page 223.

You'll find ideas for negotiating menus in restaurants in Eat Out with Savvy(page 212), help for those moments of weakness in If You're Craving (page 219), and more information in Further Reading and Resources. (pages 323 and 339).

TODAY IS THE FIRST DAY OF THE REST OF YOUR LIFE. SIX WEEKS DOWN THE ROAD YOU ARE LIKELY TO REJOICE AS YOUR BODY GROWS LEANER, MORE VITAL AND MORE BEAUTIFUL AND YOUR ENERGY LEVELS SOAR. ENJOY.

Carbs At A Glance

Eat up to 3 cups of good (low glycaemic) carbohydrate foods each day. These carbohydrate foods are high in fibre, vitamins, minerals and phytonutrients and low in simple carbohydrates. Make them the focus of your salads and stir frys.

Alfalfa	Green beans
Asparagus	Kale
Bok choy	Lettuce
Broccoli	Mushrooms
Cabbage	Onions
Capsicum	Parsley
Cauliflower	Radish
Celery	Silverbeet
Coleslaw	Sprouts
Courgette	Turnip
Cucumber	
Garlic	

Fruits

If you want to eat fruits, half a cup a day is OK. But then you will need to cut one cup from the 'carbohydrate foods' list above for every half cup of fruit you eat. These low glycaemic index fruits are the best for reducing blood glucose and insulin responses:

Apricots	Raspberries
Blackberries	Melons
Grapefruit	Strawberries

GREAT CARBS
(Less than 3g of usable carbohydrate per serving)

6 fresh asparagus spears (2.4g)
1 cup raw beetroot tops (1.8g) or 1 cup cooked
1 cup blackberries (2.9g)
1 cup chopped raw broccoli (2.2g)
1 cup chopped capsicum (2.4g)
1 cup cauliflower florets (2.6g)
1 medium cucumber (3g)
1 cup chopped leeks (2g)
1 cup boiled sliced marrow (2.6g)
1 cup sliced raw mushrooms (1.1g)
1 cup cooked mushrooms (2.3g)
5 whole enoki mushrooms (2g)
1 cup chopped raw spring onions (2.5g)
1 cup chopped parsley (1.9g)
1 tablespoon chopped raw shallot (1.7g)

INSULIN BALANCE CARBOHYDRATES
Poor Choices

Vegetables, Cooked
Acorn squash
Baked beans
Beetroot
Butternut pumpkin
Carrot
Corn
Lima beans
Parsnips
Peas
Pinto beans
Potato, baked
Potato, boiled
Potato, chipped
Potato, mashed
Refried beans
Sweet potato, baked

Grains, Cereals and Breads
Bagel
Biscuits
Breadcrumbs
Bread, whole-grain or white
Breadsticks
Buckwheat
Bulgar wheat
Cereal
Cornflour
Couscous, dry
Crackers
Croissant
Croûtons
Doughnut
English muffin
Granola
Melba toast
Millet

Condiments and Treats
Barbecue sauce
Cake
Cocktail sauce
Honey
Ice cream
Jam or jelly
Molasses
Plum sauce
Relish, pickle
Sugar
Sugar, icing
Sweets
Syrup, Golden
Syrup, maple
Teriyaki sauce
Tomato sauce

Alcohol
Beer
Spirits
Wine

PART FOUR:
NEW LIFE

21ST-CENTURY HUNTER-GATHERER

Now that you've seen how both Ketogenics and Insulin Balance work, you're ready to live the X Factor way. But before you head for the supermarket, delicatessen, whole food emporium or local farm store, it's a good idea to clear your cupboards of all the low-fat-high-carb foods you have been collecting. That includes jams and jellies, rice cakes, popcorn, flour, grains, pasta, pretzels, low-fat salad dressings, raisins, fruit-flavoured yoghurts and confectioner's sugar.

Let's Go Shopping
What you will want to keep around is some ordinary granulated sugar to serve to friends who drink sweetened drinks as well as some brown rice, which you can add three or four tablespoons of to thicken a soup once you have passed on from Ketogenics to Insulin Balance. Most people find the process of clearing out your pantry and refrigerator of foods that play no part in low-carb meals a salutary experience. It gives you the sense that you're starting a new life – as indeed you are.

The most important foods you will be buying regularly are low-density vegetables which are also low on the glycaemic index, and protein foods such as meat, seafood, eggs and game, as well as soya proteins such as tofu. One of the most surprising things that happens to some people when they enter a supermarket in search of low-carb foods is they find that most of what exists in a supermarket is not worth eating. A good general rule when choosing healthy food is this: foods with a long shelf life don't belong in your body. Processed high-carb foods often have a very long shelf life. This makes them great sales material for food manufacturers and retailers because they can sit on the shelves for a very long time, and are cheap to make with high profit margins. But most of them are whipped up out of white flour and white sugar plus a lot of junk fats, chemical additives and salt. Avoid them.

Go To The Edge
The healthiest, freshest, and the most natural foods are usually found around the outside edges of the supermarket. These include crunchy fresh vegetables and fruit, fresh game and meats, seafoods, eggs and low-fat cheeses. Such natural, wholesome foods are perishable and therefore have to be replaced

often, unlike the ready-in-a-minute, jiffy pre-made stuff that you find in the inner isles. You will be shopping 'at the edge' in another way too: you'll be looking for foods as close as possible to those our ancestors ate. You'll need to choose a wide variety of vegetables, especially leafy green ones which are low in carbohydrate, if you are doing Ketogenics, and a selection that's moderate in carbohydrate once you have entered the Insulin Balance phase. In this phase, you can even very occasionally select a few high glycaemic foods such as rice, potatoes, bananas and maize – provided, of course, that you only eat it in small quantities, and monitor both how you feel and how it affects your fat loss. In either case, however, most of the vegetables you buy need to be those that are low glycaemic index and low carbohydrate density. Here are some of the foods that are particularly good to look for:

- Asparagus
- Bok choy
- Broccoli
- Capsicums
- Cauliflower
- Celery
- Chinese cabbage
- Cos lettuce
- Courgettes
- Endive
- Fresh herbs such as coriander, basil, mint, parsley and dill
- Hot peppers
- Lambs' lettuce
- Radicchio
- Rocket
- Romaine lettuce
- Silverbeet
- Spinach

Check out the list of usable carbohydrates on page 303-21, which gives a measure of the carbohydrate density, and get to know how many carbs there are in each kind of food. It is a nuisance to begin with, but within two weeks you will be pretty savvy about it all. You will want, too, to look for vegetables that are particularly health-enhancing, such as garlic – which lowers blood pressure and triglycerides, shifts cholesterol balance and lowers blood glucose – and onions, which have many of the same health-enhancing properties but to a lesser degree.

Organic Is Best

Whenever possible, go organic. Not only do organic vegetables taste better, the organic matter in healthy soil is nature's factory for biological activity. Organic vegetables therefore supply us with an excellent balance of minerals, trace elements and vitamins which we cannot get any other way. The organic matter in soil is built up as a result of the breakdown of vegetable and animal matter by the soil's natural residents – worms, bacteria and other micro-organisms. The presence of these creatures in the right quantity and type – which you never find in factory farming – gives rise to physical, chemical and biological properties which create fertility in our soils and make plants grown on them highly resistant to disease. This resistance to illness and degeneration is then passed on to us when we eat the foods. Destroy the soil's organic matter through chemical farming and, slowly but inexorably, you destroy the health of the people and animals living on the foods grown on it.

Organic methods of farming help protect against distortions in mineral balance. This balance is vital because an increase in one or more minerals, say, can alter the body's ability to absorb as much of another mineral. Conventionally grown fruits and vegetables are sprayed with pesticides – petrochemically derived compounds which behave like low-dose synthetic oestrogens in the body. Many fruit and veg are also treated with fungicides or wax. Each one of these chemicals contributes to the toxic load that puts pressure on your liver, stresses your body as a whole and encourages free radical damage associated with degeneration. When it comes to maintaining good insulin balance, you particularly do not want this to happen. A stressed liver has trouble managing glucose levels and controls insulin poorly. Natural food emporiums are great places to find good organic vegetables and other produce, as well as eggs, meat, dairy products and fish, from animals that have not been stuffed full of antibiotics, dipped in chemicals or treated with hormones. Try to shop as much as possible in stores that offer organic produce and untreated food.

But just because you buy something in a health food store or natural food supermarket does not mean that it will be helpful in reversing insulin resistance and promoting fat loss. These stores are chock-a-block with high-carb treats, often full of sugar. And organic sugar and organic flour can still upset the insulin/glucagons apple cart. Although they may look great in their packages, most of these 'treat' foods are the last thing you want to promote good insulin balance. Read labels as carefully here as in the supermarket. Make sure that any foods you buy contain no hidden sugars such as honey or fruit juice concentrate.

Get Into Protein

When selecting meats and fish, there are two major considerations: make sure it's fresh and as unprocessed as possible. Buy fresh fish and seafood instead of processed forms such as smoked fish, crab cakes and breaded fish. There's no harm in having the odd slice of smoked salmon, especially if it is naturally smoked. But the more a fish is processed, the less quality it brings you in terms of high-level health and fat loss. (And these days, most smoked salmon has sugar added to it.)

If at all possible, add oily fish to your diet once or twice a week, as it's rich in pre-formed omega-3 fatty acids DHA and EPA. This means that the omega-3s in wild salmon, mackerel, sardines, tuna and herrings can be absorbed by the body without conversion to make it usable. Omega-3 fatty acids are known to reduce the levels of triglycerides in the body – the blood fats characteristic of Syndrome X, which put you at risk of heart disease. Omega-3 fatty acids also help spur on fat burning and weight loss, as well as lower blood pressure and improve overall heart function. I have recommended flaxseed oil as a rich source of the omega-3 fatty acids, and it's often promoted as such. But it does differ from fish oil in a couple of significant ways. Flaxseed contains a great deal of linolenic acid, which is the precursor to DHA and EPA, but the problem is that your body needs to convert the linolenic acid to DHA and EPA. Some people can't make this conversion, especially if they have eaten a lot of trans fatty acids and an overabundance of omega-6 fats in the past. Also, omega-3 from flaxseed oil is a kind that in some people can change into arachidonic acid (see page 228-9). In excess, this can cause inflammation as well as interfere with fat loss. By contrast, EPA and DHA in fish oils cannot.

If you are overweight and insulin-resistant, it is very likely that your body has some difficulty making that conversion, possibly because you have (like most of us these days) favoured omega-6 fatty acids over omega-3s. In such a case your ability to handle fats may have become compromised, and fish oil will bring much better results.

Get Ultra Fresh

They key to good fish is to buy it fresh. Always ask the person serving you which fish is the freshest and what days of the week different kinds of fish arrive in the shop. You can tell a lot about the freshness of fish just by its smell and look. Really fresh fish does not smell like fish at all. It smells more like the salty bite of a sea breeze. If it's a whole fish you are looking at, pull back the gills. They should be bright red. The moment they go pale pink or grey you know the fish has been sitting in the shop too long. Try poking the flesh of the fish with your finger as well. If it springs back instead of forming an indentation then you're likely to have a piece of fresh fish on your hand. Check out the eye

203

of the fish. It should be dome-shaped and clear and not sunken and murky. Because I live a fair way from the centre of the city where I buy my fish, I always protect it when I buy in quantity by taking a chill-box with me. That way it stays ultra fresh until I can get it home, bag it and freeze whatever I am not going to use immediately.

Go For Organic Meat

The meats we get today are a far cry from those our paleolithic ancestors ate. Probably the closest you can get to those today is by buying wild boar, rabbit, buffalo, venison or kangaroo. These meats are higher in protein and lower in fat, which makes them healthier. Where a piece of meat from wild game boasts about 22g of protein in each 100g portion, domestic meat contains as little as 15 or 16g. Wild meat is also much lower in fat: on average, only 4g of fat in the same 100g portion compared with almost 30g in domesticated meat. The ordinary meat that you buy in the supermarket is six times as fatty and only about three-quarters as rich in protein as game meat. That being said, all organic red meats like beef and lamb are excellent sources of zinc, a mineral that's enormously important not only for insulin balance and weight loss but also for skin and the reproductive system. Free-range and organic meat is far better than factory farmed in every way, including the protection it offers from BSE.

Whatever meat you buy, always choose the leanest cuts you can find. Organic meats are guaranteed to be free of antibiotics, steroids, herbicides and pesticides. One exciting development in some countries such as the United States is that some farmers are beginning to feed their animals on foodstuffs rich in omega-3 fatty acids, so within a few years we may have meat available with a healthier fatty-acid profile than the meats we have today. (It may well cost a fortune too!)

The same is true of chicken feeds. In some countries you can now buy chickens that are labelled as having been fed with an omega-3-rich fishmeal or flaxseed. The eggs from these chickens have a much better ratio of omega-6 to omega-3 fatty acids. But it may take some time before this practice is widespread. In the meantime, choose eggs from free-range chickens or organically fed chickens which have open access to grubs and worms and greens.

When choosing dairy food, it is good to remember that butter, although it is not a source of essential fatty acids, is a perfectly respectable food – far better than any margarines, no matter how fancy or how sophisticated their formulation. When choosing other dairy foods, try to go low fat. Look for low-fat cottage cheese, ricotta, mascarpone and unsweetened yoghurt. Eat a bit of cream or sour cream as a special treat now and then. It will not interfere with weight loss but you don't want too much saturated fat. Stay away from flavoured cottage cheeses, yoghurts and other dairy products which are almost always chock-full of sugar or other kinds of sweeteners, as well as questionable flavourings.

Shop The Inner Circle

Once you leave the perimeters of your supermarket and move into the inner circle, you need to be particularly savvy about what you're buying. Read labels: check the fat and protein content as well as the carbohydrate content. Remember that the carbohydrate content listed for any food on its package includes the fibre. So if there is a fibre content listed on a food package, you need to subtract the fibre from the carbohydrate in order to determine the carbohydrate density of the food – how much 'usable carbohydrate' it contains (see pages 303-321). This is the only information you need for Ketogenics and Insulin Balance. Most of the products you find in the inner sanctum of the supermarket are made from junk fats, refined sugar, refined flour and partially hydrogenated oils. If you're in the market for low-carbohydrate whole-grain crackers, read each label carefully. If you don't find what you are looking for in the supermarket – crispbreads or crackers with less than 5g and preferably 2 or 3g of carbohydrate per cracker – then look in natural food emporiums or gourmet food shops where you are more likely to find them.

When you're buying nuts and seeds, go for raw nuts which have not been roasted using yet more oils rich in omega-6, and always store them in the refrigerator. As far as drinks are concerned, the best you can find is pure water. Buy it plain, sparkling or even flavoured, so long as there are no artificial sweeteners and no calories in the product (the calories will tell you whether or not fruit juice or a sweetener has been added). These days you can find a huge selection of good herbal teas, as well as organic green tea, which is better than black tea. Both green and black tea boast many antioxidants and can help lower glucose and triglyceride levels. Coffee with caffeine in it, by contrast, raises blood glucose and can interfere with insulin balance and weight loss. Therefore it is best avoided.

Secrets Of The Coconut

When it comes to sauces, you are probably better off making your own, although if you are a careful label reader you will probably find some that are no more than 3 or 4g carbohydrate per half cup serving. As far as oils are concerned, extra-virgin olive oil is best for salads. You can also use it for wok frying. Coconut fat is good for this too, and for searing meat or fish, since being a saturated fat it is very stable. But coconut oil has some other attributes to recommend it for fat loss. American biochemical researcher Ray Peat, who has spent his life focused on understanding the endocrine system, insists that coconut fat both supports thyroid function and activates metabolism. He says 'the anti-obesity effect of coconut oil is clear in all of the animal studies, and in my friends who eat it regularly...I have found that eating more coconut oil lowered my weight... and less caused it to increase.'

Peat's observation is echoed in the experience of livestock breeders. Back in the 1940s they tried to use coconut oil as a cheap method of fattening livestock. However, the opposite effect occurred. Adding the oil to their feedstuffs produced more active, leaner animals. Other animal research shows that feeding animals coconut oil regularly reduces their white fat stores – this is the kind of stored fat that you are trying to get rid of from your body – as well as lowering total and LDL cholesterol in people who have elevated cholesterol levels. This may be one of the reasons why many Pacific countries, who rely heavily on coconut oil for their cooking, experience little heart disease. Sri Lanka, for instance, where coconut oil is the main source of dietary fat, has the lowest death rate due to heart disease. Coconut oil is rich in a certain kind of fat known as medium chain triglyceride (MCT) which has been shown to reduce body fat, reverse arteriosclerosis, improve glucose metabolism, and even lower serum and liver cholesterol, while raising HDL, the good cholesterol. Coconut oil is the richest natural source of MCT – over 50 per cent of its fat is made up of MCTs.

Flavour Is Everything

When it comes to seasonings, on the X Factor Diet the more the better. I love fresh herbs best but when I can't get them I use a wide variety of dried herbs. Buy organic whenever you can, since herbs and spices in a supermarket are most often irradiated in order to give them a longer shelf life, and you want to avoid irradiated foods whenever possible. Irradiation can be a cover-up for spoilt food. As far as canned foods are concerned, most are not worth bothering with. The exception to these are vegetables such as water chestnuts and bamboo shoots, which you can only get canned, as well as water-packed tuna and water-packed anchovies and sardines, and sugar-free coconut cream, all of which can be useful. I often carry a tin of sardines with me in my handbag that I can open any time when I get stuck wanting something to eat and either don't have time to prepare anything, or can't find something nearby that is low carb and provides a good protein snack. There are a wide variety of other wonderful foods – from Indonesian fish sauce to Mexican chillis – that you may not be used to eating, most of which are available in natural food emporiums and really good delicatessens. Get to know them, experiment and see how many can make Ketogenics and Insulin Balance even more delicious and fun.

SWEET NOTHINGS

Following the X Factor Diet may mean saying goodbye to chocolate, honey and sugary cakes, biscuits and puddings, but it doesn't condemn you to a bitter future. Let's take a look at the alternatives to sugar.

Artificial Non-Intelligence

Many people on a low-carb diet tend to replace the sugar which they long for – at least in the beginning, before their bodies have made the metabolic shift – with one of the chemical artificial sweeteners: saccharin, cyclamate, acesulfame-K or aspartame. Don't. The artificial sweeteners we have become used to in our diet drinks, diabetic jams and 'sugar-free' foods are increasingly shown to be not particularly safe for long-term use. Many of them make blood sugar rise and encourage insulin resistance, thereby stimulating the pancreas to release yet more insulin. This is not what you are looking for.

Take saccharin. Three hundred times sweeter than sugar, saccharin, which is stable in liquids and in cooking, has been shown in animal studies to bring about a significant increase in the incidence of bladder tumours. Of course, the amount of the stuff fed to these animals was major, much more than we would consume ourselves in the daily course of drinking saccharin-sweetened drinks and eating saccharin-sweetened foods. But saccharin, like most of the artificial sweeteners, is an *excitotoxin*. This means it is a substance which causes metabolic shifts and can lead to neurological, mental and emotional shifts in some people which may be highly unpleasant and can distort their perceptions of reality. Never willing to accept anything unless I try it myself, I once, 30 years ago, experimented with saccharin and some of the other artificial sweeteners in sweetened drinks for a week. I found myself in the most extraordinary mental state. It made me understand why so many kids who live on diet-colas often feel so disconnected from reality. That was exactly the effect it had on me. Belgian researchers discovered that saccharin is one of the artificial sweeteners that stimulates the pancreas to release insulin. It can also interfere with fat loss and lower overall vitality. So – don't use it.

Chemical Accident

Most other artificial sweeteners are not much better. Cyclamate was discovered in the United States in 1937 when a technician laid his cigarette near a pile of powdery residue and found when he put it back into his mouth that it tasted sweet. Recent looks at the possible negative effects of this sweetener have raised questions about its potential for causing bladder and other cancers, as well as its safety over long-term use. Cyclamate was banned from the United States in 1970, but is still used in Britain and Canada as well as other countries throughout the world.

Aspartame, discovered by researchers at the pharmaceuticals company G.D. Searle & Co., while looking for a treatment for ulcers, is different in chemical composition from the others. It's a molecule created by putting together two amino acids. In effect, it's a tiny protein fragment that can enter the blood intact and be carried throughout the body. Some scientists believe this artificial molecule may even enter delicate areas of the brain by passing through the blood-brain barrier. Once there it may stimulate the brain abnormally, resulting in excitotoxicity, very much as MSG (monosodium glutamate), the food additive in cheap Chinese foods, does. Medical reports suggest that people who eat a lot of foods containing aspartame may end up with weird symptoms such as headaches, dizziness, loss of short-term memory, sleep disturbances and mood shifts.

I know this all seems enormously depressing if you use artificially sweetened foods and don't know how you are going give up. But the X Factor Diet is not just a means for losing weight. They are pathways to looking good and feeling great. You don't want anything to interfere with that. There are two things I suggest you look at as alternatives to sugar, honey, malt extracts and those artificial sweeteners.

Meet Sucralose

One is a new sweetener called sucralose. It is used more and more in proprietary foods and is now available in many countries. It sometimes comes in a sprinkle-on form called Splenda. This sweetener has been on the market in Canada for more than a decade. It is about 600 times sweeter than sugar and is derived from the sucrose molecule itself. What technicians have done is replace two of the parts of the sucrose molecules – the hydroxyl groups – with chlorine molecules. This manipulation of the sugar molecule not only enhances its sweetness dramatically, it also makes the sucrose molecule unrecognisable to your body's metabolic machinery. In other words, it is not broken down and absorbed as sugar is. So you perceive a sweet taste when you eat the stuff, but your body can't absorb it. This means that Splenda, unlike the other artificial sweeteners, doesn't cause the rise in blood sugar and insulin. Splenda is stable and works well in cooked food. You can measure it like sugar and it has no detectable aftertaste. It also contains no calories. So far, it is the most promising of artificial sugars.

I doubt very much that it is perfect, however. For if you are putting anything into the body which the body is unable to recognise, there is always the possibility that you may also not have the enzymes to be able efficiently to eliminate this foreign substance from the body with ease. The body's inability to eliminate foreign substances is what causes many of the side effects of drugs. Drugs tend to be unique molecules that the body does not handle well. In fact, drugs have to be unique molecules, as otherwise pharmaceuticals companies cannot patent them. At this point in time we have no idea what the possible long-term side effects of sucralose or Splenda are. So far, however, so good. It is unquestionably the best alternative if you decide to use an artificial sweetener.

Splenda is readily available on the supermarket shelves of most countries, it is found in the same area where you find baking products and sugar. In the United Kingdom however the Foods Standard Agency has been slow to grant approval of Sucralose in the UK. By the time this book is published it is likely to be making its way onto supermarket shelves.

Stevia – The Good One

A South American plant, *Stevia rebaudiana*, is incredibly sweet. Stevia has been used for generations, primarily as a sweetener. In its natural fresh or dried leaf form, stevia tastes from 10 to 15 times sweeter than common table sugar, or up to 300 times sweeter when you use it in extracted form. Extracts of stevia are relatively stable during heat processing. The plant has been used widely in Japan for decades. As far back as 1987, a total of 1700 metric tonnes of stevia leaves were harvested each year to yield almost 200 tonnes of stevioside extract. Before long, stevia took over more than half of the sweetener market in Japan. So it is hardly untested. In the United States, the FDA, in one of its many misguided attempts to 'protect' Americans, refused to make stevia legal. After many years of public pressure, however, stevia began to be allowed to be sold as a herb, not as a sweetener. This is still the situation in the United States.

Stevia is readily available in most other countries of the world including Canada, New Zealand and Australia. In the United Kingdom however it is not. The European Commission looked at an application for its use a couple of years ago. The EUC Scientific Committee for Food was presented with rather bogus data and concluded that a test tube derivative of stevia know as steviol 'might produce adverse affects in the male reproductive system and damage DNA'. The EC Standing Committee for Foodstuffs decided that stevia, the plants and dried leaves of *Stevia rebaudiana*, should not be approved 'due to lack of information supporting the safety of the product'. Since no adverse affects in people have ever been associated with stevia in its long history of use I am forced to conclude that yet another unjust attack on this natural non-caloric sweetener used for centuries in South America and for over a quarter of a century in Japan has taken place here. It is nothing less than another poorly thought out attempt to discredit a beneficial herb. Stevia poses no threat whatever to human health. It does, however, pose a potentially very big threat to corporate projects of companies producing artificial sweeteners. Thankfully stevia is easy to order by post for your own use in many different forms from the USA (see Resources).

Many Options

Stevia comes in many different forms. You can buy the plant and grow it yourself, then use the leaves, either fresh or dried if you like. You can buy the stevia leaves dried and powdered. They sweeten powerfully. And like cyclamate, saccharin and acesulfame-K, they can leave a bitter aftertaste if you use too much of them.

Each leaf of stevia contains phytochemicals called *stevioside* and *rabaudioside* – the sweet glycosides in stevia – as well as lots of other plant factors, vitamins and minerals. I use stevia leaves in all its forms, from fresh to ground powdered form, to extracts and powders for sweetening such things as hot drinks, shakes, smoothies and desserts. You can add dried stevia powder (10 to 20 times the sweetness of sugar) directly to your recipes, or you can make it into a syrup by dissolving a teaspoon into two cups of filtered water, bringing it to a boil, lowering the heat and simmering until it is reduced to a slightly thickened syrup. This you can store in the refrigerator in a small bottle for a week or two. (Be warned, however, that in this form it will turn anything you add it to a greenish colour.) For more serious cooking, most people prefer a water extract or even the white stevia or a clear liquid stevia extract. It is this white stevia powder that is mostly used in Japan. In contains from 85 to 95 per cent of the plant's sweet glycosides, which makes it almost 300 times as sweet as sugar. In Japan, you find powdered stevia in little packets on restaurant tables, served together with tea. The extracts and white powder have the least aftertaste. Researchers in Canada are currently working on a new extraction process which completely eliminates any aftertaste.

Dilute It

It is important to be aware that not all brands of stevia products that you buy from health food stores – which is where they are mostly available at the moment – are the same. Some stevia powders are so intensely sweet that I prefer to mix them with water and use them by the drop. Others have a flavour that I don't care for. So shop around. Stevia also comes in a dark liquid concentrate. You can make the concentrate yourself by putting a couple of cups of clean water in a saucepan and bringing it to a boil, and then reducing the heat to a simmer and adding half an ounce of crushed stevia leaves. Cover up and let simmer for three minutes, then remove the pot from the heat and allow the liquid to steep. Once cool, strain it though a cheesecloth and refrigerate in a covered container. This form of stevia has been used for generations for its medicinal effects. It has anti-bacterial and anti-fungal properties and is used to treat burns and wounds and internally to strengthen the pancreas. When sweetening any recipe with stevia it is important to experiment. Everyone has a different threshold for sweetness. Some people like things very sweet. I, for one, am put off by that, so when mixing up any recipe for a dessert or smoothie or anything else with stevia, put a little bit in and taste it to see if you want more. Remember – it is very sweet, so you have to go easy. You can always add more later. You will find that any recipe in this book that calls for sweetening either calls for stevia or sucralose (Splenda). Experiment and see what works best for you. Naturally, if you wish, you can substitute one of the artificial sweeteners for any of them, but if you do I would advise you to go easy. The diet that you are on works to help raise levels of well-being, and you don't want to interfere with that process by undermining any of its potential.

EAT OUT WITH SAVVY

You might think the X Factor Diet is going to make it well-nigh impossible to eat out. Not true. Navigating your way through restaurant menus is not as difficult as you would imagine. But once you walk through the front door and are making your way through the complex world of foods and snacks out there, there are a few tricks which can be really helpful. If you are in the habit of drinking a cup of coffee and munching biscuits at 11 am and 3 pm, that's easier to kick when you have had a good breakfast of, say, a protein drink, scrambled eggs or fish to hold you over. Or there's the ever-useful microfiltered whey protein. See 'Shaker Travel' on page 217 for how to use this instant snack.

Packable Protein

I carry a tin of sardines everywhere with me, just in case I get hungry in muffin and bagel land. This has occasionally caused me some embarrassing moments. I remember the first time I used my store of sardines. I opened them just before a university lecture. Since I didn't have a fork with me, I ate them with my fingers. Unfortunately, I had no place to wash my hands before entering the lecture hall. On my way up the steps I heard one of the girls in front of me commenting on the strange 'fishy' smell of the lecture theatre. I didn't have the courage to take credit for it. Since then, I have learned to carry a plastic fork with me and to wash my hands later. But sardines are a great snack to walk around with since they open easily and are pure protein as well as being rich in precious omega-3 fatty acids.

Check out the cafeteria at work to see if they have good low-carbohydrate foods. If not, take your lunch. The easiest way to do this is to cook a little extra the night before. Say you're having some roast lamb or chicken. In the morning you can pop some leftovers in a plastic container, add some sprouted beans or seeds with a little salt and curry powder and you have an instant lunch to carry with you. (I find salad dressings don't work well unless you are willing to carry them in a separate container and I can never be bothered.)

Great Restaurant Food

Unlike life on a slimming diet, a low-carb lifestyle is easy to follow if you need to eat a lot in restaurants, even on Ketogenics. That is, provided you don't enter a pizzeria (although see my exception on page 214). In restaurants, see if you can get friends dining with you to keep rolls and muffins to their side of the table. Don't be afraid to ask questions of the waiter. It is essential that you avoid most sauces, as so many are based on flour. Stay away from breadcrumbs or batter on any of your food, and other hidden extras too. Choose your main course from any kind of animal protein: fish, seafood, turkey, chicken, game, or lean red meat. Eat them grilled, baked, steamed, stewed, sautéed or poached and then go for two or three servings of vegetables and/or salad. There are some delicious possibilities. I think I have explored most of them, like salmon with a macadamia nut crust (watch that no flour has been added), grilled lobster, veal à la triestina, and even crispy duck, provided you make sure the chef has not added sugar to the glazing.

Remember that many vegetables raise glucose levels so quickly that you will need to avoid them completely on Ketogenics. These include baked potatoes, corn, peas, carrots and beetroot. On Insulin Balance, if you want to order vegetables that are high glycaemic and high density, you need to count one serving of them as two servings. Otherwise you are likely to push your carbohydrate levels too high. Certain vegetables are ideal, both for Ketogenics and Insulin Balance. Green beans, for instance, broccoli, cauliflower, a huge green salad (make sure there are no croûtons), asparagus, mushrooms, sprouted seeds and sprouted grains on Insulin Balance. The protein you eat should cover about one-third of your plate and the vegetables should take up at least two-thirds.

Ask Questions

Connect with your waiter. In any good restaurant this is easy. You need to explain to him that you do not eat carbohydrate foods. Ask him to check if the soup you are ordering as an appetiser has flour in it, or if the salad dressing has sugar in it. Naturally, he will have to go back to the chef to find out. A little trick I discovered years ago which is useful in a low-carb way of eating is this: people always take you seriously if you tell them that the *doctor* has put you on a specific regime for your health. In the case of low-carb eating, it can even be helpful to tell a white lie – namely, that you are diabetic and therefore you have to make absolutely sure that there is no sugar or flour in anything or other hidden carbohydrates in anything you are eating. The outside world takes whatever the 'doctor ordered' far more seriously than anything else.

The best restaurants for low-carb eating are invariably the *best* restaurants, in the sense that these restaurants cook their foods to order in contrast to fast food restaurants, where foods are all prepackaged and come whatever way they happen to be served. In a restaurant where foods are cooked to order, you can pretty much write your own ticket. You might have green beans or asparagus with a spinach side salad to go with sea bass steamed or grilled with a little butter and garlic, instead of served (as it states on the menu) smothered in a questionable sauce. Don't be afraid to ask for a 'doggy bag' to take any extra foods you don't eat in a restaurant home. These leftovers make wonderful snacks for the next day.

The toughest restaurants, apart from fast-food chains, are those that are known as 'health food' restaurants. This means their dishes are chock-full of low-fat-high-carb dishes riddled with flour, honey and raw sugar. If you get stuck in one of these it's generally best to go for a salad and see if they have some tofu you can eat with it. If you find yourself in a fast-food restaurant with no other choice (but I wouldn't get stuck here too often), here are some suggestions:

- At McDonalds, you might order a McGrilled Chicken Classic Sandwich and get rid of the bread.
- At Wendy's, you might order chilli or a grilled chicken sandwich, again throwing away the bread.
- At Burger King, you might go for a BK Broiler without the mayonnaise.
- In all of these cases, it's best to ask for whatever you are ordering without mayonnaise, as commercial mayonnaise is full of trans fats – aka junk fats – which you don't want to make part of your diet.

Italian – But Hold The Pasta

These are easy. I go for calamari (not battered) or an antipasto plate, followed perhaps by chicken piccata, veal cutlets, grilled fish or grilled chicken. I then order some sautéed or steamed vegetables, like courgettes, aubergine or perhaps capsicums sautéed in olive oil with lots of beautiful herbs. Avoid pasta dishes like the plague and remember that even a small piece of bread can contain more than 14g of carbohydrate.

But what about pizza? Believe it or not, provided you don't eat dairy products too often, and are not allergic to milk products, pizza is do-able. I have it about once a year. Order whatever pizza you like with as much topping as possible. When it comes, eat the topping and leave the crust.

Choose Indian

Not an easy task here since Indian dishes are a mixture of so many different kinds of food. This is one of the reasons it causes digestive disturbances for a lot of people. But it is do-able. I order tandoori lamb, chicken or beef or a lamb curry without the rice. I also like chicken tikka and chicken masala. I eat this with a cucumber salad perhaps, or some spinach with paneer (fresh Indian cheese). Steer clear of all dishes made with rice, wheat or potatoes.

The Chinese Way

Stir-fries are good so long as you make sure the chef leaves out the monosodium glutamate and any sugar. Chinese chefs have a way of putting sugar in just about everything. But a good stir-fry based on snow peas and ginger, bean sprouts, bamboo shoots and broccoli and green onions and garlic is great. Water chestnuts, bok choy, and Chinese cabbage are also great low-carb vegetables to be used in hot dishes or in a salad. Chinese restaurants usually have a beautiful steamed fish on the menu which is also worth ordering. What you want to be careful of are things like noodles, mu-shu pancake, egg rolls and anything deep-fried, since they tend to stuff their deep-fried foods with sweet and sour sauces and sugar.

Out Of Japan

I love eating in Japanese restaurants, first because I find the food is so good in general and secondly, because it is one of the easiest places in the world to get simple low-carb foods. Order sashimi if you like it. But make sure you are eating at a *good* restaurant and that the raw fish is very fresh. You can eat as much raw fish as you want and never even worry about getting out of ketosis if you are on Ketogenics. Most of the fish the Japanese serve are rich in omega-3 fatty acids. If you have any doubts about the fish being served in a restaurant, do not under any circumstances eat it raw. There is always a risk of parasite contamination. This makes me very careful about the Japanese restaurants I choose, particularly when in the northern hemisphere. In the southern hemisphere, the fish is often so fresh that I don't need to worry about it. Teppenyaki – Japanese flash-grilled meat or fish and vegetables – is an ideal dish on Ketogenics or Insulin Balance, but watch for sugar in sauces to go with it. So is teriyaki chicken, or beef and salad (again, ask that the sauce be made without any sugar), seaweed broth, miso soup and tofu. Stay away from tempura of any kind since it is breaded and fried.

In Old Mexico

Like Indian food, Mexican food tends to be a bit of a hodgepodge, most of it high carb. There are some excellent ways to go, however. You can order a tostada or taco salad, but don't eat the tortilla shell. Grilled fish, beef, pork medallions, chicken, as well as shredded beef, chicken and pork are great, served with a tossed salad. Mexican restaurants often have a good selection of fish served Vera Cruz style, foods with tomatoes, peppers and onions. I adore red snapper prepared this way. *Camarones al mojo-de ago*, which is a sautéed dish made from shrimps riddled with garlic, is another excellent low-carb main course. Stay away from high-fat cheeses and too much sour cream, and ask for a salsa or a guacamole made with olive oil on the side – since much guacamole tends to be made with cheap vegetable oils. Gaspacho is a great soup to start.

When In France

French restaurants are easy. You can always go for their gorgeous vegetables, spinach, cauliflower, asparagus and marrows, as well as grilled or poached fish or any kind of roasted game. Make sure that any of the sauces that the dishes come with in your main course are not made with flour (less and less are these days). Stay away from heavy cream sauces in particular. They often contain a lot of carbohydrate from the flour used to make them. Avoid French bread like the plague and shun potatoes and rice. Some of my favourite dishes in French restaurants are *poulet aux fines herbes* (roast chicken smothered in herbs), bouillabaisse (my absolute overall favourite since it is a fish soup with everything high in protein and omega-3s), steamed mussels and poached salmon. In French restaurants, stay away from glazed foods such as duck à la orange.

Going Greek

Souvlaki – skewered lamb, beef, chicken or shrimp kebabs with vegetables – is great. You can even get it in fast food shops, where it comes stuffed inside a piece of pita bread. I throw the pita bread away and eat the innards. What you have to be careful of in these restaurants are the pastries, breads and the pastas and of course the honey-based sauces that garnish so many Middle Eastern and Greek dishes. Their salads are wonderful, particularly those full of feta cheese with olive oil and red wine vinegar dressing. Tzatziki, the yogurt, mint and garlic mix they serve as a meze, is also delicious.

Come For Dinner

What worries low-carb initiates most is how to handle an invitation to come to someone else's house for dinner. I have looked at this issue from just about every angle and have come to the conclusion that the best approach is simply to tell the truth. After all, if you were diabetic and therefore restricted about what you eat, your hostess would have no problem with handling that information. What I do is suggest to my hostess that I bring a low-carb dish which I can eat, plus maybe a low-carb dessert that I and anyone else can eat if they happen to be interested. What I find is that more often than not, 30 per cent of the people at any dinner party are fascinated by a low-carb dessert made without sugar and want to sample it.

The problem is that you may get asked a lot of questions, and I, for one, hate answering anything more than a very few. What you can do is tell people what diet you are on, and recommend that they read the book themselves – 'It would be a little difficult for me to explain in detail right here.' It's easy to get over an explanation when you say that you are experimenting by putting into practice some of the wonderful research that's come out during the last 10 years and you are returning to a diet more in keeping with what our paleolithic ancestors ate. You just wanted to find out for yourself if it can enhance energy and good looks. Tell them you never believe anything unless you try it and so you have jumped in and are having a go. Tell them, too, how wonderfully understanding your hostess has been about your eccentric experiments. That usually does the trick and I have to report that I have certainly been invited back to dinner afterwards.

Food To Go

Airlines are still a big hassle. You would think that none of the catering directors of any of the airlines (despite their dozen or more 'special meals' including kosher, vegetarian, vegan and the lot) has ever heard of low-carb eating. Since I travel a great deal and many of my travels are long-haul flights, some of which take more than 24 hours, I plan this part of my life pretty carefully. If you are on a short flight, or the first leg of a long flight, you can always cook chicken breasts without the skin and put them into separate plastic containers, taking one out and eating it whenever you feel hungry. Some of the food on airlines of course you can eat. The simpler it is the better it is. Things like steamed fish and cheese are manageable. If you order a kosher meal in advance you are less likely to get some silly high-carb sauce poured over your fish or meat. Often you can explain to the cabin crew (if you are not sitting in business class or first class) that you are on a special diet, but unfortunately the airline was not able to help you with it. Then you can ask if it is possible for them to gather together some fish, meat, salads and other low-carb foods from the first class menu for you.

Shaker Travel

The other thing I do whenever I'm travelling, in airlines, in the car, or simply out for the day, is carry a plastic shaker and a couple of little plastic bags with me into which I put a good dose of microfiltered whey protein, plus some psyllium husks for fibre. Then all I need to do is pour clean water into the shaker, add my fibre/protein powder mix, shake it up and drink it. When stuck in a long meeting without food, I have even been known to go to the ladies room to mix up my drink. It also serves as a special back-up, so that I am not ever forced to eat food that I don't want. Whatever else happens, I know at the very least that microfiltered whey protein will carry me through to the next decent meal.

These are just suggestions to help you navigate your way into your own low-carb life. Everybody is different, of course. I would love to hear suggestions from you about what you do, that we can then share with other people. Do by all means e-mail me (see Resources page 339) and let me know of any inspirations you have come up with that can help others.

It's Easy

The truth is, once you get used to living low-carb, it becomes really easy to do. Only in the beginning do real adjustments need to take place. For we human beings are creatures of habit. Whatever habits we're following at the moment, whether they serve us in the highest possible way or not, they are always the ones we tend to fall back into. I find it takes about two weeks for someone beginning Ketogenics or Insulin Balance to adjust themselves to thinking ahead, and gain confidence about what to do in any circumstances. The most important thing of all low-carb living is just that – thinking ahead.

As I've said elsewhere in this book, I worked with a group of people recently on a television documentary on ageing. They were experimenting with a low-carb lifestyle – with fantastic results by the way – to lose weight, restore insulin balance and enhance overall health and good looks. The thing that every one of them found most challenging was simply organising themselves and their foods to start with. One member of the group was a film director, Danny Mulheron, who was used to getting on set by 6 am. He found himself getting up an hour early to do some weight training so that he could arrive on set on time, then taking aerobic walks late at night. He also organised his meals, since most of the crew meals on shoots are so appalling that just about nobody would want to eat them, whether they're on low-carb diets or not. What he did was cook an extra protein meal the night before, and take that in together with a lot of lovely salad vegetables that he could call on when mealtime came. He reported he had more energy, was less stressed and enjoyed life more than ever.

So like Danny and the other participants in the project, you'll probably find that the major challenge of switching to a low-carb lifestyle is simply one of organisation. Once you get organised, everything will run smoothly.

IF YOU'RE CRAVING

We eat, not just to live, but for the sheer pleasure of it. Whether or not you are on a low-carbohydrate diet, you're likely to get the odd craving for creamy or crunchy foods, for bread, potatoes, pasta, chocolate and ice cream. With Ketogenics, most of the fun solutions for cravings which follow do not apply. But once you are well into ketosis and burning fat well – provided you keep track of your ketone levels to make sure that you stay there – they work a treat. They are also excellent for anyone on Insulin Balance.

Crunchy Foods
My favourite foods have always been crunchy. I love to bite into a really crisp piece of toast or some corn chips. When you're in a crunchy mood, try these:

■ *Crunchy Potato Skins:* (see page 283).
■ *Spicy Nuts:* These make great appetisers and are loved by everybody. You can tuck a packet in your pocket and munch 25g or so whenever you want a good and delicious snack (see page 286-7).
■ *Pork Rinds:* They may seem like all fat, but they are actually just about all protein and you can eat as many as you want, even on Ketogenics, for they contain no carbs whatever. Look for them in delicatessens and specialist cookery shops. In some countries you can even find them on the road in petrol stations.
■ *Parmesan Wafers:* An Italian invention, these crispy wafers are irresistible. In Italy they are made with Montasio cheese, but I prefer to use Parmesan, not only because it's more readily available, but because it is more delicious (see page 286). As a savoury treat, they're hard to beat.

'Pizza'
As we saw in the last chapter, while eating pizza has become almost an international pastime, the conventional form does not work on a low-carb diet. There are some fun substitutes, however. You can grill aubergine slices, for instance, cover them with a low-carb pasta sauce, sprinkle on some fresh garlic and oregano, add a slice of mozzarella or ricotta and cook under the grill. It's not the real thing, but it sure tastes great.
■ *Portobello Pizza:* You can also make mini-pizzas by steeping giant Portobello

mushrooms in a little olive oil and cider vinegar with minced garlic and chilli powder and salt for 20 minutes, then grilling for 15 minutes. Cover with sauce and low-fat cheese and continue grilling until it melts. You can even use Portobello mushrooms prepared this way as bread substitutes for sandwiches. But after grilling you need to pop them into a 200°C oven for 15 minutes to dry them first.

Pasta

Occasionally you can find low-carb pastas but they're still grainy and not viable on Ketogenics. You can eat them occasionally when you're on Insulin Balance, however. But why not try one of these instead:

- *Spaghetti Squash with Pesto:* spaghetti squash is a member of the pumpkin family, but its flesh is unusual, naturally separating into long, spaghetti-like strands. These are a delicious alternative to wheat spaghetti. First cook the squash whole by baking for an hour in a medium-hot oven, after piercing it in a few places with a skewer; or by boiling it for 20 minutes. Cool the squash for half an hour, then cut it in half, scrape out and discard the seeds and, using a large fork, pull out the long strands of flesh. Serve while still hot with homemade pesto (see page 253-4).

- *Courgette Pasta:* using a mandolin, julienne courgettes lengthwise so you get long spaghetti-like strips. Parboil for 5 minutes or serve raw. Cover with a delicious low-carb sauce and serve.

- *Silverbeet Lasagne:* substitute silverbeet or cabbage leaves which have been boiled in water for half a minute, then dried. Use them in place of noodles. Layer with ricotta and a low-carb lasagne sauce and bake as usual.

Sweets

- *Low-carb Amaretti:* These delicious almond macaroons are a great favourite everywhere (see page 290).

- *Protein Fudge Treats:* Wonderfully low-carb, these sweet treats are a favourite of chocolate fanatics (see recipe page 291)

Creamy

Creamy foods are some of the most delicious. Happily, you don't have to do without them when you are eating low-carb. Here are some of my favourite solutions when I'm craving creamy.

- *Ice Cream:* Mix a good-flavoured protein powder together with mascarpone or full-fat ricotta cheese in a blender, then pour into an ice-cream maker or put into the freezer until chilled. Serve with a sauce of fresh berries, either unsweetened or sweetened with stevia or sucralose.

▓ *Avocados:* Nothing is more satisfying to a creamy-craving palate than dishes made with avocados. Mash them into a guacamole, make an avocado curry dip or stuff them with a creamy sauce – they are luxurious, satisfying and full of essential fatty acids (see page 257-8 for a great dip recipe)

▓ *Coconut:* Cans of unsweetened coconut cream are a must for turning a simple stir-fry into a delicious Thai curry, for making creamy drinks and even for ice cream (see pages 277-8 and 280 for ideas).

Bread

This is the biggest craving that most low-carb eaters experience in the beginning, probably because we have spent so much of our lives stuffing ourselves with bread. Sadly, most of the high-protein/low-carb breads are pretty tasteless. If you must have bread, look for 100 per cent rye bread and count the carbs carefully in each slice. Ryvita 100 per cent rye crackers are another option, in small quantities. Although low-carb diet cookbooks are full of ersatz bread recipes, most don't work very well. And because wheat is so high on the glycaemic index, for some people, even a taste or two is enough to set you off craving more – especially if you happen to be wheat-sensitive. It is my guess some 75 per cent of the population to some degree is wheat-sensitive. So bread is the one area that, if possible, it is best to avoid. But if bread is a must in your life, look for ultra-low-carb breads of almost any description and eat as little of them as possible.

Potatoes

Potatoes are the other big one in terms of the foods that we love to eat and hate to let go. The good news is, unlike bread, you can eat potatoes – as potato skins, crunchy (see above) or otherwise. And cauliflower makes a brilliant substitute for potatoes in many recipes.

▓ *Baked Potatoes:* Don't be scared of ordering them in a restaurant. Just clear out the white fluffy centre and eat the skin itself, seasoned and smothered in olive oil and crushed garlic, in butter or even in sour cream and chives if you must. They're delicious, carry most of the nutrients in potatoes, and can be very satisfying.

▓ *Mock Potato Salad:* (see page 250-1).

■ *Mashed Cauliflower:* This is actually so delicious, you might find it hard to believe you are not eating mashed potatoes. You can mash broccoli and pumpkin, too.

TROUBLESHOOTING

Every journey has its pleasures and its challenges, and the X Factor Diet is no exception. Along the way you may hit a plateau – a common experience when anyone is shedding fat. Or at some point you may need some extra help from specific nutrients or natural substances. And at the beginning of the programme you may find yourself craving carbohydrates. Here are some frequently asked questions complete with suggestions on how to handle difficulties when they arise.

Carb Cravings
Be patient. These are likely to be strongest during the first 48 hours of Ketogenics. If you are a real carb lover who adores chocolate, biscuits and cups of coffee, be gentle with yourself. It takes a while for your metabolism to switch over from relying on glucose from carbohydrate foods and caffeine for energy to getting it by burning fat stores. It also takes a little time for your enzymes to adjust themselves. Most people find that craving and hunger largely disappear within 48 hours. If your hunger does not disappear rapidly, there are two things that you can do. First, increase the number of fats that you are eating. Sear your meats and fish in coconut oil – an excellent saturated fat with protective properties which also encourages fat burning in the body. Add a little coconut fat or flaxseed oil to your protein drinks along with 1 to 2 teaspoons of ground psyllium husks – a good fibre which slows down the rate of absorption. Second, try taking some L-glutamine on an empty stomach. L-glutamine is a natural amino acid with no known side effects. It works best when taken on an empty stomach between meals or whenever cravings arise. You can buy it in powder form which you mix with water. It's deliciously sweet. Alternatively you can buy it in capsule form. It is available in most health food stores or can be ordered over the net.

Oops, I Blew It
Don't worry. Everybody falls off the low-carb wagon every now and then. Sometimes it is when you are particularly tired. At other times it's all about organisation – you may have forgotten to have at hand foods that you can eat.

What happens if you suddenly have a high-carb meal? You will find that your body retains water to deal with the carbohydrate load. In fact, it retains quite a lot of water. This is because carbohydrates encourage the kidneys to hold extra water and salt. Afterwards, you may feel slightly sluggish, tired and bad-humoured. You might even feel you are not thinking as clearly as usual, for a low-carb diet really sharpens the senses and mental clarity. The trouble with blowing it is that afterwards there is the temptation to keep on eating carbohydrate foods and make yourself feel miserable. I wouldn't. If you get stuck and find that you have eaten a single high-carb meal, you will do very little damage to the process of fat loss. The weight you gain right away is mainly water and by returning to Ketogenics you can lose it within a couple of days. So don't feel bad about yourself or waste time and energy being upset. Just get back onto Ketogenics, drink lots and lots of water and forget about it.

Bad Breath

A detox sign. Particularly at the start of Ketogenics, some people find they experience halitosis, or bad breath. This happens seldom and usually only occurs as your body is adjusting to a ketogenic way of eating. It is nothing more than an indication that your body is detoxifying itself through the lungs, as stored fat in your body is burnt. I like to use parsley oil capsules for this, or simply chew fresh mint leaves. Most of the proprietary breath fresheners are made from questionable chemicals which I wouldn't want to put into my mouth and I don't suggest you put in yours. Parsley oil capsules are different. They are derived from parsley itself. They work best when you take them just after a meal, but you can always pop one whenever you feel you need it. The amount of oil per capsule varies a lot from brand to brand, so it's best to follow the labels. Parsley oil capsules are available from a pharmacy or health food store. Breath sprays can also help – go for the natural ones, as the others are chemicals and you don't want to put them in your body. If you are going to use sugar-free gum, read the labels carefully, since sugar-free does not mean carbohydrate-free. Finally, drinking lots of water really helps neutralise bad breath. So does making sure that the measure on your ketone strips stays in the 'trace' to 'small' range.

I've Hit The Wall

Everybody does. Plateaus are always part and parcel of shedding fat from the body. Many people lose as much as 4lb a week for the first two or three weeks and then settle down to a steady ½ to 2lb a week for months. Then all at once, weight loss seems to stop. So far as I know, no one has ever been able to figure out the exact cause of plateauing. If it happens to you, there are many things you need to check out.

▧ **Are you *really* stuck?** It may be that your body is recomposing itself and you are continuing to shed fat although, at the same time, you are gaining muscle. Muscle – lean protein tissue in the body – is much heavier than fat. When you are gaining muscle your size becomes smaller but your weight on the scales won't change. So check out whether or not your size has shrunk before assuming that you are plateauing at all.

▓ **Take a look at how much energy you are burning.** The energy or calories that you need to maintain your weight can be figured by looking at three factors. 1. How much energy you expend. 2. The thermal effect of whatever exercise you get during the week. 3. The thermal effect of your foods. An easy way to estimate this is simply to multiply your body weight in pounds by 15.5 calories if you are a woman and 16 calories if you are a man. This will give you the level of calories needed to maintain your weight where it is right now. Don't get obsessed about calories, but it can be useful for the next three or four days to chart the number of calories you are eating and find out if by any chance you are eating more than your body actually needs to maintain its weight. If this is the case, you might want to reduce the number of calories you are eating to below the level needed to maintain your current weight.

▓ **Are you drinking coffee?** Even a little? Even decaf? As I've said elsewhere – stop. Every doctor I know who works with Ketogenics reports that coffee is the single most common block to fat burning. As yet no one is sure why – probably because it raises insulin levels. What few people know is that even decaffeinated coffee contains three per cent caffeine.

▓ **Are you on course?** One of the reasons why it is valuable to keep a journal on Ketogenics is so you can go back and carefully examine the exact number of carbohydrates that you are consuming at any particular time. This is important – don't guess at it. The remarkable transformation that Ketogenics brings about depends entirely on a metabolic process that occurs only when your carbohydrate levels are low enough to trigger ketosis. It is easy for any of us to find, without being aware of it, that our carbohydrate levels have gone up. Check out what you have been eating. A little piece of gingerbread can yield as much as 60g of carbohydrate, a banana 30g – not all that different from 60g of pure sugar, which yields 50g of carbs. If you are eating any of these foods every now and then, they are likely to trigger plenty of plateaus without your even being aware that it is happening. Make sure that you read labels carefully so that you are not getting any hidden carbs in the foods that you are eating. If necessary, buy yourself a little book to help you count the exact carbohydrates. Always subtract the amount of fibre from the carbohydrate count in order to get the significant level of usable carbohydrate in a food. This is all you need to concern yourself with. This process of record keeping and checking can be extremely tedious but it is very worthwhile – especially at first. For after two weeks of looking at every single food you will find that your awareness of how many carbohydrates are in everything has become acute. (And don't forget the kind of vinegar that you are using for your salads, or that piece of sugar-free chewing gum which although it may not have sugar in it, it still has carbs.) After two weeks, you will be pretty savvy about carbohydrates and much less likely inadvertently to allow more carbohydrate into your diet than your body can handle. Try cutting your carbohydrates way down to between 10 and 20g a day for three days to get things moving again.

▓ **Drink more water.** Simply increasing the amount of water you are drinking can help many people burn fat rapidly.

▓ **Check out food allergies.** For many people, Ketogenics seems to reduce dramatically any food sensitivities or food allergies. So if, say, you are allergic to milk, you can get away with a bowl of yoghurt every now and then with no after-effects. But if you are genuinely sensitive to a particular food that you're eating, this can halt fat loss. Try to identify what it is and cut it out of your diet. It is likely to be something that you find yourself craving.
We tend to be addicted to the foods that we are sensitive to.

▓ **Don't obsess over weighing yourself.** For years we have measured success in fat loss by weight on scales alone. As a result many people – especially women – weigh themselves every morning, horrified to find that they are half a pound heavier than they were the morning before. This is not only silly, since it focuses all the time on the fear that you will not be losing weight, but it is also not a very efficient way of measuring progress. Instead, try weighing yourself once a week. Measure your waist, your hips and your thighs. You are likely to be surprised to find that they are shrinking in size much more rapidly as you gain muscle mass and lose fat. The more muscle you make the more fat you will burn.

▓ **Check out drug interference.** Lots of drugs – including oestrogens used for hormone replacement and birth control – have an effect on the body's hormonal system. So to some degree they can counteract the processes set in force by Ketogenics. Steroid drugs can be big problem makers. So can non-steroidal anti-inflammatories, although to a lesser degree. Look out for oestrogens, ibuprofen, hormone replacement therapies, blood pressure medications and antidepressants. You must never stop the use of any drug without your doctor's guidance and knowledge. But it would be worthwhile talking to him or her should you hit a plateau on the X Factor Diet. You may find that the levels of the drug you are taking can be reduced. Otherwise settle yourself into being a little bit more patient about the weight loss. It will happen, but probably more slowly than otherwise.

▓ **Make sure you are eating enough.** If you are not eating enough this too can slow down your weight loss, for your body senses it is not getting enough calories and thinks it is starving. It therefore tries to preserve energy by slowing down your metabolism. Never be tempted to skip meals. It doesn't work for you. It actually works *against* you. Make sure you have protein snacks with you and – at least within the first month of Ketogenics – have three meals and two snacks a day. After that you can play it by ear. You will need three meals a day at the very least.

■ **Cut out artificial sweeteners.** A few people are extremely sensitive to the sweetness in artificial sweeteners. It can actually trigger the release of insulin, probably very much the way in which the bell triggered Pavlov's dogs to salivate. See page 209-11 for information on stevia, a natural alternative.

■ **Check your thyroid.** Read *Hyperthyroidism: The Unsuspected Illness* by Broda Barnes MD and Lawrence Gayton (Boston: Little, Brown, 1997). The best way to find out if your thyroid is functioning properly is using the basal temperature method developed by Barnes, a pioneer in the work of thyroid hormone research. Here's how:

Put a thermometer by the side of your bed before you go to sleep. For the next four days, before you get up in the morning, before you even stir, reach over and place the thermometer under your armpit for 10 minutes. If you are female, the best time to do this is day two, three, four, and five after the beginning of your period, since hormone shifts can affect the reading. If your temperature is below 98.2, this is considered low, and is taken as a sign of hyperthyroidism.

■ **Consider adding supplements.** Try 100mg of Co-Enzyme Q10 per day, 400mcg of chromium picolinate a day, and/or some L-carnitine, a nutrient which carries the fatty acids to the mitochondria in cells to be burned off. Too much insulin interferes with this process. This is why L-carnitine, amongst other things, works well on a low-carb diet where the insulin levels are lower. In addition to promoting fat burning in the body, L-carnitine enhances brain function and boosts the immune system, lowers cholesterol and triglyceride levels and relieves PMS. Robert Crayhorn, author of *The Carnitine Miracle* (New York: M.Evans & Co., 1998), says that our paleolithic ancestors probably got 500 to 2000mg of carnitine a day, whereas we get very little because of the way the animal products we eat have changed in their consistency. Crayhorn believes that obesity itself is nearly always a functional carnitine deficiency. He recommends taking 1000 to 4000mg of L-carnitine a day, in two doses before breakfast and lunch, together with either flaxseed oil or a supplement of omega-3 fish oil. You can buy carnitine in two forms – L-carnitine, which is the natural form, and a less expensive form which works perfectly well. You can also buy acetyl-L-carnitine. This is a great deal more expensive. It stimulates the release of acetylcholine – a neurotransmitter useful for enhancing learning and memory. Unless you are concerned about this, ordinary L-carnitine is a perfectly effective form to help with fat burning. It should not be taken in the late afternoon or evening as it does enhance energy in the body and might therefore, in some people, interfere with sleep.

▓ **Add more omega-3s.** Literally hundreds of studies have been done which demonstrate how powerful an effect fish oils rich in omega-3 fatty acids can exert on insulin resistance, obesity, cardiovascular health, glucose intolerance, Type II diabetes, auto-immune conditions and chronic inflammatory diseases. Most of us are deficient in omega-3 fats and get far too many omega-6 fats, which come primarily from vegetable oils. If the balance of omega-3 to omega-6 in your body is not good (it should be 1:1 or 1:2 omega-3 to omega-6, whereas people on a Western diet get a balance of 1:22), then your weight loss can be impeded. For many people, flaxseed oil rich in omega-3 fatty acids can help. Studies show that flaxseed oil has a protective effect against cardiovascular disease similar to that of fish oil. It's also delicious and has a buttery taste. You must never heat it, but you can pour it over steamed vegetables and use it as a salad dressing. You have to be very careful with flaxseed oil, as with the fish oil omega-3s, since it easily oxidizes and becomes rancid. It should always be bought from a shop where it is kept in the refrigerator with a sell-by date of no more than two months ahead, and you must always keep it in the refrigerator once you get it home. Check the taste as well as the sell-by date. If there is an acrid bite to the back centre of your tongue, the oil is rancid – throw it away. The difference between the omega-3s in flaxseed oil and those in fish oil is that the former are shorter-chain fatty acids that can be changed in the body to arachidonic acid (more about this in a minute), unlike the longer-chain omega-3s in fish oil, EPA and DHA. So some people who are sensitive to arachidonic acid should stick to fish oils. Fish oil with EPA and DHA is expensive (they too need to be kept refrigerated at all times) and in buying them you generally get what you pay for. Try adding a couple of extra teaspoons of flaxseed oil to your meals each day, or eat more fish and also take three to four 1000mg omega-3 fish oil capsules a day.

▓ **Are you arachidonic-acid sensitive?** Arachidonic acid (AA) is a long-chain unsaturated fatty acid – a principal fat of the omega-6 family found in the brain. In a developing foetus, arachidonic acid is taken from the mother to encourage brain development and then continues to be supplied to the child through the mother's breast milk. After that, arachidonic acid appears to be no longer important in the body for health. It is found in chicken, turkey, beef and pork, and also to some degree in peanuts, cod-liver oil and a few species of seaweed and algae. For most people, arachidonic acid causes no problems. In fact, we can make our own from linoleic acid. For others it can not only block fat loss but also help create inflammation in the body. Here's how. Arachidonic acid is a precursor to many highly inflammatory substances including prostaglandin E2, leukotrine, prostacyclin and thromboxane A2. These in turn can produce pain, swelling and inflammation in the body, causing symptoms such as arthritic and rheumatic pains as well as a sense that you are infected with a virus or bacteria when in fact no infection is present. Because the levels of omega-3 fatty acids to omega-6 fatty acids in the Western diet have become so askew, there are some people who tend to produce too much arachidonic acid.

SENSITIVE TO ARACHIDONIC ACID?

The main symptoms associated with too much AA (or sensitivity to it) are:

- Chronic fatigue
- Trouble sleeping
- Difficulty awakening or grogginess upon awakening
- Split ends or unhealthy hair
- Thin or brittle nails
- Constipation
- Dry, flaking skin
- Minor rashes.

If you find yourself plateauing, try dropping red meat and eggs from your diet and see what happens. You can also take fish oil rich in EPA and DHA as recommended above, which will help prevent excessive arachidonic acid from accumulating in the tissues. In fact, many doctors trained in functional medicine give these omega-3s therapeutically as a way of reducing arachidonic acid in the body. If you find any sort of inflammation or aches and pains seem to go along with your plateauing, you might like to try making some of these changes and see if weight loss resumes within a few days.

Digestive Problems
The X Factor Diet is likely to correct them for you. But here are some of the common causes of trouble.

WHAT CAUSES DIGESTIVE TROUBLES

- Eating too much
- Eating before the previous meal is completely digested
- Drinking iced drinks often (especially before or during meals)
- Too much alcohol
- Eating 'on the run'
- Eating at irregular times
- Eating heavy meals at night
- Infections from yeasts or parasites or bacteria
- Dysiosis (low levels of Lactobacillus acidophilus and Bifidobacteria adolescentis)
- Food allergies or sensitivities
- Nutrient deficiencies (eg. zinc, iron, vitaminA)
- Low stomach acid
- On-going physical, emotional or mental stress
- Medications:
  Antibiotics (even when used for as little as one day)
  Non-Steroidal Anti-Inflammatory Drugs (NSAIDs)
- Low-protein diet
- Increased demand for protein owing to:
  Trauma
  Surgery
  Excessive exercise
  Illness
  Fasting
- Too little fibre

PART FIVE:
SHEER
PLEASURES

BOUNTIFUL BREAKFASTS

In the beginning, when switching over from conventional eating to low carbs, breakfast is a big challenge. I guess it's partly because we get set in our ways. Most have come to think of breakfast as a natural high-carb meal – a glass of fresh orange juice, a muffin, packaged muesli – or worst of all – one of those highly refined packaged cereals every kid in American movies pours into a bowl before dashing out to school. Not to mention muffins, bagels, pancakes and all those gooey jams and syrups we get used to spreading on them.

New Ways

It is mostly our passion for high-carb breakfasts which has us reaching for another sticky bun or cup of coffee mid-morning to keep going. Unless you happen to be a long distance cyclist setting out on a 70-mile cycle for the day, a high-carb breakfast raises blood sugar far too high and causes insulin imbalances.

It is time to take a breath and open wide the doors of possibility. You might be surprised at just how simple and delicious it can be to make a great morning meal. I'm not into breakfasts which take a long time to prepare. There are more interesting things to do at the beginning of the day. That's why this section is full of easy to make but delicious ideas for everything from breakfasts on the run where you grab a tub of low-fat cottage cheese or toss a few things into the blender to produce a smoothie, to instant omelettes and low-carb pancakes. My mother had an attitude towards breakfasts that I used to think kind of weird. Now I've come to embrace it fully. She could never figure out why anybody wanted to eat conventional foods at breakfast time. Her idea of a delicious breakfast was some spicy Italian dish or left-over bouillabaisse from the night before. I've recently taken to heart her fascination with unusual breakfasts. I find myself preparing a salad rich in phyto-nutrients, based on sprouted seeds and grains. I crush a clove of garlic, and chop some rocket or radicchio, then add some cubes of left-over chicken or fish cooked the day before. If I am really in a hurry, I toss it all into a square plastic container, pour on the olive oil, squeeze some lemon juice, season with a dash of Worcester sauce, salt and pepper. Then I put the lid on and give it a toss within the container. I either eat it immediately or take it with me wherever I am going. When my 20-year-old son Aaron saw me doing this recently he found it curious but one morning thought he'd try it. Like me, he found these strange breakfasts so refreshing and uplifting – not to mention that it takes you through the whole morning without being hungry – that he has since begun making them himself. But let's look at more conventional fare. Here are some of my favourite breakfasts:

Quick Shake
Serves 1

If you like chocolate, this is one of the fastest recipes I know for breakfast. I use it often. Because it is so low in carbohydrate (this does depend somewhat on which brand of whey protein powder you are using) it gives you the best quality protein breakfast yet leaves you a lot of carbs to play with. This means you can add a handful of berries to add flavour and texture. You can also make it with vanilla-flavoured powder or any other flavoured whey.

What You Need
1-4 scoops of mircrofiltered whey protein or whey protein isolate powder – enough scoops to yield 20-30g of protein
1 tsp flaxseed oil
250 ml (8 fl oz) cold water
2 tbsp unsweetened organic cocoa
3 ice cubes
1-2 heaped tsp ground psyllium husks (optional)
artificial sweetener to taste (optional)

Here's How
Pour all ingredients into a blender or food processor. Blend until smooth. Serve immediately.

Protein 20-30g
Usable carbohydrate 1-7g (depending upon the protein powder you are using, so do read labels)

Vanilla Nutmeg Smoothie
Serves 1

This breakfast in an instant is based on the traditional egg-nog that people used to drink at Christmas. In fact the egg is optional, you can make it with or without. If you decide to put the egg in – I like to do this because it gives more flavour – make sure your egg is free-range or organic. You don't want to mess around with battery-laid eggs eaten raw. There is always the danger of salmonella.

What You Need
200 ml (6½ fl oz) cold filtered or spring water
6 ice cubes
1-2 scoops of natural or vanilla-flavoured microfiltered whey protein or whey
    protein isolate powder – enough scoops to yield 30 grams of protein
1 egg (optional)
1 tsp vanilla essence or several drops of natural vanilla oil
a pinch of freshly grated nutmeg to taste
artificial sweetener to taste
1 heaped tsp psyllium husks (optional)
1 tbsp flax seeds (optional)

Here's How
Place all the ingredients in a blender and blend vigorously until combined. Be careful not to blend more than 20 seconds, however, since this can change the nature of the microfiltered whey protein. Sprinkle a little extra grated nutmeg on top and serve immediately.

Protein 38g
Usable carbohydrate 3g

Berry Bliss Smoothie
Serves 1

What You Need
50g (2oz) fresh or frozen raspberries, strawberries, blackberries, loganberries
    or a mixture
1½ tbsp cold filtered or spring water
2-3 scoops microfiltered whey protein or whey protein isolate powder to yield
    30g
artificial sweetener to taste
2 tbsp flax seeds (optional)
3 ice cubes (optional)
tsp lemon zest (optional)

Here's How
Put all ingredients into a blender and blend well but not more than 20 seconds. You can add more or less water if you want a slightly thicker or thinner shake. Serve immediately.

Protein 32g
Usable carbohydrate 10g

Sweet Nothing Soufflé
Serves 2

Soufflés usually take a long time to make and are a lot of trouble. This one is virtually instantaneous if you are using a microwave and is just as much fun for breakfast as it is as a sweet at the end of a meal.

What You Need
6 egg whites
1 tbsp vanilla protein powder
3 egg yolks
3 tbsp shredded unsweetened coconut
artificial sweetener to taste (optional)
pinch of ground cinnamon

Here's How
Put your egg whites in a mixing bowl and beat until thick peaks form. In a separate bowl, mix together egg yolks and protein powder, beating until they are smooth. Gently add the egg yolk mix to the beaten egg whites, at the same time folding in the shredded coconut. Pour into a soufflé dish or two individual ramekins and pop into a medium heat microwave for about three minutes, until the soufflé rises and peaks on top. Be careful not to overcook this soufflé, otherwise it will lose its fine texture. Add the artificial sweetener if you want a sweet soufflé. I personally find that this soufflé is sweet enough without any extra sweetening. Sprinkle with cinnamon and serve immediately.

Protein 30g per serving
Usable carbohydrate 1g per serving

Omelette On The Run
Serves 1

I don't know why people make such a palaver out of making an omelette. It's about the easiest thing in the world. I learned this from Paul, the father of my youngest son who turned out omelettes to die for in less than two or three minutes. The key is having the right pan to cook it in. Years ago I bought myself a French crêpe pan – a cast iron flat round pan which is about the best thing in the world for omelette making. You can make this omelette either with whole eggs, or with one whole egg and 3 egg whites, depending upon how fluffy you like to go. I make mine with whole eggs.

Eat it on its own, or fill it with grated cheese, salsa or simply chopped garlic, tomatoes, onions and green peppers. This way it turns into what I call a salad omelette, namely an omelette full of beautiful fresh crunchy vegetables. You can even fill it with left-overs from the day before.

What You Need
1–2 tsp of extra virgin olive oil
50g (2 oz) left-over ham or chicken, finely chopped
1 medium tomato
2 cloves crushed garlic
½ green or red capsicum
1 whole egg plus 3 egg whites beaten until light and fluffy or alternatively, 2
    whole eggs
1 tbsp grated cheese, eg. Parmesan, ricotta, mozzarella (optional)
cracked pepper to taste
dash of Cajun seasoning
Maldon sea salt to taste

Here's How
Oil the pan and sauté the stuffing ingredients – ham, chicken, tomatoes, garlic, what have you – until they are warmed through. Pour the egg mixture over the top. Let it set, using a spatula to tilt the liquid egg to the edges of the pan. After it has set completely, sprinkle the surface with cheese (if you are using cheese) and fold in half. Cover with cracked pepper and Cajun seasoning and serve immediately. If you are making a stuffing-free omelette, then simply pour your eggs directly into the pan once the oil has heated. Use a spatula to tilt the liquid egg to the edges of the pan. When almost set, roll up and serve sprinkled with Maldon sea salt and other seasoning.

Protein 28g
Usable carbohydrate 5g

Phyto-Nutrient Eggs
Serves 1

This is a recipe I make from low density low glycaemic carbohydrates that I've cooked the night before. Spinach works well, so does kale, Chinese leaves or just about any other leafy green vegetable except lettuce, which doesn't work at all. You can make this for one person or for many, depending upon how much vegetable you have left over. You will need 60–120g or a bit more per serving. Amounts here are for one serving which you can pour into an individual ramekin. If you want to make more than one serving at a time, either use more individual ramekins or do as I do, make it in a non-stick ceramic loaf pan. I like to squeeze a little lemon on the green vegetables. Here are the ingredients that you'll need for each serving.

What You Need
2 tsp extra virgin olive oil or butter
60-120 g (2½-4 oz) of leafy green vegetables eg. spinach, kale, Chinese leaves
    etc. squeezed dry
2 large eggs
Maldon sea salt to taste
black pepper to taste
1 tbsp grated Parmesan cheese (optional)
1 tbsp chopped parsley (optional)

Here's How
Preheat the oven to 160°C (325°F) Gas 3. Butter the ramekin or loaf pan and then lay the cooked vegetables on top and pop into the oven to heat through. Break your eggs into a small bowl, then slide them into the ramekin. Season with salt, pepper and herbs and sprinkle the cheese on top. Then pop back into the oven, covering lightly with a layer of aluminium foil and let cook for 5-6 minutes. The whites will go firm. The yolks may look underdone still but don't worry, by the time you get them to the table the heat from the ramekin will finish the job.

Protein 22g
Usable carbohydrate 0g

Light As Air Pancakes
Serves 2

This is a recipe I developed for my family long before I was aware of low-carb eating. I used to make masses of it on Sunday morning. My kids loved them. It makes very light and fluffy pancakes rather like pancake soufflés. They need to be eaten immediately for it is the egg white that gives them their fluff and that very quickly gets lost once they have been cooked. They can be served with a delicious strawberry or blueberry syrup, some butter or some low-carb jam.

What You Need
4 eggs
100 g (3½ oz) creamed cottage cheese
2 tbsp soda water

30 g (1 oz) soya flour
pinch of Maldon sea salt
½ tsp baking powder
1-2 tbsp coconut oil
artificial sweetener to taste

Here's How
Separate the eggs and beat the whites until almost stiff. In another bowl,
combine the egg yolks with the cottage cheese, soda water, soya flour, salt and
baking powder. Blend thoroughly. Gently fold in the egg whites. Heat coconut
oil in a frying pan or crêpe pan. Pour out individual dollops of the mixture.
Cook until the underside turns a light golden brown. Flip each pancake only
once. Take off the heat. Serve immediately topped with a dollop of artificially
sweetened plum spread or butter and some low-carb berry syrup or low-carb
jam.

Protein 24g per serving
Usable carbohydrate 2g per serving

Scrambled Tofu
Serves 1

*Lighter and more delicate in texture than scrambled eggs, tofu works well for
breakfast provided you season it richly, for tofu has almost no flavour of its own.
If you add a pinch of turmeric, you will create a 'vegan scrambled egg' in a rich
yellow colour just like the real thing.*

What You Need
1 tbsp extra virgin olive oil
2 spring onions, chopped fine
2 cloves of garlic, crushed or chopped
200g (7oz) tofu
pinch of turmeric (optional)
Maldon sea salt to taste
fresh ground black pepper to taste
Mexican chilli powder to taste
½ tsp curry powder
½ tsp cumin powder
4 tbsp grated Parmesan cheese (optional)

Here's How

Heat the oil in a heavy frying pan and sauté the spring onions and garlic until they are soft (2–3 minutes). Mash the tofu then stir it into the pan with the turmeric. Add your other seasonings and any other herbs you want to add. Cook over high heat, turning frequently until tofu goes firm. This takes about 2 or 3 minutes. Sprinkle on the cheese if you are using it. Season with salt and pepper and serve immediately.

Protein 40g
Usable carbohydrate 4.5g

Blueberry Curds And Whey

Serves 1

This is an old-fashioned recipe, just about as old-fashioned as you can get, but with a new twist: it is enriched with microfiltered whey protein and almonds. You can substitute walnuts, pecans, or even macadamias if you prefer to make a highly satisfying one-bowl meal that is refreshing, sweet and delicious. You can also add 1 teaspoon of flaxseed oil for extra omega-3 support.

What You Need

1 tbsp chopped almonds or other nuts that have been toasted over a high
   heat in a dry frying pan
100 g (3½ oz) creamed cottage cheese
1-2 scoops of whey protein (enough to yield 20g of protein)
artificial sweetener to taste
1 tsp flaxseed oil (optional)
50 g (2 oz) fresh blueberries, strawberries or raspberries

Here's How

Chop and toast your nuts beforehand. Store toasted nuts in a refrigerator for use in this recipe or any other recipe where you want to use them as a topping or a crust. (Toasted chopped nuts will keep for 2-3 weeks in a fridge.) Using a food processor or a hand blender mix all ingredients except nuts and berries together with creamed cottage cheese. Fold in the sliced berries. Sprinkle with the toasted nuts and serve immediately.

Protein 35g
Usable carbohydrate 14.5g

Raspberry Syrup
Serves 4

This you can make with blueberries, strawberries, loganberries or blackberries – whatever happens to be in season. It's great on pancakes or cottage cheese for breakfast or over mascarpone as a dessert or snack.

What You Need
225 g (8 oz) raspberries or other berries
125 ml (4 fl oz) filtered or spring water
1 tsp grated orange or lime zest
artificial sweetener to taste
a pinch of nutmeg

Here's How
Bring the berries with a little water to the boil and gently simmer over a low heat. Add the other ingredients and cook very gently until the syrup thickens slightly. Then remove from the heat. Either you can put this syrup into a blender to purée it or you can leave it chunky and serve it as is. The syrup will keep well in a fridge for a week.

Protein 0g per serving
Usable carbohydrate 4.5g per serving

Blueberry Jam
Serves 16

This is another method for delicious low-carb jam which you can make with blueberries, blackberries, loganberries, raspberries, strawberries or wild strawberries. You don't have to have the fresh berries, you can use frozen ones instead.

What You Need
juice of 1 lemon
500 ml (17 fl oz) filtered or spring water
450 g (1 lb) berries, washed and sliced
artificial sweetener to taste
1 sachet unflavoured gelatin

Here's How
Put the lemon juice, water, berries and sweetener into a non-stick saucepan and simmer over a medium heat until the berries soften. This usually takes about five minutes. Pour the hot liquid through a strainer into a food processor or blender. Place the strained berries in a glass jar. Empty the gelatin sachet into the blender and pulse blend until the gelatin dissolves completely. Pour this mixture over the berries in the glass jar. Cover and refrigerate. This recipe, which makes 16 servings – about half a litre (or nearly a pint) – will keep for up to two weeks.

Protein 0g per serving
Usable carbohydrates 2g per serving

Hand-Made Sausage
Serves 4

I adore sausage. Yet the sausages that you buy are full of all sorts of artificial flavouring and colourings, not to mention carbohydrate 'stuffers' which you don't want to eat. This is an old-fashioned pattie sausage which you can vary, depending upon your taste, and what herbs and meats you have available. You can make it with pork, venison, chicken, lamb, beef or wild boar. I mix the ingredients together the night before, then put them in the fridge to chill and absorb all flavours. Eat within three days.

What You Need
350 g (12 oz) lean minced pork, chicken, lamb, beef, venison or wild boar
1 tsp Maldon sea salt
2 tbsp oat bran
4 cloves of garlic (optional)
2 tbsp chopped fresh parsley, coriander or sage
½ large onion chopped fine

Here's How
Combine all your ingredients in a big mixing bowl and mix thoroughly with your hands. Refrigerate until well chilled, then separate into four patties and cook in an oiled pan until crunchy on the surface and cooked through.

Protein 23g per serving
Usable carbohydrate 0.5g per serving

CRUNCHY FEASTS

The quickest and easiest way to get a phyto-chemical-rich diet is to eat a delicious nutrient-dense salad a couple of times a day, complete with lots of top quality protein. Forget the limp lettuce leaves and tomato fare. I'm talking green mesclun and bright flowers, wild herbs, fennel, rocket, ruccola, colourful Swiss chard, almonds and bright peppers, as well as vegetables that most people don't even think to put into a salad, cauliflower and broccoli, for instance. These vibrant gifts of nature are chock full of phyto-nutrients to protect you from premature ageing, detoxify your body and energise your life.

Preparing a gorgeous salad is more an art than a science. For me it is like meditation. I set aside ten minutes as a break from my busy work life to see what I can create from the freshest ingredients I happen to have in my fridge or in my garden. Often people say to me, 'I'd love to eat more salads but I don't have time.' I know they still have a lot to learn about how easy and quick salads are to make. I can make a protein-rich salad that is a whole meal for four people and have it on the table in ten minutes. Even better than popping something in the microwave. It's all about knowing how.

Shop For Beauty

Great salads start at the shopping stage. Buy what's most beautiful. Forget the rest. Bring home your vegetables, wash and dry them thoroughly. Put them in the vegetable tray in the refrigerator. When you shop once or twice a week for fresh vegetables, do this as soon as you get home, then you are all set for instant salad meals. The key to keeping your vegetables fresh for a whole week once they've been washed is always to store them in the plastic trays in the fridge and cover with big plastic bin-liner bags. This keeps things fresh and crisp for so long it always surprises me. When it comes to fresh herbs, such as basil, parsley and coriander, I place them in a bowl full of cold water in the refrigerator. This way they too will last a week.

It is important to have all your vegetables ready to use, for preparation is what takes all the time. Then when you come into the kitchen you can simply pull out two, three or four trays full of lovely bright-coloured, fresh foods and dive into salad making. I love working with whatever is there. You can make a fabulous salad from a bunch of rocket with some gorgeous black olives, and fresh slivers of Parmesan cheese. Delicious and nutrient-rich salads are especially easy to make. Use shredded raw broccoli and cauliflower, red and yellow capsicums, chopped red onion, and slivers of Chinese leaves, smothered in a creamy home-made mayonnaise made with extra virgin olive oil or an irresistible curried avocado dressing.

Mandolin Magic

The one piece of kitchen equipment I never want to be without is a mandolin. These remarkable vegetable shredders are so different from the usual graters you find in most stores. The tiny knives they contain make perfect slices of whatever vegetable you like. Stainless steel mandolins are not only expensive, they are virtually useless. The best are cheap and made from plastic. They have a V-shaped blade, into which plastic inserts fit, each of which has different size knives. You can julienne, make chip-size chunks, slice thin or thick. Unlike the conventional grater which mashes vegetables and fruits, a mandolin slices them clean and sharp. Be sure to use the hand protector device which comes with every model. If you don't – and I know this from bloody experience – what you end up with is shredded fingers instead of shredded cabbage.

I try to mix between two and five vegetables together to make a salad. Not only do I combine varieties of vegetables, I also mix textures, using fine julienned celeriac, for instance, together with a coarsely grated red cabbage, plus slivered spring onions. It's the mixture of colours and textures that makes it all work. Let your imagination take over. Feel and taste the ingredients you are using. Treat the whole process of salad making as you would that of painting a picture or making a sculpture. Have fun. Make it a delightful experience and you can't miss.

Phyto-nutrient Delight

Any salad can be chock full of all of the flavonoids, carotenoids and sulforaphanes – the phyto-nutrients that offer the best you can get for high level health as well as protection against premature ageing. Sounds like it should be a salad that tastes bad, but which you eat knowing that it's going to do you good? Just the opposite is true. For a long time I was troubled by how to make salads tasty when using vegetables which are particularly rich in phyto-nutrients like broccoli and cauliflower. Then I discovered the way to do this: simply shred them very very fine using a mandolin, so that you get small crunchy pieces. This adds texture and richness, while giving your salad great nutrient density. At first when I began experimenting with this, I thought that no-one but me would eat my offerings. I soon discovered otherwise. My friends love them – especially when they are tossed with a rich home-made mayonnaise or avocado dressing. Now I grate broccoli and cauliflower into many of the salads I make day after day.

Lazy Cook

Lazy about salad dressings, I usually make my salad in a large flat bowl. Then, instead of mixing the salad dressing separately, I dress the salad right then and there. A few tablespoons of extra virgin olive oil, some chopped fresh herbs, crushed raw garlic, a dash of Worcester sauce, some Maldon sea salt, the juice of a lemon or a couple of tablespoons of wine vinegar or balsamic vinegar, some home-made Cajun seasoning from the fridge or a dash of the powdered variety from the market. To top it off I use some freshly ground course black pepper. I like to grind peppercorns with a mortar and pestle because it tastes so much better that way. I sprinkle this all on top and toss. Ready in an instant. Sometimes I top off salads with seeds, like pumpkin, sesame or sunflower. Others, I scatter with chopped fresh garlic or shredded wild garlic leaves when they are growing down the path near where I live. When they are to be found in the garden, I even add some fresh edible flowers like marigold petals or heartsease.

Go With What You've Got

Of course you need none of these things to turn a simple salad into a masterpiece. What you do need is a child's sense of experimentation, plus plenty of love. For it is that ingredient which makes every meal a joy: not just what you make matters and how you make it that matters, but it's also your attitude to what you are doing in the kitchen. Years ago in India I discovered that the best foods are those you buy in the cheapest cafés. They have been made with love and joy, sometimes with humour too. The word café is really a euphemism for these places which are often little more than a few stones within which a fire has been built for cooking. Yet the foods they sell are infinitely better tasting, more nourishing and safer – less likely to cause Delhi Belly – than all the fancy foods you can get in expensive restaurants. It doesn't matter how skilful or how knowledgeable and important a cook is, if he doesn't invest the food he gives you with affection, then it's dead food, not energy food. This affection cannot be faked or disguised. Have fun, experiment with the energy and colour of living foods. You can't help but create something wonderful and infinitely nourishing. Here are a few of my own suggestions to help inspire you:

Caesar Salad With Hard-boiled Croûtons
Serves 2

When it comes to low-carbs, croûtons can be killers but there are alternatives. You can use rashers of lean organic bacon, diced and fried crisp, then drained on a kitchen paper towel. My preference is a couple of hard-boiled eggs. The good thing about the bacon is it gives that crunchy texture that only crisp bacon and croûtons carry. But the eggs are also delicious. So take your pick. Anchovies are a great source of omega-3 fatty acids as well as being rich in the nucleic acids, DNA and RNA, which some experts in human biochemistry believe may help prevent premature ageing. To this Caesar salad you can also add slices of left-over chicken or fish or turkey to create a delicious whole meal in a bowl.

What You Need

For the Salad
1 head of cos lettuce
6-12 anchovy fillets, drained and cut in thirds
300g (11 oz) cooked chicken in chunks (optional)
Maldon sea salt to taste
freshly ground black pepper to taste
50g (2 oz) Parmesan cheese, shaved, not grated

For the Croûtons
2 rashers of lean bacon, diced, fried and drained or
2 hard-boiled eggs, quartered

For the Dressing
1½ medium-sized lemons, juiced
2 cloves of garlic, chopped fine or crushed in a mortar and pestle
2 tbsp extra virgin olive oil
several dashes of Worcester sauce
1 free-range organic egg

Here's How

To Prepare the Dressing
In a small bowl mix together the lemon juice, garlic, olive oil and Worcester sauce, break the whole egg into the bowl and whisk with a fork to blend well.

To Prepare the Salad
Wash and dry the lettuce leaves, then tear them into chunky morsels. Wrap them in a clean towel and chill in the fridge until you need them. Place the lettuce leaves in a large flat salad bowl, add the cooled 'croûtons' and pour the freshly-made salad dressing all over, add the anchovies and season. Toss and serve up with shaved Parmesan.

Protein 19.5g per serving
Usable carbohydrate 3g per serving

Chef's Salad
Serves 2

A chef's salad is one of those perfect low-carb meals you can not only order in a restaurant, but also make yourself – provided you have plenty of leftovers.

What You Need
1 head of the most beautiful lettuce you can find (any kind) torn into bite size pieces
½ cucumber, cubed
1 small tomato, cubed
2 cloves of garlic, crushed or chopped fine
3 tbsp fresh parsley, basil or coriander, chopped
2 tbsp extra virgin olive oil, or half olive oil and half flaxseed oil
2 tbsp lemon juice
1 tbsp of balsamic vinegar
4 hard-boiled eggs, halved
100 g (3½ oz) ham, sliced in strips
100 g (3½ oz) cooked chicken, sliced in strips
150 g (5 oz) Parmesan cheese, in julienne strips
Mexican chilli seasoning as a garnish

Here's How
Arrange lettuce, cucumber and tomato in a big flat salad bow and sprinkle on the fresh herbs and garlic. Pour the oil, lemon, and vinegar over the top, season and toss. Arrange eggs, ham, chicken and cheese on the top of the salad. Shake Mexican chilli seasoning over all and serve immediately.

Protein 35g per serving
Usable carbohydrate 5g per serving

Greek Salad
Serves 2

So simple, this salad is such a delight. It, too, is pretty readily available in restaurants. But I prefer to make my own.

What You Need
100 g (3½ oz) of dark lettuce leaves, spinach or rocket torn into bite-size pieces
1 small Spanish onion, sliced in rings

80 g (3 oz) feta cheese, cubed
a handful of fresh, black olives, drained
1 small tomato, wedged
½ green capsicum, julienned
3 tbsp extra virgin olive oil
3 tbsp balsamic vinegar
juice of half a lemon
Maldon sea salt to taste
freshly ground black pepper to taste

Here's How
Lay all ingredients in a large salad bowl and pour over the olive oil, vinegar and
lemon. Toss well, season and serve immediately.

Protein 7g per serving
Usable carbohydrate 7.5g per serving

Mesclun And Flower Salad
Serves 2

*Mesclun is that wonderful mixture of delicate salad leaves, including such things
as curly endive, romaine, radicchio, flat-leaved parsley, dandelions – even
purslane. All are brimming with phyto-nurtrients. These leaves are not only easy
to grow, you harvest them by cutting a few leaves at a time and letting the plants
go on reproducing yet more beautiful leaves. Nowadays mesclun is pretty easy to
find in supermarkets, often washed and ready to eat. I like to serve this salad with
a fish soup, roast or lobster because it is so light and uplifting. The flowers are not
absolutely necessary but they add such beauty to the dish that I can never resist.*

What You Need

For the Salad
50-75 g (2-3 oz) three or four mesclun leaves: cos lettuce, dandelion leaves,
    radicchio, rocket, lambs' lettuce, oakleaf lettuce, purslane, curly endive
½ ripe avocado, sliced
handful of fresh mushrooms, sliced
50g (2oz) of celery, finely sliced
10-12 bright coloured nasturtium flowers (optional). You can also
  use marigolds or heartsease, the gorgeous little pansy-like
  flowers that have a reputation for easing heartache.

For the Dressing
2 cloves of garlic, chopped fine
½ tsp Dijon mustard
3 tbsp walnut oil
1 tbsp white wine vinegar
1 tbsp lemon juice
1 tbsp chervil, chopped fine
1 tbsp flat leaved parsley, chopped fine

Here's How
Put all of the mesclun leaves plus the other salad ingredients into a big bowl. I like to use glass bowls because the leaves are so beautiful, it's a shame to conceal them. Then, for the dressing, put all the ingredients into a screw top jar and shake vigorously to blend. Sprinkle delicately over the leaves, toss lightly and serve.

Protein 1g per serving
Usable carbohydrate 10g per serving

Crunchy Broccoli Salad
Serves 6

This is a salad which you can make either with fresh broccoli, raw – the way I prefer it – or by trimming the stalks and florets of steamed broccoli while it is tender and crunchy. If you are using fresh broccoli, grate it on a mandolin nice and fine. If you are using steamed broccoli, then rinse it with cold water after cooking and drain.

What You Need
450 g (1 lb) fresh broccoli
1½ tsp mayonnaise (preferably home-made)
3 tbsp sour cream (optional)
3 tbsp fresh lemon juice
¼ tsp dried tarragon, crushed
1 tbsp mild American mustard
2 tbsp finely chopped green peppers (or spring onions)
Maldon sea salt to taste
freshly ground black pepper to taste

Here's How
Prepare your broccoli if you are going to cook it, then chill. Place broccoli either cooked or raw, in the bowl. Add mayonnaise, sour cream, lemon juice, tarragon,

mustard, green peppers (or spring onions) and season. Toss your salad until everything is evenly combined.

Protein 2g per serving
Usable carbohydrate 7g per serving

California Sprouted Salad
Serves 2

This salad relies heavily on sprouted seeds and grains. Sprouts are vegetables which grow in any climate, mature in 3-5 days, can be planted any day of the year, need neither soil nor sunshine, and are some of the richest sources of anti-oxidant vitamins, minerals and phyto-nutrients in the world. Grow them in jars in your kitchen or the airing cupboard. Buy them in the supermarket. They are the perfect compromise between the agriculture of years gone by and the 'just add water' mentality of the 20th century. Sprouts are full of anti-cancer properties and anti-ageing properties. The vitamin content of a seed increases phenomenally when it germinates. The vitamin C in soya beans, for instance, multiplies five times within three days of their germination. In fact, a mere tablespoon of soya bean sprouts contain half the recommended daily adult requirement of vitamin C – provided of course that they are fresh. Sprouts are also rich in chlorophyll, known to have anti-cancer and anti-ageing properties. Researchers have discovered when they expose bacteria to carcinogenic chemicals in the presence of extracts taken from lentil sprouts, mung bean sprouts and wheat sprouts, that cancer development is inhibited by 99 per cent. To top all this off, sprouts taste delicious and make absolutely wonderful California-type health salads.

What You Need
75 g (3 oz) crunchy lettuce
½ small tomato, sliced
1 tbsp spring onions, chopped fine
2 cloves of garlic, crushed or chopped
1 avocado, sliced
½ bulb fennel, sliced
25 g (1 oz) alfalfa sprouts
75 g (3 oz) sunflower seeds
Maldon sea salt to taste
freshly ground pepper to taste

Here's How
Wash and shred your lettuce and place in a serving bowl. Place the tomato,

onions, garlic, avocado and fennel over the lettuce. Top the salad off with alfalfa sprouts and sunflower seeds and pour over your favourite dressing. Season.

Protein 4g per serving
Usable carbohydrate 5g per serving

Salmon Salad
Serves 4

My favourite salads are whole meal salads where you pick your vegetables and then add to them ready cooked protein foods: tofu, which has been fried in coconut oil and seasoned with Cajun seasoning, cooked salmon, flaked, cooked chicken, small cubes of left-over lamb roast, left-over wild duck, even hard-boiled eggs. This salad is ready in a minute, easy to prepare and is delicious.

What You Need
500 g (17 oz) cooked wild salmon, flaked
4 large stalks of celery, sliced thin on a diagonal using a mandolin
3 tbsp fresh coriander, chopped fine
½ small red onion, chopped fine
small finger of fresh ginger, shredded fine
2 tbsp fresh lemon juice
4 tbsp mayonnaise (preferably home-made)
4 glorious lettuce leaves

Here's How
Combine the flaked salmon (or whatever else you're using) with the celery, coriander, onion and ginger. Drizzle with lemon juice and mix in the mayonnaise with a fork. Place the lettuce leaves on four plates and spoon over the mixture. Chill for half an hour before serving.

Protein 34g per serving
Usable carbohydrate 1 gram per serving

Mock Potato Salad
Serves 4

You might be amazed at what a great substitute for potatoes cauliflower makes. Not only can you cook it, mash it and add a bit of butter and flavour, cauliflower also works beautifully for making a non-potato potato salad.

What You Need

For the Salad
1 cauliflower, divided into florets
1 chopped red onions
4 stalks of celery, finely sliced diagonally on a mandolin
½ red capsicum, chopped fine
4 tbsp chopped, large-leaved parsley
3 cloves of fresh garlic, crushed or chopped fine
Maldon sea salt to taste
freshly ground black pepper to taste

For the Dressing
200 ml (6½ fl oz) mayonnaise (preferably home-made)
2 tbsp balsamic vinegar
2 tsp dry mustard
1 tbsp fine lemon zest
3 hard-boiled eggs, grated
Mexican chilli seasoning as a garnish

Here's How
Steam the cauliflower florets until crunchy tender, drain and put aside to cool.
Put the other ingredients in a big salad bowl and season with salt and pepper.
Make the dressing by mixing all the ingredients together in a small bowl until
smooth. Once the cauliflower is cool, chop it and add it to the vegetables,
mixing with enough dressing to coat the lot. Stir in the eggs, cover and allow
to sit in the refrigerator for 2 hours for the flavour to develop. Sprinkle with
Mexican chilli seasoning and serve.

Protein 9g per serving
Usable carbohydrate 6g per serving

DRESSINGS, DIPS AND SAUCES

This area of Ketogenics and Insulin Balance eating is unmistakeably self-indulgent. You can make the most wonderful dressings for salads, dips for crudités and sauces of all sorts — things you would never dream of being able to eat on a high-carb/low-fat diet. When it comes to dips, dressings and sauces, provided you have an understanding of the basic principles of cooking low-carb foods, virtually the sky is the limit. Here are some of my own favourite recipes.

DRESSINGS AND SAUCES

Coconut Curry Sauce
Serves 4-6

This sauce I learned from my friends from the Cook Islands who seem to use coconut for everything, with marvellous results. The sauce is easy to make and will turn meat, fish or chicken into a delicious meal. If I'm feeling really energetic, I serve it over a bed of unsweetened hand-shredded coconut in place of rice.

What You Need
½ onion, chopped fine
3 cloves of garlic, crushed
1 tbsp coconut fat
1 can of unsweetened coconut cream
2 tsp mild, medium, or hot curry powder
1 pinch of artificial sweetener
pinch of turmeric (optional)

Here's How
Place the onions and garlic in a pan. (I often use the pan that I have stir-fried whatever meat, fish or chicken that I'm going to use in the curry so that after I have cooked the protein and removed it from the pan, the crispy crunchy bits and pieces carry the flavour over into the curry sauce.) Add the coconut fat to the frying pan and brown the garlic and onions, picking up any left-over residue from protein foods you have cooked. Pour on the coconut cream and add all the other ingredients. Bring to a gentle simmer, and simmer for a minute or two, then it's ready to serve. This recipe makes enough sauce for a curry to feed 4-6 people.

Protein 0g
Usable carbohydrate 2-1.5g per serving

Japanese Teriyaki Marinade
Makes approx 125ml (4 fl oz)

*I love teriyaki but so often the marinades that are made for soaking fish, chicken
and meat to get a teriyaki taste are full of sugar and saké, both of which raise
insulin far too high. This is my alternative. It's equally delicious, easy to make and
very low in carbs.*

What You Need
100 ml (3½ fl oz) tamari or soya sauce, with no sugar added
2 tbsp soy oil (or olive oil in a pinch)
2 tbsp spring or filtered water
2 tsp wine vinegar
1 finger of fresh ginger, grated fine
2 cloves of garlic, crushed or chopped
¼ tsp artificial sweetener

Here's How
Combine all your ingredients in a flat, low pan then marinate your beef, pork,
chicken or tofu before teppenyaki grilling or stir-frying or barbecuing. If you
are stir-frying, you can pour the remainder of the sauce into the pan once the
meat and vegetables are cooked to further season the food. This recipe makes
about 125 ml (4 fl oz).

Protein 8g
Usable carbohydrate 9g

Winning Pesto
Makes approx 500ml (17 fl oz)

*Probably my favourite sauce of all time is Italian pesto. I grew up eating it over
pastas and for a time missed it terribly when I wasn't eating pasta. Then I realised
that the same sauce, which is low-carb, goes brilliantly on fish, green beans, squash
– even a salad of buffalo mozzarella and thin sliced tomatoes. I make this sauce
in a blender, store it in the fridge and use it up within two days. I am notorious
for buying huge bunches of fresh basil and making masses. When I want to freeze
pesto, I make it without the cheese and then add the cheese to it when I defrost it.
It keeps very well this way.*

What You Need
200 ml (6½ fl oz) extra virgin olive oil plus 250 ml (8 fl ozs)
  flaxseed oil or 250 ml (8 fl oz) extra virgin olive oil
4-6 cloves of garlic, crushed or chopped
huge bunch of fresh basil leaves, about as much as you can
  gently pack into three big cups
70 g (3 oz) pine nuts, macadamias, or even almonds
70 g (3 oz) freshly grated Parmesan cheese

Here's How
Put the olive oil and flaxseed oil (if you're using it) into a blender. Add everything except the cheese. Blend until smooth. Pour into a bowl and stir in the cheese.

Protein 37g
Usable carbohydrate 3g

Hollandaise Sauce
Makes approx 150ml

I adore hollandaise sauce. For years I did not eat it because I, like so many people, was afraid of the fat it contains. This recipe is easy to make, low in carbs and tastes great over cooked spinach or asparagus. Use it as a dipping sauce for artichokes as well.

What You Need
100 g (3½ oz) butter
4 egg yolks, beaten
juice of 1 lemon
Maldon sea salt to taste
freshly ground black pepper to taste
1 tsp Dijon mustard (optional)
sprinkling of Mexican chilli powder (optional)

Here's How
Melt one third of the butter in a bain-marie, then remove from the heat. Beat the egg yolks in a bowl, using either a hand-held electric beater or a whisk. Very slowly add the melted butter to the egg yolks, continuing to mix all the time. Pour this mixture into the bain-marie and put back over simmering water. Gradually add the rest of the butter, little by little, all the while continuing to whisk. Once the butter is completely melted and integrated with the sauce, remove it from the heat, stir in your lemon juice, salt, pepper and other additions.

Protein 13.5g
Usable carbohydrate 1g

Easy Mayonnaise
Makes approx 500ml (10fl oz)

Mayonnaise is not as difficult to make as everybody makes out, particularly since the advent of high-speed blenders and food processors. It does take a little bit of patience and a little bit of practice. If by any chance you don't succeed with your first emulsion, simply wash out and dry carefully your blender or food processor then use the 'unemulsified emulsion' to drop back, drop by drop, into a new supply of egg yolks as though it were oil itself. Go through the process all over again. Naturally you will have to add a bit more seasoning as you'll end up with a bit more mayonnaise. If at first you don't succeed, try again. You will.

This mayonnaise is made with extra virgin olive oil. You can make a proportion of the oil flaxseed oil instead. You can add all sorts of wonderful things to it, like nuts, garlic, herbs, mustards. The sky is virtually the limit once you get the basic principles of how to do it under your belt. Commercial mayonnaise – the kind you buy in jars in the supermarket – is something you want to avoid as much as you can. These products are full of trans-fatty acids and made from the cheapest, nastiest forms of hydrogenated junk fats. Mayonnaise you make yourself will keep for 4-5 days in the coolest part of the refrigerator. Here's my basic recipe plus some suggestions on how to vary it.

What You Need
2 yolks from large eggs
275 ml (9 fl oz) extra virgin olive oil
2 tbsp cider vinegar
2 tbsp lemon juice
½ tsp dry mustard
Maldon sea salt to taste
freshly ground black pepper to taste

Here's How
Put the egg yolks in a blender or food processor and begin to blend on a low setting. Very, very gradually add your oil – literally drop by drop – as the blender is running until you see an emulsion beginning to happen. When this begins you will no longer be seeing liquid swirling round and round, but something thicker with the consistency of a light face cream. Continue slowly to add oil to the mixture in a thin stream, all the while keeping the blender low, until you have added half the contents of the oil. Then put in the vinegar, lemon juice, mustard, salt and pepper, all the while continuing to blend. Finally, slowly add the remaining olive oil. Taste and adjust seasoning.

Protein 0g
Usable carbohydrate 5g

Other Ways To Go

Flax It
Replace a quarter of the olive oil with flaxseed oil.

Go For Garlic
Add 2-4 crushed cloves of garlic when you are adding the lemon juice for an intense garlicy mayonnaise – excellent with fish soup.

Nuts Are Great
Add 70g (2½ oz) chopped almonds, macadamias or walnuts when putting in the lemon juice.

Orange Zest
Take 250 ml (8 fl oz) of your home-made mayonnaise, leaving out the garlic and mustard, and add to it 2 tsp of grated orange zest as well as 1 tbsp of fresh orange juice and 2 tbsp of finely chopped fresh mint leaves.

Curried Mayonnaise
Take 125 ml (4 fl oz) of your home-made mayonnaise and add to it 1 tsp of mild-to-medium strength curry powder as well as 1 tsp of finely grated fresh ginger.

Tofu Mayonnaise Lite
Makes approx 150ml

This mayonnaise, instead of being made with oil, is made with tofu. You can use it for salads and dips as well as sauces to go on cooked vegetables. It's easy to make and light as air to eat. Like conventional mayonnaise, you can vary this recipe by adding garlic, Cajun seasoning, mustard or fresh herbs to give a totally different look and flavour to your mayonnaise.

What You Need
450 g (1 lb) soft tofu, drained
50 g (2 oz) of granular lecithin
3 tbsp lemon juice
a small pinch of artificial sweetener (optional)
1 tsp vegetarian stock powder
3 tbsp flaxseed oil or extra virgin olive oil
Maldon sea salt to taste
freshly ground black pepper to taste
1 tsp fine lemon zest

Here's How
Put the tofu into a blender and add the lecithin granules, lemon juice, artificial sweetener and stock powder as well as half of the oil. Blend well until thoroughly mixed. Now slowly, drop by drop, add the remaining oil and blend again for 2-4 minutes until the mixture grows thick and creamy. Season. Finally stir in the lemon zest. This mixture will keep in the refrigerator for 5-6 days.

Protein 36g
Usable carbohydrate 10g

Basil And More Basil Dressing

Makes approx 150ml

Since basil is my favourite herb I'm occasionally accused of overdoing it, but so far as I'm concerned there is nothing more uplifting than a basil dressing on a magnificent salad of green leaves. My favourites are rocket – especially wild rocket – and lambs' lettuce or mâche as the French call it.

What You Need
100 ml (3½ fl oz) extra virgin olive oil
3 tbsp fresh lemon juice
25-50 g (1-2 oz) fresh basil, chopped
1 tsp vegetable bouillon powder
freshly ground black pepper to taste

Here's How
Mix all the ingredients in a food processor until smooth. Adjust flavour as necessary. Use immediately or store in a container in the refrigerator for up to two days.

Protein 0g
Usable carbohydrate 5g

DIPS AND SPREADS

Curried Avocado Dip

Makes approx 250ml (8 fl oz)
This dip is great for crudités. I serve it together with a platter of fresh phyto-nutrient vegetables such as chicory, bulb fennel, crunchy lettuce, celery, slices of red, green, and yellow capsicum and anything else I happen to have around. It's a huge hit with everybody. If you make it a little thinner by adding a bit of water to it, you can also use it as a dressing on a salad.

What You Need
2 large ripe avocados, peeled and cubed
3 cloves of garlic, chopped
3 tbsp lemon juice
1 tsp vegetarian stock powder
⅛ tsp of Cajun seasoning
Maldon sea salt to taste
freshly ground black pepper to taste
1 tsp mild-to-medium strength curry powder
1 tbsp lemon zest

Here's How
Add chunks of avocado plus garlic, lemon juice, stock powder and other seasoning to the food processor – everything except the lemon zest. Blend until creamy and add lemon zest and serve.

Protein 0g
Usable carbohydrate 8g

Fish Dip Or Paté
Serves 6

I discovered this recipe one night when I happened to cook too much fish for my son Aaron and myself, and didn't know what to do with it. So I put it into a blender and began adding various ingredients. I ended up producing a fish paté or dip so delicious that the whole thing disappeared before I had a chance to store it overnight for the next day's lunch. You can make it with just about any kind of light tasting fish you can find. I even use smoked salmon but if you do this make sure you buy a form of smoked salmon that doesn't have sugar in it.

What You Need
450 g (1 lb) of cooked white fish or smoked salmon
50 g (2 oz) mayonnaise (preferably home-made)
handful of chopped fresh parsley, coriander or basil
1-2 tsp vegetable bouillon powder (to taste)
2-5 tbsp of filtered or spring water (play this by ear, watch the consistency)
dash or two of Worcester sauce
2 tbsp extra virgin olive oil or half olive oil and half flaxseed oil
2-4 cloves of fresh garlic, crushed

Here's How
Place all the ingredients in a blender and blend until smooth. If you need a little more water, add it here, remembering that once you have chilled the paté it's going to go firmer in the refrigerator so you need to make allowances for

this. If you are using it as dip, naturally you will use more water; if you are using it as a paté you will use less. Turn off the blender and adjust flavouring. Be creative about this. Put anything else in that you think might be flavourful such as part of a chopped onion perhaps – this is best blended in by hand afterwards to keep the onions from going liquid, for their crunchiness is a wonderful part of the texture of the paté itself. Remove from blender and pour into ramekin dishes. Cover and chill. This will keep in the fridge for 4-5 days.

Protein 16g per serving
Usable carbohydrate 0g

Energy Salsa

I adore salsa. It's such a great way to add zing to anything from cooked vegetables to fish and crisp potato skins. You can eat this salsa hot or cold. I like to spoon it onto omelettes for brunch or breakfast and to eat it with crudités. This recipe is all raw. It makes the best possible use of the phyto-nutrients in the herbs and vegetables that go into it. I like to cut my salsa rougher than most so you get a great mixture of textures as well as flavours. Make them in the food processor, as far as I'm concerned, and you turn a salsa into a gaspacho which is all very well if that's what you are after.

What You Need
2 cloves of garlic, finely chopped
½ red onion, finely chopped
handful of fresh coriander, chopped
handful of fresh basil, finely chopped or 2 tbsp fresh mint, chopped
handful of broadleaved parsley, chopped
green or red chilli pepper, roughly chopped (after removing the seeds)
1 large tomato, roughly chopped
1 large green pepper, roughly chopped
Maldon sea salt to taste
freshly ground black pepper to taste
3 tbsp extra virgin olive oil
3 tbsp lemon or lime juice

Here's How
Mix everything together in a bowl and chill in the refrigerator. It takes this chilling process to let the ingredients in salsa meld properly. I like to keep my salsa fresh and would never keep it in the fridge for more than 48 hours.

Protein 0g
Usable carbohydrate 9g

THE MAIN THING

It may be surprise you just how luxurious Ketogenics and Insulin Balance cuisine can be. Main dishes, vegetable dishes, even crunchy, rich and delicious snacks are easy to make and loved by everybody. It's simple to modify your usual cooking style and turn your favourite recipes into low-carb wonders too. Most main courses are easy to modify because they are already protein based. So are many sauces.

All Change
You can use cauliflower instead of potatoes to thicken your soups or sauces. Try egg yolks instead of flour, or soya flour instead of wheat flour to thicken sauces. For your favourite recipes which call for vegetables, check out the list of low-carb varieties and try substituting the vegetables you are used to using – say, potatoes and carrots – for a low-carb variety. This is essential in Ketogenics. If you want to dredge any of your fish or chicken dishes in flour, try instead some soya flour, ground almonds or macadamias. Follow the quick and easy low carbohydrate list of foods (see page 174-5). When making dips and dressings use whole leaves of chicory, hard-boiled eggs, celery or capsicums cut into wedges – even pork rinds – instead of savoury biscuits and bread. You can still make flans: instead of using a flour for the crust, try the almond and flaxseed crust (see page 294-5) or do without a crust altogether by buttering your pan well and pouring the eggs directly into it. Explore sugar substitutes (see page 208-11). Both Splenda and stevia are good for cooking and baking since they don't lose their sweetness when they are heated.

Know Your Carbs
Never assume that any food is low carbohydrate. Always read labels. It's a good idea to invest in a good carbohydrate counting book for Ketogenics as well – especially right at the beginning until you get to know what works and what does not work. Tiny mistakes here can make a huge difference to successful fat loss. Finally, beware of any *hidden* carbohydrates as often they will not even be listed on the labels. Here are some common foods you will find them in:

- sweeteners such as mannitol, sorbitol, hexitols as well as any other sweeteners that bear the suffix *'ose'* – read labels carefully and be aware that 'no sugar added' does not mean that these products don't include natural sugars like fructose or honey

- prepared sauce, gravies and stock powders laden with starches to thicken them or sugars as sweeteners
- spices from the supermarket which contain sugar and other chemicals
- luncheon meats
- margarines (don't eat these anyway)
- 'low fat' varieties of mayonnaise, ketchups, pickles and relish
- 'diet cheeses'
- bottled salad dressings
- chewing gum, breath mints, cough syrups – these often contain sugar and other carbohydrates so be careful
- dairy products – if you are going to use them, you are better to have cream rather than skimmed milk – but not too often. Choose sour cream rather than yoghurt. Generally the higher the fat content, the lower the carbohydrate content.

Be Eccentric

In traditional societies, breakfast is often a large meal, while tea, dinner or supper are light and eaten early. I find that this way of eating works extremely well. You have energy when you need it and don't end up going to bed at night with a heavy stomach hoping that you will be able both to digest your food and sleep at the same time. What appears below are some of my favourite recipes for main meals, snacks and vegetable dishes. Don't get hamstrung into believing you should use them at the meal that seems most politically correct. Make a big pot of protein rich chicken soup or fish soup filled with low density low glycaemic vegetables, which you can keep in the refrigerator for two or three days to heat up whenever you happen to be hungry. The best recipes are the ones that you make up yourself. Here are some of mine to give you some ideas.

MAIN DISHES

Teppenyaki Tofu Strips
Serves 4

Tofu, a great vegan form of protein, is something that all of us should have in our diet on an ongoing basis. The problem with tofu or soya bean curd is that it has no flavour of its own. So you need to marinade it well before cooking it. I like to cook tofu in strips or chunks which I can then eat immediately at one meal and store to be used the next day at another, or even to eat cold as a snack. You can add these tofu strips to a low-carb stir fry or a phyto-nutrient rich salad as well.

What You Need
450 g (1 lb) firm tofu

Marinade
4 tbsp tamari or soya sauce (without sugar)
1 tbsp extra virgin olive oil or coconut fat
4 cloves of garlic, crushed
1 small finger of fresh ginger, shredded fine
1 tbsp lemon juice
½ tsp wasabi or 1 tsp mêaux mustard
a pinch of artificial sweetener

Here's How
Slice the tofu into long strips. Separate them and lay them in a shallow baking pan. Mix together the marinade ingredients and pour over the tofu. Allow to marinate for an hour or two (best overnight). Remove the tofu strips and fry on a teppenyaki grill or in a heavy frying pan using coconut fat or extra virgin olive oil, turning gently until lightly browned on all sides.

Protein 12g per serving
Usable carbohydrate 6g per serving

Pizza If You Must
Serves 4

If you are a pizza lover, chances are you are going to miss it more than any other food on a low-carb diet. Here's my own version of pizza sauce which you can spread on teppenyaki tofu strips (cut them wider than usual) or over grilled slices of aubergine (although take note that if made with aubergine, this will not be a high-protein meal). It ain't the same as all of the gooey dough you will find in pizza, but it's quite delicious in its own right and lots of fun to make.

What You Need
450g of teppenyaki tofu slices or aubergine, cooked and cooled (best made
    from ultra firm tofu)
2 tbsp extra virgin olive oil
Maldon sea salt to taste
freshly ground black pepper to taste
handful of fresh basil leaves, chopped
2 tbsp of fresh oregano
200 g (7 oz) shredded mozzarella
anchovies and/or olives to garnish

Sauce
1 tbsp of extra virgin olive oil
1 tin chopped tomatoes
4 cloves of garlic, crushed
1 tsp vegetarian stock powder
Maldon sea salt to taste
freshly ground black pepper to taste
pinch of cayenne pepper
1 tbsp fresh oregano, chopped fine or ½ tsp dried oregano

Here's How
Make the sauce by heating the oil in a frying pan and adding all the other ingredients, then allowing the sauce to reduce until it becomes thick. This usually takes about 5 minutes. Now place the slices of the pre-cooked tofu on an oiled baking sheet, sprinkle with seasoning and spread the pizza sauce over the slices, topping off with basil leaves and fresh oregano as well as the cheese and garnishes. Place under the grill for 3 or 4 minutes until the cheese melts. The sauce will keep for 3-4 days in the fridge if you make extra, and this recipe makes a delicious snack which you can eat the next day.

Protein 25g per serving (made with tofu)
Usable carbohydrate 11g per serving (made with tofu)

Sautéed Sea Bass With Garlic
Serves 2

Great for any fish – sole, halibut, cod, salmon, tuna, whatever, this recipe is quick and easy to prepare.

What You Need
1 tbsp coconut oil
450g (1 lb) sea bass fillets or other boneless white fish
4 cloves of garlic, chopped
¼ red onion, diced fine
2 tbsp fresh coriander or broad-leaved parsley, chopped fine
juice of 1 large lemon

Here's How
Melt coconut oil on a teppenyaki grill or heavy frying pan. Add the fish and sauté for 5 minutes, turning over only once. Remove the fish from the pan and pour in all the other ingredients, allowing them to heat through. This takes

about a minute and a half, then pour these other ingredients over the fish and serve immediately.

Protein 64g per serving
Usable carbohydrate 4g per serving

Nut Crusted Tuna
Serves 1

This is a wonderful way of cooking fish steaks, whether they be salmon, swordfish, tuna or any other kind of large fish. You can use almonds, pecans, walnuts or macadamia, whatever you prefer.

What You Need
2 tbsp melted coconut oil
2 tbsp melted butter
120 g (4 oz) chopped nuts (the best way to do this is in a coffee grinder)
Maldon sea salt to taste
freshly ground black pepper to taste
150 g (5 oz) boneless fish steaks
2 tsp fresh chopped parsley

Here's How
Pre-heat the oven to 220°C (425°F) Gas Mark 7.
Grease a baking sheet. Melt coconut oil and butter in a pan. Remove from the heat. Mix the chopped nuts together with the seasoning and put them onto a plate. Dip the fish in the oil/butter mixture and then into the nut mixture, pressing down to make sure the nuts hold. Place the nutted fish steaks on the baking sheet and pop them into the oven for 6-10 minutes until cooked through. Garnish with parsley.

Protein 52g
Usable carbohydrate 4g

Salmon Delight
Serves 2

Another recipe from my friend Belinda Hodson, a fellow traveller in Ketogenics: 'Salmon is such a delightful fish with a unique and delicate flavour. I was pondering one day what marinades I could invent for my two superb fillets and stumbled across the idea of using lemon as a base. I really love this dish because it is easy to prepare and very tasty. The marinade enhances the natural flavours of the fish and the spring onion really gives it its own special zest.'

What You Need
2 large spring onions
juice of 4 medium sized lemons
pepper and salt
2 fillets of salmon
1 dsp coconut oil
zest of 1 lemon
2 lemon wedges
chopped parsley (for garnish)

Here's How
Finely chop spring onions and place in a mixing bowl. Add lemon juice, pepper and salt and blend. Place salmon fillets in the marinade (pink side faced down) and leave for 45 minutes. Turn fillets onto the other side and leave for a further 15 minutes.

Heat coconut oil in a fry pan. Drain fillets and place in pan. Sauté fillets until tender then garnish with lemon zest, wedges and parsley.

Protein 28g
Usable carbohydrates 3g

Chicken Curry
Serves 4

Curry is a dream to make low-carb. It comes creamy thick, full of spices, with a rich fragrance and flavour. I often prepare it using left-over pieces of chicken, tossing them into a frying pan, mixing in all of my sauce ingredients, and then serving over a plate of lightly steamed broccoli or cauliflower florets. Another way I make curry – the real lazy way – is to take a chicken cut in pieces, and put it into a large cast iron pot with a lid. I then toss in all of the ingredients (I leave out coconut oil however). Pop them into the oven with the lid on, and cook for about an hour at 200°C (400°F) Gas Mark 6. Turn the chicken so that the sauce covers it and cook for another 15 minutes. This way you end up with curried chicken pieces rather than a true curry but it is so quick to prepare – in all it takes about 5 minutes – and once it's done you have got a dish to use any time you want for snacks or main courses. Here is my recipe for a more conventionally made chicken curry.

What You Need

2 tbsp coconut oil

3 tbsp chopped chives

6 cloves of garlic, chopped

1 good sized finger of fresh ginger, sliced fine

2 tsp mild-to-medium strength curry powder

pinch or two of cayenne pepper

pinch of turmeric

2 tbsp chopped spring onions

1 large chicken, skinned and de-boned and cut into bite size pieces

1 large tin of coconut milk

Maldon sea salt to taste

freshly ground black pepper to taste

chilli powder

handful of fresh parsley, chopped

artificial sweetener

Here's How

Melt your coconut oil in a heavy pot. Add chives, garlic, and ginger and lightly brown. Toss in curry powder and spices. Put in chicken pieces and coat them with the sauce, allowing them to cook lightly for 2-3 minutes. Now cover and turn the heat down until the chicken pieces cook through, stirring every 5 minutes to make sure that nothing burns. Finally, pour on the coconut milk, add a little water if you need more juice, bring to a sizzle and cook gently for another 4 minutes, season with chilli, parsley and artificial sweetener and serve.

Protein 27g per serving
Usable carbohydrate 6g per serving

Meatballs

Serves 4

Meatballs are a traditional New Zealand favourite from Belinda Hodson for people of all ages. This recipe is simple to prepare, tasty and the meatballs will go well with a number of different sauces. These meatballs are also great for picnics and barbecues.

What You Need

750 g (1½ lb) lean mince (beef or lamb)

½ tsp garlic powder

pepper and salt

4 cloves of garlic, finely chopped

1 egg
1 large onion, diced
1 tbsp fresh parsley, finely chopped
1 tbsp fresh thyme, finely chopped
1 tbsp fresh marjoram, finely chopped
1 tbsp fresh sage, finely chopped
1 dsp coconut oil

Here's How
Heat oil in a frying pan. Mix remaining ingredients together in a large mixing bowl, spoon balls of meat into the frying pan and cook gently for 20–25 minutes. Drain the meatballs on kitchen paper towels then serve with your favourite sauce.

Protein 43g
Usable carbohydrates 0g

Stir-fry It

There is no better way to cook Ketogenic and Insulin Balance meals than stir-frying them. Not only is it quick, it is also an excellent means of preserving as many of the phyto-nutrients, vitamins and minerals that come in fresh organic vegetables. The trouble with most stir fries is they are high-carb, full of things like sugar, cornstarch, oyster sauce and hoisin sauce. Stay away from these, using instead some sugar-free tamari or soya sauce. Stir-frying is about the easiest thing in the world. All you need to do is to cut up the ingredients until they are about the same size. You can do this by dicing or shredding them – I use a mandolin for mine – and making sure you have a wok or frying pan on the stove. Get everything ready first. Make sure you use a high heat. Coconut oil works best for stir-fries since it is highly stable, even at high temperatures. It's a good idea to heat the work or frying pan for 30–60 seconds before adding your oils. A wok is ready to take the vegetables and meats as soon as a hint of smoke begins to rise. Don't wait longer than this or you will get too much heat. At this point, toss in your meat, onions and garlic and sear quickly on all sides, then add your vegetables, anything from Chinese cabbage, Chinese leaves and spinach to spring onions, cauliflower, broccoli, beans – just about anything you have – as well as your garlic, ginger and other seasonings. Then let it all cook for 2–3 minutes, stirring quickly. Finally, add your seasonings and cook for another minute. Serve immediately.

Go For Broke
Don't be afraid to experiment with main dishes. You can make beef stroganoff, for instance, which you serve over puréed cauliflower instead of the usual noodles. Barbecued steaks, pork and lamb chops can be marinated in the

marinade in the teppenyaki tofu recipe or any similar marinade. Make sure any sauces you make are sweetened either with artificial sweeteners instead of sugar and that you don't use any ingredients which themselves carry a lot of hidden carbs. Roasts are always great for a low-carb way of eating. You can even make fried chicken cooked in coconut oil, using crumbled pork rinds mixed with some egg and a little soya or spelt flour to roll your chicken pieces in before frying them. The sky is virtually the limit as to what you can create in the way of delicious tasting protein-based main dishes, so let your imagination run wild.

GREAT VEGETABLES

I never met a vegetable I didn't like. But it took me a long time to realise this. Like a lot of people, I grew up with the mushy Brussels sprouts, canned spinach and revolting beetroot salads plus other nameless horrors served in school meals. It was only when I began to make exuberant salads and to cook my own vegetables (instead of massacring them) that I discovered just how delicious vegetables can be in their many incarnations.

Cook Pleasure

From the humble turnip to the light-filled leaves of radicchio, vegetables are also sources of light energy from the sun – the same light energy that 15 billion light years ago created the universe – the same energy from which the living body is made. Their beauty is the beauty of the life force itself. When they are grown organically in healthy soils and eaten either raw or with as little cooking as possible this energy, which cannot be measured in chemical terms and whose potential for enhancing health probably goes far beyond even that of the newly discovered phyto-nutrients, becomes our energy.

For a long time cooked vegetables had a bad rap. Some of this, I suspect, is the result of our not being able to buy good quality organic vegetables during the last 20 or 30 years. So people have come to think of vegetables as rather flavourless things that everyone knows you're supposed to eat because they're good for you, but nobody can be bothered. When vegetables are cooked properly they have a marvellous flavour of their own. There is nothing quite as comforting as the pleasure of a crunchy potato skin stuffed with a well-dressed living salad, or the light, crisp taste of stir-fried mange touts spiked with almond slivers. And there is little more beautiful to serve with a fish, meat or tofu dish than brightly coloured vegetable purées of broccoli, pumpkin or spinach. Steam them, stir-fry them, bake them, purée them, eat them raw – however you go, vegetables are not only some of the most important foods in relation to health, they are also some of the most delicious.

Baked Asparagus

Serves 4

Not only does asparagus appear in early spring with a very short growing season – which makes it seem ultra-desirable – it is also a powerfully healing vegetable. Asparagus has long been used in ayurvedic medicine as a remedy against indigestion. Not long ago researchers compared the therapeutic effect of asparagus with a commonly used drug in the prevention of nausea and hiatus hernia, heartburn and gastric acid reflux. They discovered that asparagus was just as effective as the common drug remedy, yet had no side- effects. Asparagus also has great diuretic properties. It stimulates the digestion and has long been used to alleviate rheumatism and arthritis. And it has sedative properties. A member of the lily family, asparagus was used by the ancient Greeks to treat kidney and liver troubles. It's one of the best natural remedies for PMS-related bloating and a top source of folic acid, the antioxidant glutathione, and vitamin C. All three are associated with reduced risk of cancer, age-related degenerative diseases and heart disease. Finally, asparagus contains good amounts of potassium and zinc, vitamins A and B complex. When shopping for asparagus, look for bright green, straight, fresh-looking spears with compact tips. Stay away from the woody, stringy or streaked spears and those with spreading tips. These are sure signs that they're not really fresh. Bring the asparagus home and rinse it in cold water. Then trim off the bottoms or woody portions. If you end up with very large spears that look tough, peel the outside before cooking. You can use raw asparagus in salads by cutting it into 1 cm (½ inch) pieces, and also as crudités with dips. But the thinner asparagus is better for this. And it must be very fresh and crunchy if you're not going to cook it. Because the tips of asparagus cook much faster than the tails, it's a good idea to steam it in a tall, lidded pan designed specially for that purpose, but don't worry if you don't happen to have one. You can also cut it into pieces and pop them into the steamer – the heavier ends first and the little tips afterwards. I like to serve steamed asparagus with wedges of lemon and shaved Parmesan, plus a little garlic salt and pepper. You can also use any of the dips, pestos or mayonnaise including aïoli and serve asparagus hot or cold. I'm also fond of baked asparagus.

This recipe makes a great starter to a formal meal, but I like to eat it on its own as a meal in itself.

What You Need
3 dozen asparagus spears, trimmed and peeled if necessary
2–3 tbsp melted butter, or olive oil
Maldon sea salt coarsely ground pepper to taste
1 lemon, divided into 6 wedges

Here's How
Preheat the oven to 220°C (425°F) Gas Mark 7.
Place the asparagus side by side in a flat, rectangular baking dish and drizzle with butter or olive oil. Season with salt and pepper. Cover with a lid or with tin foil. Then bake for 20–30 minutes, depending upon the thickness of the asparagus – that is until the spears are browned and tender. Add a little extra melted butter just before serving if it is needed, and a wedge of lemon to each plate. Serve warm or cold.

Protein 3.6g per serving
Usable carbohydrate 6.25g per serving

Mangetout And Almond Stir Fry
Serves 4

Quick and easy as well as ultra-healthy, stir-frying vegetables sears the flavour and the nutritional value within. This way you cook your vegetables very quickly in a minute quantity of light oil, or if you're a low-fat freak, you don't even need the oil. You can substitute stock boiled down to be very thick, or a little water mixed with vegetable bouillon in its place. If you're in a hurry, prepare all your vegetables in advance – chop them up and leave them in the refrigerator so you're ready to cook them – although the preparation itself is so quick that it's hardly worth the trouble. I stir-fry just about any vegetable (except the starchy ones) that I can find in the refrigerator. With larger vegetables like cauliflower florets and broccoli, the trick is to cut them fine enough so they can cook fully within a three-minute period. Here are a few of my suggestions, but don't be afraid to create your own combinations.

This is great combination of crunchy almonds and delicate green mangetout.

What You Need
250 g (9 oz) mangetout
2 tbsp soy oil or reduced stock
50 g (2 oz) almond slivers, toasted or raw
2½ cm (1 inch) finger of fresh ginger, shredded fine
125 g (4 oz) mushrooms
1 tsp tamari

Here's How
Top and tail the mangetout. Heat the oil or reduced stock in a wok or large frying pan. When hot, add the almonds and ginger and stir-fry for 3–5 minutes. Now add the remaining ingredients and continue to stir-fry for another 2–3 minutes. Serve immediately.

Other Ways To Go
Great candidates for stir-frying include Chinese leaves with cashews, sprouts with tofu, cauliflower florets with fresh parsley, and cabbage with onions.

Protein 10g per serving
Usable carbohydrates 7g per serving

Char-Grilled Capsicums
Serves 4

Another great way of cooking vegetables is to char grill them with a little olive oil. They make a good vegetable accompaniment to a main course or, as I like to do, you can eat them as a meal on their own, hot or cold, some afternoon or evening when you're not terribly hungry but want to nibble on something delicious. Many vegetables lend themselves to char grilling. Although this recipe is for peppers, you can carry out the same procedure with red onions, tomatoes, courgettes, aubergines, fennel, celery, cauliflower and broccoli. Even Brussels sprouts, which are by no means my favourite vegetable, come out well when you char grill them.

Capsicums go back at least 7000 years in their many forms: bell peppers, pimentos, cherry peppers, paprika, piquin, anaheim, jalapeno, chilli, cayenne and aji to name a few. They became part of European fare when Columbus returned from their native New World and introduced them to the Court. By mid-sixteenth century they were being cultivated widely in Spain and Portugal. All capsicums are rich in vitamin C, E and the carotenoids which help protect against degeneration and the damaging effects of toxic chemicals in the environment. The hotter peppers are rich in the alkaloid capsaicin which appear to decrease pain, enhance digestion and even detoxify the body, protecting it from flu and colds. Eat them raw as crudités, bake them, add them to soups and stews. Their magnificent colour and their health-enhancing capacities are a wonder to behold.

I serve char-grilled vegetables just as they come, marinated in the sauce that I use to baste them while they are under the grill or on the barbecue. Sometimes I squeeze extra lemon over them.

What You Need
8 capsicums, red, yellow or green
1 red onion, chopped
4 cloves of garlic, sliced fine

For the Dressing
8 tbsp olive oil
½ tsp tamari
juice from 1 lime
zest from 1 lime (use lemon if you can't find lime)
2 cloves of garlic, chopped fine
2 tsp bright red peppercorns, ground in a mortar and pestle
2 tbsp shallots, chopped fine
For the Garnish
A small handful of finely chopped fresh herbs. Choose from tarragon, basil, coriander, flat-leaved parsley or fennel.

Here's How
Combine the ingredients of the dressing or marinade and mix well. Pour into a flat pan. Cut the peppers in half, remove the seeds and plunge into the marinade. Allow them to sit for between 15 minutes and 2–3 hours, turning occasionally so that they soak up the marinade. Now you're ready to cook – either on a cast-iron char-grill pan, a teppenyaki grill (my favourite method), underneath the grill of your oven or atop the barbecue. It is important that your grilling surface is extremely hot. If you're using a pan or teppenyaki grill, you check this by splashing on a bit of water. The water drops should jump high and then disappear all together. Place onions and garlic, and then the backs of the vegetables facing the heat first on your grill or pan and cook until brown, turning them over as necessary and brushing on more of the marinade as you go. Finish off on the open side, filling the centre of the peppers with more of the marinade. Finally, just before serving squeeze on some lemon and sprinkle with fresh herbs. Alternatively serve them in a little pile on each dish so that people can sprinkle on the garnish themselves. Add freshly-ground red peppercorns and serve with ribbons of lemon peel around the vegetables on each plate.

Protein 1g per serving
Usable carbohydrates 6g per serving

Perfect Peppers
Serves 4

Another recipe for peppers from my friend Ariana Te Admorere, a fellow traveller in Ketogenics.

Our caterer at the first meeting of the documentary group prepared a beautiful meal for us. These peppers were part of the feast. I've made some changes, so here's my version:

What You Need
2 dsp olive spread
4 peppers, all red, or mixed colours look fabulous (cut into halves)
4 tbsp shredded sweet basil
4 small tomatoes, cut into halves
225 ml (7 fl oz) ricotta cheese
1 crushed clove garlic
1 tbsp extra virgin olive oil

Here's How

Preheat the oven to 200°C (425°F) Gas Mark 7.

Place olive spread in the bottom of the peppers, then put shredded basil on top. Layer with tomato halves, then ricotta cheese and garlic. Next drizzle with extra virgin olive oil. Roast for 40-60 minutes. I love putting them in the pan with roast lamb or roast beef during last 60 minutes. Try serving them with roast pumpkin and salad. Hot or cold, these are scrumptious.

Protein 7g
Usable carbohydrates 13g

Red Peppers On The Run

Serves 2

Red peppers are also one of Belinda Hodson's favourite vegetables because of their stunning colour and because they look so good on just about every dish you put them into. Here is her recipe and what she has to say about them:

'I was running late one day when preparing a dinner for my guests. Looking for something really colourful to go with my green salad and fish I reached for two large fresh red peppers and invented a stuffing for them on the fly.'

What You Need

1 small onion, diced
3 cloves garlic, finely chopped
4 large mushrooms, chopped
2 tbsp of olive oil
pepper and salt
2 tsp parsley, finely chopped
½ tsp grated ginger
dash of chilli powder or Tabasco sauce
1 tbsp of Parmesan cheese
1 tomato
2 large fresh red peppers

Here's How

Preheat the oven to 180°C (350°F) Gas Mark 4.

In a saucepan sauté onion, then garlic, then the mushroom in olive oil. Add pepper, salt and parsley. Sauté for a minute longer then remove from heat. Add remaining ingredients, except tomato, and mix thoroughly.

Cut the tops off the peppers and remove seeds. Dice the tomato and place in the bottom of peppers. Fill the rest of the peppers with the mushroom mixture. Place the tops back on the peppers, drizzle with olive oil and bake in the oven for 45 minutes (turning every 15 minutes).

Protein 6g
Usable carbohydrates 15g

Flying Soup
Serves 4

Another recipe from my friend Ariana Te Admorere who, like me, loves the beauty and comfort of a good soup. She says:
*   'This came about through incorporating micro-filtered whey protein into diet. I've called it flying soup because of the speedy energy it gives you. You'll swear you're flying.'*

What You Need
1 chopped red onion
1tbsp olive oil
2 crushed cloves garlic
1 l (1¾ pt) vegetable stock
2 chopped spring onions
400 g (14 oz) tin chopped Italian tomatoes
250 ml (8 fl oz) chopped watercress
225 ml (4 fl oz) chopped sweet basil
225 g (8 oz) chopped pumpkin
Maldon sea salt
freshly ground pepper

Here's How
In a saucepan sauté onions and garlic in oil for 5 minutes. Add all remaining ingredients, cover pan with a well-fitting lid and simmer for 1 hour.
     This is the flying factor: to every serving dissolve 2 scoops of micro-filtered whey protein in the hot soup. The energy this gives you will amaze you. It's excellent in a Thermos – add the micro-filtered whey protein before you eat it.

Protein 6g
Usable carbohydrates 9g

Perfect Purées

Serves 4

I've never been able to figure out why the most common puréed vegetable is mashed potatoes, when there are so many other low glycaemic carb vegetables like swede, spinach, cauliflower, broccoli and celeriac, which purée equally well. The secret of great vegetable purée lies in what you add to it. You can either cook the vegetables and purée them on their own, or you can mix them with mashed potatoes to make bright-coloured complements for fish, poultry and meat dishes. Of course, every root vegetable makes a great purée. One of my favourites is celeriac, which I think goes beautifully with any kind of game or fish. Broccoli, too, makes a wonderful purée, as do spinach and cauliflower.

What You Need
2 scoops of plain microfiltered whey protein powder
125 ml (4 fl oz) filtered water
450 g (1 lb) low glycaemic carb vegetables
75 g (3 oz) butter
2 cloves of garlic, chopped (optional)
1-1½ tsps vegetable bouillon powder
3 tbsp chopped parsley
handful of raw almonds
Maldon sea salt to taste
freshly ground black pepper

Here's How
Mix the protein powder with water to make a cream of it. Cut off the top and bottom of the vegetables and wash thoroughly, but do not peel, as much of the nutritional value in vegetables is in the skin itself. Slice each vegetable about 1 cm (½ inch) thick and cut each slice into 4–8 pieces. Place them in a steamer over boiling water. Bring to the boil and steam for 15–20 minutes until they grow tender. Put the cooked vegetables into a food processor or blender. Add the butter, garlic, vegetable bouillon powder, parsley and almonds and blend, adding enough of the protein powder to give your purée the consistency you want. This usually takes about 2–3 minutes. Taste and season accordingly.

You can make these purées the day before and then gently reheat them with a knob of butter on top.

Protein 7g per serving
Usable carbohydrates 4g per serving

Roast Them
Serves 4

Roasting vegetables not only helps them to maintain their natural flavour, it brings a quality of richness and comfort to any meal. There's something charming to me about serving a whole baked onion at a meal – amusing as well as delicious. Roasting vegetables is a good method for preserving their vitamins and their minerals too.

You can either put them in the oven on their own or mix them together in a kind of hotpot. If you are lucky enough to have a wood-burning oven (unfortunately I am not – at least not yet), then you will get a special flavour that can't be had any other way. The best vegetables to roast are the ones like swedes, celeriac, turnips, capsicums, summer marrows and courgettes, plus, of course, t he perennial broccoli and cauliflower. You can slice them, dice them (I like to cut them into 1-cm/ ½-inch cubes), quarter them or – provided they are small – cook them whole.

What You Need
500 g (17 oz) vegetables, sliced, diced, quartered or whole, depending upon size
3 tbsp olive oil
Maldon sea salt to taste
freshly ground pepper to taste
fresh chopped herbs – chives, parsley, rosemary, thyme, sage

Here's How
Pre-heat the oven to 200°C (400°F) Gas Mark 6.
Place the vegetables in a roasting pan and pour the olive oil over them, seasoning with salt and pepper and mixing with your fingers. Spread them out so that they are in a single layer in the pan. Put into the oven and cook uncovered, stirring occasionally, until they are just beginning to take on a caramel colour. (But beware here – caramelised vegetables taste sweeter, but they are very easy to burn, and if they get too dark they grow bitter.) Now sprinkle with the fresh herbs and serve immediately.

Protein 3g
Usable carbohydrates 3g

Coconut Cream Sauce
Serves 4

When I think of the traditional sauces that used to be served on meat, fish and vegetables in my mother's time, they make me cringe. They were so full of flour and so complicated to make. I prefer simple sauces you can whip up in a minute, which are bright and clear in flavour, and spiked with herbs and spices. This is a sauce you can use just about anywhere and it works. This recipe uses the spice turmeric, which has wonderful health properties. I frequently add turmeric to vegetables and fish just because I love the brilliant yellow colour. I also like, as often as possible, to get the benefits of this splendid spice into meals I prepare.

Coconut cream sauce is easy to make and works beautifully over steamed cabbage, broccoli, cauliflower, spinach, fish, chicken or lamb – in fact over just about anything. You can make it with fresh coconut liquid, in which case you need to mix it with a bit of arrowroot in order to thicken, or you can make it – as I usually do – with tinned coconut milk.

What You Need
3 tbsp cold pressed sesame oil
1 small onion, chopped fine
2 cloves of garlic, chopped fine
300 ml (10 fl oz) tin of coconut milk
1 tsp Cajun seasoning
½ tsp of ground turmeric
2 tbsp broad-leaved parsley or fresh coriander, chopped fine
Maldon sea salt to taste
freshly ground red peppercorns to taste

Here's How
Put the sesame oil into a pan and fry the onions and garlic until very light brown. Now add the coconut milk, Cajun seasoning, turmeric and other ingredients except the chopped herbs. Cook for 2-3 minutes until heated through, then remove from heat. Add the fresh herbs, reserving a teaspoonful as a garnish, and pour the sauce into a bowl or directly over the vegetables or fish. Garnish with the rest of the chopped fresh herbs. If you prefer your sauce thicker, thicken with a little arrowroot or cornflour.

Protein 4g per serving
Usable carbohydrates 30g per serving

Sign Of The Cross Specials
I always think the word 'cruciferous' sounds like some kind of a crunchy salad.

In fact it is used to identify vegetables, including the brassicas, which get their name from the fact that they carry cross-shaped flower petals. These same vegetables – including Chinese leaves, mustard greens, collards, turnips, swedes, broccoli, kale, cabbage and cauliflower, boast high levels of all sorts of phytochemicals and vitamins, plus special kinds of fibre for long-lasting good looks and high-level well-being. For a start they are rich in indoles, especially indole-3-carbinol, which has the remarkable ability to increase your body's production of detoxifying enzymes. This is one of the reasons why women who eat a lot of the crucifers – say four or more times a week – have a very low incidence of cancer of the breast and of the ovaries. Indole-3-carbinol, and probably other plant factors too, in cruciferous vegetables both help clear the body of the forms of oestrogen that have a negative effect on it, as well as dramatically decreasing the body's production of these forms of oestrogen. But beware – indoles are highly heat-sensitive. To get the best from them both in flavour and in their health-boosting powers, it is good to eat them raw, lightly steamed or wok-fried, maybe with a mild coconut cream sauce.

Another phytochemical in broccoli – sulforaphane – also stimulates the production of anti-cancer and anti-ageing enzymes in the body. As nature would have it, it comes packaged with folic acid, a vitamin which few of us get in adequate quantities. It has excellent preventative and protective properties of all sorts. In terms of both useful fibre and the well-known antioxidants, vitamin C and vitamin A, you would be hard-pressed to get more of these important nutrients from other fruits and vegetables. Even half a cup of broccoli contains two-thirds of the recommended daily allowance for vitamin C. Steam it in a beautiful Chinese steam basket. Then serve it hot, or chill and use in salads.

Here are two of my favourite broccoli recipes:

Broccoli Soup
Serves 4

What You Need
1 tbsp coconut oil
500 g (17 oz) firm tofu, cut into small chunks and browned in coconut oil or olive
1 onion, chopped
4 fat garlic cloves, chopped
1 l (1¾ pt) organic vegetable stock (use cubes or powder to make)
1 large bunch broccoli, about 500 g (17 oz), stems peeled and chopped fine, florets chopped
500 g (17 oz) chopped cauliflower florets

salt and pepper to taste
1 tsp red pepper flakes, optional
2 tbsp French parsley
50 g (2 oz) chopped pine nuts

Here's How

In a heavy pot, heat the coconut oil or olive oil over medium heat and add the tofu chunks. Sauté with onion until golden. Add the garlic and cook for 1 minute. Add the stock, cover, and bring to the boil. Add the broccoli and cauliflower pieces and return to the boil, then lower to a simmer and cook, uncovered, 10 minutes or until the vegetables are tender. Blend in the food processor. Season. Ladle the soup into warm bowls and add a pinch of hot pepper flakes if you like. Sprinkle with parsley and chopped pine nuts and serve immediately.

Protein 23g
Usable carbohydrates 8g

Coco-almond Broccoli

Serves 4

Great with fish or chicken, this dish makes something really special from good old broccoli.

What You Need

1 bunch of broccoli florets
250 ml (8 fl oz) tinned coconut milk
a pinch of Maldon sea salt
a pinch of Mexican chilli
1 tbsp sliced almonds, toasted in a heavy pan

Here's How

Steam the broccoli uncovered until still crunchy, about 3 minutes or so. Drain and season. Meanwhile, warm the coconut milk over medium-high heat until it boils. Let it evaporate by about half. Pile the broccoli in a serving dish and drizzle it with coconut milk. Season. Scatter the almonds on top and serve.

Protein 6g
Usable carbohydrates 2g

Aubergine Curry
Serves 4

This recipe was given to me by my friend Vic Armstrong, a fellow traveller in Insulin Balance, who in the beginning had 'serious reservations about being a guinea pig for somebody's theory.'

'Well I dunno about spinning a yarn as good as Leslie might in describing how I came about this recipe, but an old school mate of my old man fought in the Second World War in the Khyber Pass in India. He developed a passion for the genuine article in Indian cuisine and used to regularly make interesting meals. It completely smelled the neighbourhood out, long before it was a clever thing to "do" ethnic food!'

This recipe comes from a book he showed me back in the 1970s, before it was easy to purchase the many excellent spices and condiments we have available today. I last referred to this book when I did a dinner party about 15 years or so ago, and that went down a treat, but I then moved on to other food tastes. Now I'm very interested in spicing up my cooking again. I'm also looking forward to seeing how much conversion will be required to adapt the recipes to fit within the Insulin Balance diet. (I used chickpea flour in coating the aubergine in the following recipe, instead of wheat flour, and it worked a treat.)

What You Need
2 medium size aubergine
chickpea flour
1 egg
15 g (½ oz) butter for frying
2 large onions
4 fresh chillies or 1 capsicum
2½-cm (1-inch) piece of ginger
2 cloves garlic
½ tsp turmeric
250 ml (8 fl oz) water, with 1 beef stock cube added
25 g (1 oz) unsweetened frozen coconut cream (I used unsweetened coconut
   cream out of a tin)

Here's How
Wash and salt the aubergine and cut them into 1-cm (½-inch) slices. Coat the slices in seasoned flour, then dip them into the beaten egg. Heat the ghee and fry the aubergine slices until golden brown on both sides. Keep warm in a low oven. Slice the onions and chillies or capsicum. Mince finely the ginger and garlic.

In the same pan fry the onions, garlic and ginger. When they begin to brown, add the turmeric, chillies or capsicum and the beef stock. Bring to the boil, then cover and simmer for about 15 minutes Add the coconut cream to dissolve in the gravy. When it has melted, add salt to taste and carefully put the aubergine slices into the gravy and heat gently.

Protein 5g
Usable carbohydrates 9g

ON THE SIDE

Ketogenics and Insulin Balance cuisine clear the way for delicious snacks and side-dishes. Fun to make and fun to eat, either with a meal or on their own – spicy nuts, crunchy potato skins, little almond macaroons and even cheese wafers are so irresistible that friends who know nothing about low-carb eating ask for the recipe. If you are a potato lover and will miss your potato salad, there is a way of getting round this. Use cooked cauliflower florets instead of potato chunks, mixing them together with parsley, capsicums, olives, home-made mayonnaise and hard-boiled eggs. You can create a non-potato potato salad with less than 5g of carbohydrate per serving.

Crunchy Potato Skins
Serves 4

Most of the carbohydrate in a potato lies in the fluffy white stuff on the inside. Yet most of the fun of eating a potato – for me at least – is to be found in the crunchiness of the skin. That, by the way, is also where most of a potato's nutrients lie. If ever you're craving potatoes, crunchy potato skins are a wonderful way to experience the pleasures without all the carbs. The bigger the potato you cook the better, since the surface area to volume ratio is much greater and you will get a lot more skin out of a big one than you will from a small one.

What You Need
4 large baking potatoes
6 tbsp coconut oil or butter, melted
a pinch or two of Mexican chilli powder
Maldon sea salt to taste
freshly ground black pepper to taste
grated Parmesan or feta cheese (optional)

Here's How
Pre-heat the oven to 200°C (400°F) Gas Mark 6.
Scrub the surface of the potatoes and prick them with a fork to keep them from exploding. Pop them into the oven for an hour until the insides are soft and the outsides crisp. Remove from the oven to cool. Scoop out the starchy white part and discard. Place the skins themselves on a baking sheet. Cover with the

melted coconut oil or butter, add seasoning and put back in the oven for 10 minutes until they've gone golden and crispy. If you like you can also add some grated Parmesan or feta cheese to these delicious snack foods. Serve immediately.

Protein 0g per serving
Usable carbohydrates 10g per serving

Devilled Eggs

I grew up on devilled eggs. It was one of those American dishes always served at barbecues and get-togethers in the country. I associate it with beautiful summer afternoons and young girls in gingham dresses. Devilled eggs are not only great garnishes for salad dishes and make good hors d'oeuvres, they are also an excellent snack food that you can carry with you during the day.

What You Need
6 large organic or free range eggs, hard-boiled
2 tbsp minced red onion
3 tbsp mayonnaise (preferably home-made)
1½ tsp Dijon mustard
Maldon sea salt to taste
freshly ground black pepper to taste
80 g (3 oz) finely chopped celery
12 black olives, sliced
Mexican chilli powder as a garnish

Here's How
Slice the hard-boiled eggs in half lengthwise. Take out the yolks, put them in a bowl and mash them. Stir in all your other ingredients except the garnish, then spoon into the egg whites and garnish with the olive slices, lightly doused with Mexican chilli powder and serve.

Protein 9g per recipe
Usable carbohydrate 8g per recipe

Bachelor's Curried Caviar

What You Need
1 tin sardines*
1 tsp curry powder
1 or 2 tsp lemon juice

Here's How
Mash sardines with fork adding lemon juice and curry powder. Spread on daikon 'biscuits'. Adding minced onion and/or garlic is quite OK, especially if using more than one tin of sardines. I'd recommend minced spring onion, and do use some of the green foliage.

*If using sardines canned in water some drops of olive and/or flaxseed oil should be added to the mashed sardines. The only sardines that I use that are canned in oil are ones canned in olive oil otherwise I only use sardines canned in water.

Protein 30g
Usable carbohydrate 1g

Tofu Cheese
Makes 500g (about 1lb)

This recipe is from my friend Joelle Gregorius whose body was transformed in the first five weeks of Ketogenics. She says:
'I don't really enjoy tofu, as it has no taste, so when my mother-in-law passed this recipe on to me, I found not only could I use it as a spread on vegetables (like aubergine) or rye bread etc, I could also use it as a salad dressing by diluting it with lemon juice. So, Enjoy.'

What You Need
500 g (17 oz) tofu
1 tbsp apple cider vinegar
2 tablespoons lemon juice
½ small onion grated
1 tbsp chives finely cut
2 tbsp dill (I used 1 tsp dried)
½ tsp gamasio (this is just roasted sesame with salt)
1 tbsp soya oil/extra-virgin olive oil/flaxseed oil (optional)
2 tbsp yeast powder (optional – I did not use this)

Here's How
In a bowl mix half of the tofu and all of the other ingredients with a mixer until the consistency of cream. Crumble the other half of the tofu with a fork then spoon it through the cream. Season to taste. Keep in fridge.

Protein 41g
Usable carbohydrate 8g

Parmesan Wafers
Serves 12

This is a recipe I don't make often because I prefer not to eat a lot of dairy products. Parmesan is, however, one of the best cheeses if you are going to eat cheese. It is a naturally made, very hard, non-greasy cheese which is high in protein. There is no more delicious way of eating it than as these Parmesan wafers which are a dream to make.

What You Need
1 tbsp coconut oil
500 g (17 oz) Parmesan cheese, grated fine
2 cloves of garlic, chopped fine
a sprinkling of Mexican chilli powder

Here's How
Heat the oil in the bottom of a heavy frying pan. Meanwhile, mix together the parmesan with the chopped garlic and chilli powder. Using a tablespoon, drop round balls of the mixture into the hot oil. It will spread out quickly making little pancake-like wafers. Cook for 2-3 minutes until cheese has melted. Don't let it go brown, for this spoils the flavour. Turn with a spatula and cook the other side. Remove, drain on kitchen paper towels. Serve immediately or save for later.

Protein 18g per serving
Usable carbohydrate 2g per serving

Spicy Nuts
Serves 5

These are great to carry as a snack. You can make them ahead, cool them and store them in a tightly-closed jar.

What You Need
2 tbsp coconut oil
250 g (9 oz) almonds
¼ to ½ tsp Cajun seasoning
½ tsp vegetable bouillon powder

Here's How
Place the coconut oil in the bottom of a heavy frying pan – big enough to allow the nuts to sit in it side by side so that they get evenly toasted. Heat the oil until it shows a hint of smoke, toss in the nuts, turning them frequently so they don't burn. Take them out to cool on kitchen paper towels. Meanwhile, mix together Cajun seasoning and bouillon powder. While the nuts are still warm, place the nuts together with this mixture in a paper or plastic bag or jar and shake vigorously to coat.

Protein 8g per serving
Usable carbohydrate 2.5g per serving

Afghans

This recipe which was given to me by my friend Belinda Hodson who did an experiment one day to see what she could do with stevia, cocoa powder and soy flour. It was inspired by the Edmonds Cookery Book *Afghans recipe.*

What You Need
200 g (7 oz) butter
75 g (3 oz) splenda
175 g (6 oz) soy flour
125 g (4 oz) organic cocoa powder
32 drops stevia
50 g (2 oz) crushed walnuts
12-16 walnut halves

Here's How
Preheat the oven to 180° (350°F) Gas Mark 4.
Soften butter, add splenda and beat to a cream; add flour, cocoa and lastly stevia and crushed walnuts. Put spoonfuls on a greased baking tray and place a walnut half on each Afghan. Bake for about 15 minutes.

Protein 103g per recipe
Usable carbohydrate 59g per recipe

Pete's Bread And Biscuit Substitute

This idea is from my friend Peter Sim. He says:

'Having found a sugar-free liver pâté I was faced with a problem. Being on a ketogenic diet, toast or savoury biscuits were on the banned list. Scooping out the pâté with a spoon appealed but would probably upset friends and family. By chance I had some Chinese radish, or daikon, in refrigerator. Sliced rounds of radish, spread with pate were tasted and tested on friends and relatives. Consensus was very approving.

Would work equally well with turnip, swede or large carrots. The only trouble with the last two being their high glycaemic index. Turnips are round rather than cylindrical like daikon. One gets more even-sized vegetable biscuits with daikon.

Obviously anything one would spread on a biscuit could be spread on the daikon. You'll have to use your own judgement as to the suitability of various spreads.'

JUST DESSERTS

Ketogenics and Insulin Balance eating lend themselves to great sweets and desserts. The only trouble is that you may find that after living in a Ketogenic or Insulin Balance way, before long, the sweets that you once craved may have lost their fascination. Still, everybody likes something sweet every now and then and there are all sorts of delicious things that you can make. I prefer to stay away from the recipes that you find in most low-carbohydrate cookbooks for cheesecakes made with masses of cream cheese and ice cream made with dollops of heavy cream. I don't believe that large quantities of dairy products are going to do anybody much good. I also see no reason to perform some kind of overkill in consuming so many saturated fats.

So you will find only a few recipes that use rich cream for special occasions. Most are lighter sweets which call for cream cheese and cream only occasionally. There are so many delicious things you can make which don't require them – from ambrosia made by slicing naval oranges thin, sprinkling fresh coconut plus half a teaspoon of Grand Marnier per person on top (about 9g of carbohydrate per serving) to delicious amaretti biscuits made with egg whites and crushed almonds.

Sweet Dreams
What you like best? Chocolate mousse? Fresh strawberry sorbet? You can even make healthy protein bars based on microfiltered whey protein plus a little nut butter if you like. None of these sweets contain sugar. I don't recommend using artificial sweeteners such as aspartame or saccharin (see page 207-8). The one that I make an exception for is sucralose or Splenda. Made from sugar itself, this form of sweetener is modifed in its molecular structure, replacing two of the components of sucrose – the hydroxyl groups – with chlorine molecules. Splenda tastes sweet but is not absorbed by the body and does not affect insulin levels. It's quite light and behaves in many ways like sugar itself, except that it doesn't caramelise. Sucralose comes in packets, generally equal to two teaspoons of sugar, and is worth 1g of carbohydrate. You can also buy it in bulk and measure it out like sugar. The perfect sweetener? Too soon to tell – but certainly the best of the artificial ones on the market.

The sweetener I like best is the purely natural herb stevia (see page 209-11). It comes in many forms from the fresh or dried leaf to water extracts, alcohol extracts and powder. Stevia is unbelievably sweet. Become familiar with the particular form of stevia you are using and taste everything you make as you make it to make sure you get the right sweetness. Stevia extracts work better in most desserts. The dried leaves and the fresh leaves tend to turn things green. (I have yet to be seduced by the idea of a green meringue). Some people don't care for the particular sweetness of stevia. In that case Splenda is probably the best alternative.

Almond Macaroons
Makes 18 macaroons

This is my low-carb version of the delicious amaretti biscuits from Italy which simply melt in your mouth. They are easy to make, have only 1.5g of carbohydrate per biscuit and are delicious with tea or at the end of a meal.

What You Need
50 g (2 oz) finely ground almonds (best done in a coffee grinder)
50 g (2 oz) unsweetened coconut
1 tsp vanilla essence
1 tbsp almond flavoured liqueur (optional)
a pinch of salt
2 egg whites from free-range or organic eggs
50 g (2 oz) almond meal
artificial sweetener to taste
1 tbsp coconut oil or butter for greasing the baking sheet

Here's How
Preheat the oven to 150°C (300°F) Gas Mark 2.
Mix the finely ground almonds together with the coconut, vanilla, almond liqueur and salt, then lay aside. Beat the egg whites in a separate bowl. Fold in the almond meal and artificial sweetener, and mix gently with your fingers. Roll the mixture into balls the size of large marbles and place on a greased baking sheet. Bake for 20–25 minutes or until golden brown yet still soft on the inside. This recipe makes about 18 macaroons.

Protein 1 gram per biscuit
Usable carbohydrate 1.5g per biscuit

Protein Fudge Treats
Makes 20 sweets

These are tasty sweets, not only for someone on a low-carb diet but also to give to kids in their lunch boxes. They look quite a lot like the sweets that all the other kids munch and are delicious. But since they contain no sugar, they don't cause dental caries or the kind of behaviour problems that a high sugar diet can create.

What You Need
50 g (2 oz) unsweetened dried coconut
25 g (1 oz) unsweetened dried coconut for rolling
50 g (2 oz) walnuts or almonds, finely ground (use a coffee grinder if
    possible)
100 g (3½ oz) of plain or vanilla unsweetened microfiltered whey protein
    powder
1 heaped tbsp coconut fat or almond butter
60 g (2¼ oz) unsweetened organic cocoa powder
artiificial sweetener to taste
a small quantity of iced water

Here's How
Mix everything but the water and 25g (1oz) of dried coconut in a big bowl. Using your fingers, work it all together well, gradually adding the water drop by drop until you get a malleable dough, then form it into balls. Roll the balls in the extra coconut until they are completely coated. Refrigerate until chilled thoroughly (best overnight). These will keep in the fridge for 3 or 4 days.

Protein 5.5g per sweet
Usable carbohydrate 1.5g per sweet

Other Ways To Go
Instead of water, add a handful of fresh raspberries, blueberries or strawberries.

Protein Whip
Serves 4

I make toppings for low glycaemic carbohydrates such as berries or melons using microfiltered whey protein. It's the easiest thing in the world to do. I prefer to work with microfiltered whey protein that is either vanilla flavoured or with no flavour at all. This is a recipe you can also make with heavy cream if you prefer. I try to avoid cream myself – except very occasionally – since I find it lowers my energy. Here are two versions of a kind of whipped topping – take your pick.

Version 1 – Cream Based

What You Need
200 ml (6½ fl oz) double cream
1-2 scoops of microfiltered whey protein (enough to yield 20g of protein)
artificial sweetener to taste (stevia extract or the white sucralose powder
    works here otherwise you end up with green cream)
flavouring (pure vanilla, coffee, chocolate or strawberry essence or naturally
    flavoured oil)

Here's How
Whip all ingredients together, preferably using an electric mixer, in a bowl until thick and blended thoroughly. Serve chilled.

Protein 20g per recipe
Usable carbohydrate 6g per recipe

Version 2 – Pure Protein

What You Need
A few scoops of microfiltered whey protein (enough to yield 40g of protein)
artificial sweetener to taste
1 tsp pure vanilla, coffee, chocolate or strawberry essence or naturally
    flavoured oil
200 ml (6½ fl oz) unsweetened soya milk

Here's How
Mix everything together in a medium size bowl with a beater or blender. Chill and serve. Do not mix for more than 20 seconds at a time. This can denature the protein.

Protein 60g per recipe
Usable carbohydrate 7g per recipe

Raspberry Chocolate Mousse
Serves 4

This is a fun dessert that everybody seems to enjoy. You can make it with or without the heavy cream. If you don't use cream, what I suggest you use instead is enough microfiltered whey protein to yield 40g of pure protein. If you choose the non-cream route you will end up with a mousse that is high in protein.

What You Need
120 ml (4 fl oz) filtered or spring water
2 tsp unflavoured gelatine
120 g (4 oz) unsweetened baker's chocolate, grated or chopped fine
artificial sweetener to taste
240 ml (7½ fl oz) double cream
1 tsp pure vanilla extract or pure vanilla oil
225 g (8 oz) fresh raspberries

Here's How
Bring the water to the boil and add the gelatine, stirring until dissolved. Toss in the shredded chocolate and the sweetener. Mix well and remove from heat and set aside. Beat the cream in a chilled mixing bowl until almost thick. Add vanilla and beat again to mix. Fold in the chocolate mixture and pour into four serving dishes. Garnish with the fresh raspberries and chill for half an hour before serving.

Protein: 2g per serving (42g if you are using microfiltered whey protein)
Usable carbohydrate 11g per serving

Elizabeth Moxon's Lemon Posset
Serves 4 to 6.

This recipe is from my friend Peter Sims:

'I found this recipe many years ago in Robert Carrier's Great Dishes of the World *(1963). With a name like this it certainly stuck in my mind. Then only a year ago, nearly 40 years after its publication I heard a chef on a very popular local radio programme give out the very same recipe. When challenged to produce a ketogenic cooking sequence for a television documentary using stevia as an ingredient some stress set in. Desserts and sweets have never been my* forte. *Then I recalled this one.*

As it stands the recipe is great but if you have fresh berries available fold them in and enjoy! I love it when guests leave some. It means I go to the refrigerator next morning and have a great breakfast treat.'

What You Need
grated rind and juice of 2 lemons
600 ml (1 pt) double cream
150ml (5 fl oz) dry white wine
sugar*
whites of 3 eggs

Here's How
Add the grated lemon rind to 600 ml (1 pint) of double cream and whisk until stiff. Stir in lemon juice and dry white wine. Add sugar* to taste. Whisk egg whites until they form peaks and fold into whipped cream mixture. Serve in a glass serving dish or in individual glasses.

*Sugar is out! I use 1 serving sachet of stevia powder but I noticed test panel tasters adding an extra drop of liquid stevia. Start small, you can always adjust upwards later, it's rather difficult trying to get too much sweetener out!

Protein 5-3g
Usable carbohydrate 4-3g

Easygoing Piecrust

This piecrust which is made from fresh almonds and flaxseeds is healthfully rich in the omega-3 and omega-6 fatty acids. I use it for just about everything from a frozen raspberry pie to a cheesecake. I like to grind up my flaxseeds in a coffee grinder. I do the same with the almonds. I find that coffee grinders reduce things to a beautiful powder which you can easily manipulate into whatever you want.

What You Need
60 g (2¼ oz) flaxseeds, ground to a fine powder
1 tsp fresh lemon juice
2–4 tbsp iced water
artificial sweetener to taste
a pinch of salt
180 g (6 oz) almonds, ground to a fine powder
1½ tbsp coconut oil, melted

Here's How
Soak your flaxseeds in lemon juice and a couple of tablepoons of iced water for 20 minutes. Mix together with a fork and put aside. In another bowl mix together the sweetener and salt with the almonds and the melted coconut oil. Now put the seed and nut mixture together and stir with your fingers until they are mixed thoroughly. Pour into a 23-cm (9-inch) flan pan and using your fingers, press the mixture into the pan all along the bottom and the sides. Prick with a knife or fork and bake at 160°C (325°F) Gas Mark 3 for quarter of an hour. Let cool and you are ready to fill.

Protein 29.5g per recipe
Usable carbohydrate 48g per recipe

Lemon Cream Pie
Serves 8

This is one of the fillings that I use for pies. It's creamy and yummy. You can make similar recipes using pumpkin, strawberries or rhubarb. You can even make chocolate cream pies and strawberry cream pies – all it takes is a little imagination.

What You Need
120 ml (4 fl oz) fresh lemon juice
125 g (4 oz) unflavoured gelatine
450 g (1 lb) cottage cheese
200 g (7 oz) sour cream
1 tsp of finely shredded lemon zest
200 ml (6½ fl oz) whipping cream, whipped
120 ml (4 fl oz) fresh raspberries, blackberries, blueberries or strawberries, crushed and sweetened with a little artificial sweetener

Here's How
Heat half of the lemon juice gently in a saucepan sprinkling the gelatine into it and stirring over a low heat until dissolved. Mix the artificial sweetener together with the cottage cheese, blending in the sour cream, the remainder of the lemon juice and the lemon zest. Now mix in the gelatine lemon mixture and blend well. Cool in a refrigerator until the mixture thickens but does not set completely. Fold in the whipped cream. Fill the piecrust with the completed recipe. Chill for several hours and serve with the crushed berries as a topping.

Protein 9g per serving (not including the crust)
Usable carbohydrate 7g per serving

Protein Ice Cream

When I was first exploring Ketogenics I began to experiment with making ice cream since I adore cold foods. I discovered I could make such delicious ice cream from pure microfiltered whey protein plus a few things added for flavour that for a time – in the middle of summer – I found myself eating ice cream for breakfast every day. My children found this amusing. To me it was a lot of fun.

What You Need
A few scoops of microfiltered whey protein powder (enough to yield 40g of
    pure protein)
200 ml (6½ fl oz) chilled water or 200 ml (6½ fl oz) unsweetened coconut
    cream
3 ice cubes
artificial sweetener to taste
½ tsp vanilla extract or coffee, chocolate, orange or lemon
60 g (2¼oz) raspberries or blueberries (optional)
an ice cream chiller or an ice cube tray without the dividers in it

Here's How
Blend all the ingredients together in a blender that crushes the ice completely. Place in an ice cream maker or chiller for 10–15 minutes until ice cream is formed. If you don't have an ice-cream maker, you can pour the mixture into flat ice cube trays (provided you remove the dividers) and put in the freezer to chill. Remove every 10–15 minutes and mix with a fork so that it doesn't go completely hard and then chill again. This usually takes 30–45 minutes. What you end up with is a delicious ice cream which is entirely made of protein if you go for water; or which is low in carbs if you go for coconut cream.

Protein 40g per recipe
Usable carbohydrate 0g per recipe

PART SIX:
APPENDIX

GLOSSARY

Aerobic capacity How well the body processes oxygen, determined by lung capacity, the size of capillaries, the pumping action of the heart and the transfer of oxygen to target tissues.

Aerobic exercise Repetitive exercise that gets the heart and lungs moving while bringing about only a modest increase in breathing, so that the exercise may be maintained over a long period. This form of exercise facilitates adequate oxygen transfer to muscle cells, preventing a build-up of lactic acid and so avoiding the burning sensation of overworked muscle. Aerobic exercise is useful for reducing insulin levels and lowering blood glucose.

Antioxidant Any substance that helps protect against free radical damage. Some, such as vitamins A, C, E and D, the minerals selenium and zinc, as well as phytonutrients such as lipoic acid and the flavonoids from vegetable foods, are nutritional antioxidants, while others are produced in the body as enzymatic antioxidants.

Arachidonic acid An omega-6 long-chain polyunsaturated fatty acid found primarily in animal fats. Levels of this fatty acid are often too high in modern diets. Arachidonic acid can be converted into powerfully inflammatory prostaglandins, such as PGE2. High-carbohydrate diets can activate an enzyme called delta-5-desaturase, causing the body to make too much arachidonic acid and causing inflammation. The omega-3 fatty acids EPA and DHA counter the effects of arachidonic acid.

ATP Adenosine triphosphate, the primary fuel used by cells to generate the biochemical reactions necessary for life.

Blood glucose Otherwise known as blood sugar, this is the primary source of energy in the body. Raised blood glucose levels can result in accelerated ageing and in some people may cause diabetes.

Carbohydrates A macronutrient made out of carbon, hydrogen and oxygen. These can be simple sugars or bigger molecules made up of joining simple sugars together. Examples are lactose, glucose, sucrose, maltose, starch and glycogen. Fibre is also considered a carbohydrate although it is not digestible by humans and does not constitute *useable carbohydrate*, and therefore it is not important in calculating carbohydrate levels of a food for Ketogenics and Insulin Balance.

Cholesterol A waxy sterol, manufactured by all animal cells. Cholesterol is an essential component of the body's biochemistry. It is used to make steroid hormones such as cortisone, testosterone and oestrogen.

Co-enzyme Q10 Also known as ubiquitone, Co-Q10 is a nutrient with two important properties. It is a key player in the mitochondrial generation of ATP – in other words, the body's ability to burn fuel as energy. It is also a powerful antioxidant. Supplements of Co-enzyme Q10 can be helpful for some people in the fat-burning process.

DHA Docosahexanoic acid, a long-chain polyunsaturated fatty acid of the omega-3 group, and the most important omega-3 fatty acid found in high concentrations in the brain. DHA is found in oily fish such as salmon, mackerel, herring, tuna, anchovies and sardines. Some people cannot convert other essential fatty acids into DHA and need therefore to take fish oils to get enough.

DNA Deoxyribonucleic acid. The genetic material in the nucleus of every cell, which provides the blueprint for cell reproduction and all body functions. DNA is very sensitive to oxidation damage from excess free radicals.

Enzymes Proteins which bring about metabolic changes in biological systems. They help change one substance into another. For instance, delta-60 saturase helps add double bonds to fatty acid molecules, making them more unsaturated. It converts alpha-linolenic acid to EPA. Another enzyme in turn converts EPA into the brain fat DHA. Enzymes usually require minerals and vitamins to act as co-factors and catalysts for them to do their work.

EPA Eicosapentanoic acid. A long-chain polyunsaturated fatty acid which, like DHA, is found in foods such as salmon, mackerel, herring, sardines and tuna. It can be made into prostaglandin E3, a substance that helps counter inflammation.

Essential fatty acids The fats your body cannot make for itself and therefore which must be taken in via food. Essential fatty acids are the building blocks of prostaglandins. There are two groups – omega-3 and omega-6 fatty acids, each of which produces different prostaglandins.

Free radical A highly reactive molecule that has at least one unpaired electron. Free radicals interact with proteins, fats and carbohydrates in the body as well as cells and tissues and can cause free oxidation, which is associated with degenerative disease and early ageing. Problems happen when free radical production exceeds the body's ability to protect itself against them. Antioxidants help protect against free radical damage.

GLA Gamma-linolenic acid, an omega–6 family long-chain polyunsaturated fatty acid sometimes used to increase the production of the body's PGE1, which protects your body from inflammation. It should, however, be used with care, as in some people, particularly those with insulin resistance, GLA supplements can produce more arachidonic acid and therefore more inflammation in the body.

Glucagon A pancreatic hormone that causes the release of glycogen (stored glucose) in the liver to help regulate blood glucose levels. Glucagon is a fat-mobilising hormone which counters insulin – a fat-storage hormone released by exercise, a protein meal, and low levels of blood glucose/insulin.

Glucose The simplest form of sugar, which is found in some foods and also as blood sugar, which circulates in the bloodstream. In the body, glucose is produced mostly from the breakdown of carbohydrate foods during digestion. It can also be stored in the muscles and the liver as glycogen.

Glycaemic index The potential of a sugar or carbohydrate to raise blood sugar levels. Foods with a high glycaemic index raise insulin and can stimulate the conversion of omega-6 fatty acids into the inflammatory arachidonic acid. This can interfere with fat burning as well as cause many inflammatory problems in the body. Ironically, some simple sugars, such as table sugar, have a lower glycaemic index and enter the bloodstream more slowly than many complex carbohydrates such as potatoes and bread. The faster a carbohydrate enters the bloodstream, the higher its glycaemic index will be. The higher the glycaemic index, the greater will be the increase in insulin levels it brings about. Some fruits and most non-starchy vegetables tend to have a low glycaemic index, whereas pasta, grains, breads and starches all tend to have a high glycaemic index.

Growth hormone A hormone released from the pituitary, which interacts with fat cells to release fatty acids, and also with the liver to produce insulin growth factors. Exercise enhances growth hormone release, which is one of the reasons it helps clear insulin resistance, lower insulin levels and spur fat burning.

HDL Sometimes called 'good cholesterol', high-density lipoprotein is a protein and lipid particle in the blood which functions to remove cholesterol from the cells. Higher blood levels are more desirable. If insulin levels go up, HDL levels go down. The lower the HDL level the more likely you are to age rapidly and the more at risk you are of getting heart disease.

Hormones A substance formed in an organ which excites some vital process by communicating changes in cells which respond to the information they carry.

Hyperinsulinaemia A state in which the body continually maintains abnormally elevated levels of insulin. This is usually the result of insulin resistance, where the cells are not responding to insulin's call to reduce blood glucose levels.

Insulin The 'storage hormone'. A hormone secreted by an area in the pancreas, which helps shuttle glucose from the blood into the cells. Excess insulin is the primary reason for obesity and early ageing. Insulin is also one of the body's most important chemical messengers which directs the cells' activities.

Insulin resistance A condition where cells no longer respond to insulin, also known as Syndrome X. This results in the body secreting more insulin into the bloodstream in a brave attempt to lower blood glucose levels.

Insulin sensitivity The normal, healthy state where your body's cells remain receptive and responsive to insulin's action.

Ketogenic diet A diet that causes ketone bodies to be produced by the liver, shifting the body's metabolism away from burning glucose as fuel towards burning stored body fat. A ketogenic diet restricts carbohydrates below a certain level – generally below 75g per day – bringing about a series of adaptations. The ultimate determinant of whether a diet is ketogenic or not is the level of carbohydrate that it contains. The level of carbohydrate intake at which an individual enters ketosis varies greatly; it can be as low as 25g per day. Exercise increases ketosis.

Ketone bodies By-products of the breakdown of free fatty acids in the liver. Ketones serve as a fat-derived fuel for tissues such as the brain. When ketones are produced at high rates they accumulate in the bloodstream. This results in a metabolic state called ketosis, where there is a decrease in both the production and use of glucose as energy, as well as a decrease in the breakdown of protein to be used as energy – a phenomenon called protein sparing. Many athletes are drawn to ketogenic diets as a way of shedding body fat while sparing the loss of lean muscle tissue.

LA Linoleic acid, one of the essential fatty acids, which means that the body cannot make it so it needs to be ingested in food. Linoleic acid belongs to the omega-6 family and must be obtained in small quantities from the daily diet. The Western diet is far too high in it and the other omega-6 fatty acids, in relation to the omega-3 group.

LDL Sometimes called 'bad cholesterol', low-density lipoprotein is a protein and lipid particle in the blood which carries most of the blood's cholesterol. When damaged, it can be deposited in the artery wall. Lower values of LDL are more desirable.

Lean body mass The total body weight minus the fat mass. Lean body mass is made up of water, bones, collagen, muscle and organs.

Lipid Fatty acid molecules derived from the diet, including triglycerides, phospho-lipids, fatty acids and waxes. Cholesterol is often considered a lipid as well, although it is technically not a fat, but a sterol.

Macronutrients Proteins, carbohydrates and fats – the major components that make up the foods we eat.

Mitochondria Minute organelles, or specialised areas, within a cell that act as energy factories. It is here that the body takes in the fuel provided by the diet or by the body's fat reserves and converts it into energy that drives every process in the body.

Neurotransmitter A substance, often an amino acid or a protein, which makes it possible for cells in the nervous system to communicate. Neurotransmitters affect mood, behaviour, muscle contraction, hunger and sleep, as well as bringing about many other actions in the body. They are taken up by receptors in cells. Each neurotransmitter has to fit into its receptor much the way a key must fit into the a lock.

Noradrenalin Also known as norepinephrine, this is a neurotransmitter involved in concentration, alertness and self-assertion. Athletes and people who get a lot of exercise tend to have high levels of norepinephrine, sometimes called the 'feelgood' neurotransmitter. Chronically depressed people tend to have low levels. Exercise increases the levels of noradrenalin in the body.

Omega-3 fatty acids These polyunsaturated essential fatty acids are found in purified fish oils and oily fish such as wild salmon, rainbow trout, eel, tuna, mackerel and herring. We need more of these fatty acids to balance the high levels of omega-6 fatty acids we end up eating in the modern convenience-food diet. Omega-3s are especially beneficial in combating heart disease, inflammatory conditions and premature ageing, in no small part because they promote the formation of protective anti-inflammatory prostaglandins. Omega-3s are also found in flaxseeds.

Omega-6 fatty acids These polyunsaturated essential fatty acids are found in nuts and seeds. Omega-6 fatty acids can produce both inflammatory prostaglandins, such as prostaglandin E2, and also anti-inflammatory prostaglandins such as prostaglandin E1.

Omega-6 to omega-3 ratio An important comparison of the amount of omega-6 fatty acids to omega-3 fatty acids in the diet. Both fatty acids are necessary for life, but they need to be properly balanced. The paleolithic diet had a ratio of between 1:1 and 2:1 omega-3s to omega-6s. The ratio in modern diets is sometimes as high as 30:1. This balance needs to be rectified for lasting health.

Percentage body fat That percentage of your total body weight which is not lean body mass. The higher your percentage of body fat, the greater the likelihood of chronic disease, such as cancer, diabetes and heart disease. The relative level of body fat to lean body mass has little to do with how 'fat' or 'thin' you appear. Many thin people have a high percentage of body fat. Ketogenics decreases body fat and increases muscle mass.

Prostaglandins Hormone-like substances derived from fatty acids. Some, such as prostaglandin E2, made from arachidonic acid, are powerfully inflammatory, while others – prostaglandin E1 and prostaglandin E3 – are anti-inflammatory.

Receptors Sites on the surface of cells where neurotransmitters, hormones and other substances can attach to do their work, rather like keys which fit into receptor locks. Each receptor is of a specific shape and size needed to react specifically to another molecule. As soon as the molecule attaches to the receptor, a nerve signal can be sent.

Saturated fats Fat molecules which contain no double bonds. Saturated fats are not necessary. An excess of saturated fats can interfere with the production of fatty acids essential for brain function, as well as harden cell membranes.

Syndrome X A cluster of metabolic disorders which include insulin resistance, obesity, blood fat abnormalities, glucose intolerance and hypertension. Syndrome X does not necessarily mean that all these conditions are present, but they often occur together.

Trans fatty acid An unsaturated fatty acid in which the fat molecule is twisted, producing a 'junk fat'. Junk fats result when polyunsaturated fats are processed via heat or solvents to produce the oils used in almost all convenience foods. The process changes the essential fatty acid from its normal curved shape to an arrow shape. Trans fatty acids are very harmful to the body. They alter cell membrane fluidity and have been found to enter the brain in animal studies, with unknown consequences. They need to be avoided at all costs.

Triglycerides Fat molecules composed of three fatty acids attached to a glycerol molecule – the kinds of fat found in different lipoproteins in blood. High levels of triglycerides usually accompany high levels of insulin. The ratio of triglycerides to high-density lipoproteins is an important indicator of insulin levels and can be used to predict the likelihood of heart disease in the future.

Unsaturated fats Fats that contain double bonds between their carbon atoms in one or more locations. Common unsaturated fats include linoleic and linolanic acid, with two or three points of unsaturation, or double bonds. DHA fatty acid from the omega-3 group is a highly unsaturated fatty acid containing six double bonds.

USABLE CARBOHYDRATES

Food	Amount	Weight (g)	Carbohydrate (g)	Fibre (g)	Usable Carbohydrate (g)
BAKERY					
Breads					
Rye, American	1 slice	23	12.0	0.1	11.9
Rye, pumpernickel	1 slice	32	17.0	0.4	16.6
White	1 slice	23	11.6	trace	11.6
Wholewheat	1 slice	23	11.3	0.3	11.0
Cakes					
Banana	1oz*	28	16.2	-	16.2
Carrot	1oz	28	12.6	0.1	12.5
Chocolate, with uncooked icing	1 piece	74	43.8	0.1	43.7
Coconut	1 piece	87	46.3	0.1	46.2
Fruitcake	1 slice	15	9.0	0.1	8.9
Biscuits/Cookies/ Bars					
Assorted biscuits	1 avg	20	14.2	trace	14.2
Brownie	1 serv	100	48.0	0.5	47.5
Chocolate chip cookie	1 avg	11	6.6	trace	6.6
Fig bar	1 avg	14	10.6	0.2	10.4
Oatmeal cookie	indiv	13	9.2	-	9.2
Shortbread biscuit	1 avg	7	4.6	trace	4.6
Gingerbread	1 piece	117	60.8	0.1	60.7
Crackers					
Cheese	1 avg	1	0.6	trace	0.6
Rye wafer	1 avg	7	5.3	0.2	5.1
Wheat & rye thin	1 avg	2	1.3	-	1.3
Wholewheat	1 avg	4	2.7	0.1	2.6
Doughnuts					
Cake type	1 avg	32	1.4	trace	1.4
Yeast-leavened	1 avg	30	11.3	0.1	11.2
Muffins					
Blueberry	1 avg	40	40.0	16.8	23.2
Bran	1 avg	40	17.2	0.7	16.5
English	1 whole	56	28.3	-	28.3

Food	Amount	Weight (g)	Carbohydrate (g)	Fibre (g)	Usable Carbohydrate (g)
Pancakes					
Pancakes	1 avg	45	15.3	trace	15.3
Pies					
Apple	1 piece	118	45.0	0.5	44.5
Cherry	1 piece	118	45.3	0.3	45.0
Lemon meringue	1 piece	105	37.2	-	37.2
Pecan	1 piece	103	52.8	0.5	52.3
Pumpkin	1 piece	114	27.9	0.6	27.3
Piecrust	1 avg	180	78.8	0.4	78.4
Quick Breads (Miscellaneous)					
Taco shell	1 avg	11	7.6	-	7.6
Tortilla	1 avg	30	3.6	0.2	13.4
Rolls					
Bagel	1 avg	55	28.0	-	28.0
Danish pastry	1 sm	35	16.0	trace	16.0
Hard	1 avg	25	14.9	0.1	14.8
Sweet	1 avg	55	27.1	0.1	27.0
Wholewheat	1 avg	35	18.3	0.8	18.5
Rusk	1 piece	9	6.4	trace	6.4
DRINKS					
Spirits					
Ale	1 cup	230	8.0	-	8.0
Daiquiri	1 cup	240	12.5	-	12.5
Gin/Rum/Vodka/Whiskey	1 oz	30	-	-	-
Beer & Wine					
Beer	1 cup	240	9.7	0	9.7
Champagne	wine glass	120	3.0	0	3.0
Dessert wine	1 cup	240	14.0	0	14.0
Muscatelle or Port	wine glass	100	14.0	0	14.0
Rosé	wine glass	100	2.8	0	2.8
Sherry	1oz	30	2.4	0	2.4
Table wine	1 cup	100	1.0	0	1.0

Food	Amount	Weight (g)	Carbohydrate (g)	Fibre (g)	Usable Carbohydrate (g)
Non-alcoholic					
Coffee – ground	1 cup	240	1.1	0	1.1
Coffee – instant	1 cup	240	-	-	-
Coffee – decaff	1 cup	240	trace	trace	trace
Cola	1 cup	240	24.0	0	24.0
Cream soda	1 cup	240	26.4	0	26.4
Ginger ale	1 cup	240	19.2	0	19.2
Root beer	1 cup	240	25.2	0	25.2
Tonic water	1 cup	240	22.0	-	22.0
CEREALS					
Wholegrain	1 oz	28	18.2	1.9	16.3
Arrowroot	1 tbsp	8	7.0	0	7.0
Barley, pearl	1 oz	28	7.7	trace	7.7
Buckwheat, wholegrain	1 cup	100	72.9	0.2	72.7
Bulgur, dry	1 tbsp	14	10.6	3.1	7.5
Cornmeal	1 cup	238	25.5	0.2	25.3
Malt extract	1 tbsp	8	7.1	-	7.1
Millet, wholegrain	1 oz	28	20.0	0.5	19.5
Oats, wholegrain	1 cup	80	-	-	-
Quinoa	1 oz	28	19.0	1.3	17.7
Wheat					
Wheatbran, unprocessed	1 tbsp	9	5.6	0.8	4.8
Wheatgerm, unprocessed	1 tbsp	9	4.2	0.2	4.0
Wheatgerm, toasted	1 tbsp	6	3.0	0.1	2.9
Breakfast Cereals					
Cornflakes	1 cup	25	21.3	0.2	21.1
Flakes, sugar-covered	1 cup	25	22.8	0.1	22.7
Granola	1 cup	245	76.0	-	76.0
Grapenuts	1 serv	112	10.8	-	10.8
Porridge (oatmeal), cooked	1 cup	236	22.9	0.5	22.4
Puffed rice	1 cup	13	11.6	0.1	11.5

Food	Amount	Weight (g)	Carbohydrate (g)	Fibre (g)	Usable Carbohydrate (g)
Wheat, cream of, cooked	1 cup	245	21.3	-	21.3
Puffed wheat	1 cup	12	9.4	0.2	9.2
Shredded wheat	1 med	22	17.6	0.5	17.1
Flours					
Buckwheat flour	1 cup	100	72.0	1.6	70.4
Corn flour	1 cup	110	84.5	0.8	83.7
Cornstarch	1 tbsp	8	7.0	trace	7.0
Oat flour	1 cup	133	-	-	-
Peanut flour	1 cup	80	18.9	1.6	17.3
Potato flour	1 oz	28	22.4	0.4	22.0
Rye flour	1 oz	28	20.9	0.3	20.6
Soybean flour, full-fat	1 cup	72	21.9	1.7	20.2
Soybean flour, no fat	1 cup	138	52.6	3.2	49.4
Wheat flour	1 cup	110	83.7	0.3	83.4
Pastas					
Macaroni	1 cup	140	42.1	0.1	42.0
Noodles	1 oz	28	6.2	trace	6.2
Spaghetti	1 cup	146	43.9	0.1	43.8
Rice					
Bran	1 oz	28	14.4	0.4	14.0
Brown rice	1 cup	150	38.3	0.5	37.8
White rice	1 cup	150	36.3	0.5	35.8
Rye, wholegrain	1 cup	185	135.8	3.5	132.3
Semolina	1 oz	28	23.9	1.1	22.8
Sorghum	1 oz	28	20.4	0.5	19.9
DESSERTS AND SWEETS					
Desserts					
Apple strudel	1 serv	100	39.0	0.4	38.6
Banana split	indiv	411	97.0	-	97.0
Blintzes, cheese	1 serv	28	-	-	-
Bread pudding	1 cup	220	62.5	0.2	62.3
Sweets					
Butterscotch	1 piece	5	4.7	0	4.7
Chocolate-coated almonds	1 oz	28	11.1	0.4	10.7

Food	Amount	Weight (g)	Carbohydrate (g)	Fibre (g)	Usable Carbohydrate (g)
Chocolate-coated nougat & caramel	1 oz	28	20.4	0.1	20.3
Chocolate-coated pecans	1 piece	2	0.8	trace	0.8
Chocolate fudge	1 piece	25	18.8	0.1	18.7
Chocolate, sweet	1 oz	28	16.2	0.1	16.1
Fruit gums	1 sm	1	0.9	0	0.9
Licorice	1 oz	28	24.5	0	24.5
Lollypops	1 med	28	28.0	0	28.0
Marshmallows	1 avg	8	6.4	0	6.4
Milk chocolate, plain	1 bar	57	32.4	0.2	32.2
Chewing gum	1 piece	3	2.9	-	2.9
Custard, baked	1 cup	265	29.4	0	29.4
Eclairs	1 avg	110	25.5	0	25.5
Gelatin, dessert, prepared	1 cup	240	34.0	0	34.0
Honeycomb	1 oz	28	20.8	-	20.8
Honey, strained or extracted	1 tbsp	20	16.5	trace	16.5
Jams & preserves, red cherry or strawberry	1 tbsp	20	14.0	0.2	13.8
Molasses, cane, blackstrap	1 tbsp	20	11.0	0	11.0
Chocolate pudding	1 oz	28	1.6	0	1.6
Vanilla pudding	1 cup	297	61.1	0	61.1
Custard sauce	1 tbsp	18	2.3	-	2.3
Sorbet, orange	1 cup	193	59.4	0	59.4
Beet or cane sugar, brown	1 tbsp	14	13.5	0	13.5
Beet or cane sugar, granulated	1 tbsp	8	8.0	0	8.0
Beet or cane sugar, icing	1 tbsp	11	10.9	0	10.9
Maple	1 piece	15	13.5	-	13.5
Syrup, chocolate	1 tbsp	20	12.5	0.1	12.4
Syrup, maple	1 tbsp	20	13.0	0	13.0

Food	Amount	Weight (g)	Carbohydrate (g)	Fibre (g)	Usable Carbohydrate (g)
Trifle	1 serv	112	27.2	0	27.2
EGGS					
Raw, whole, fresh	1 med	48	0.6	0	0.6
Raw whites	1 med	31	0.4	0	0.4
Raw yolks	1 med	17	0	0	0
MAIN COURSES					
Beef stew	1 oz	28	1.5	0.1	1.4
Cheeseburger	indiv	105	25.0	0.2	24.8
Cheese soufflé	1 cup	150	9.3	-	9.3
Chilli con carne	1 cup	230	28.1	1.4	26.7
FISH & SEAFOODS					
Anchovy, canned	indiv	4	-	0	0
Anchovy paste	1 tsp	7	0.3	0	0.3
Caviar, sturgeon, granular	1 tsp	10	0.3	-	0.3
Clams – raw, hard & soft, meat only	1 cup	200	4.0	-	4.0
Cod	1 oz	30	0	0	0
Crab, steamed	1 oz	28	0.1	0	0.1
Crayfish	1 oz	28	0.3	-	0.3
Eel, smoked	1 serv	100	0	0	0
Flounder, with salt, baked	1 oz	28	0	0	0
Haddock	1 oz	28	0.1	0	0.1
Hake	1 oz	28	0.1	0	0.1
Halibut	1 oz	28	0	0	0
Herring	1 oz	28	0	0	0
Mackerel, raw	1 oz	28	0	0	0
Trout	1 oz	28	0	0	0
Lobster	1 oz	28	0.1	0	0.1
Mullet	1 oz	28	3.4	-	3.4
Mussels	1 oz	28	0.4	-	0.4
Oyster, raw meat only	1 med	35	2.2	-	2.2
Prawns	1 oz	28	0	0	0
Salmon	1 sm	100	0	0	0
Sardines, Atlantic, canned in oil	1 med	12	0.1	0	0.1

Food	Amount	Weight (g)	Carbohydrate (g)	Fibre (g)	Usable Carbohydrate (g)
Seabass	1 oz	28	0	0	0
Shrimp	1 med	11	-	-	-
Squid	1 oz	28	0.4	-	0.4
Swordfish	1 oz	28	0	0	0
Tuna canned in water, solids and liquid, w/salt	1 cup	200	0	0	0
FLAVOURINGS & SEASONINGS					
Allspice	1 tsp	2	1.4	0.4	1.0
Basil	1 tsp	1	0.6	0.2	0.4
Catsup, bottled	1 tbsp	15	3.8	0.1	3.7
Celery seed	1 tsp	2	0.8	0.2	0.6
Chilli powder	1 tbsp	15	8.2	3.3	4.9
Chilli sauce, regular	1 tbsp	17	4.2	0.1	4.1
Cinnamon	1 tsp	2	1.6	0.5	1.1
Cocoa, powder without milk	1tbsp	7	6.3	0.1	6.2
Coriander leaf, dried	1 tsp	1	0.5	0.1	0.4
Cocoa, mix for hot chocolate	1 tsp	7	5.2	0.1	5.1
Curry powder	1 tsp	2	1.2	0.3	0.9
Garlic powder	1 tsp	3	2.2	0.1	2.1
Garlic salt	1 tsp	5	-	-	-
Ginger	1 oz	28	2.7	0.3	2.4
Mustard, prepared, brown	1 tsp	5	0.3	0.1	0.2
Mustard, prepared, yellow	1 tsp	5	0.3	0.1	0.2
Nutmeg	1 tsp	2	1.0	0.1	0.9
Onion powder	1 tsp	2	1.6	0.1	1.5
Oregano	1 tsp	2	1.3	0.3	1.0
Paprika, domestic	1 tsp	2	1.1	0.4	0.7
Pepper, black, ground	1 tsp	2	1.3	0.3	1.0
Purslane, leaves & stems, raw	1 cup	60	2.3	0.5	1.8
Rosemary, leaves	1 tsp	1	0.7	0.2	0.5

Food	Amount	Weight (g)	Carbohydrate (g)	Fibre (g)	Usable Carbohydrate (g)
Sage	1 tsp	1	0.6	0.2	0.4
Soy sauce	1 tsp	15	1.4	0	1.4
Tarragon	1 tsp	1	0.5	0.1	0.4
Tabasco sauce	1 tsp	5	0.1	0	0.1
Vinegar, cider	1 tbsp	15	0.9	0	0.9
FOOD SUPPLEMENTS					
Seaweed, kelp, raw	1 oz	28	-	0.6	-
Yeast, brewers', tablet form	6 tabs	5	-	-	-
Yeast, torula	1 tbsp	10	3.7	0.3	3.4
FRUITS					
Apples, raw, fresh, unpeeled	1 med	150	21.2	1.5	19.7
Apricots, raw	1 med	38	4.9	0.2	4.7
Avocados, all varieties, raw, halved, without skin	1 avg	250	15.8	4.0	11.8
Bananas, common yellow, short, thick	1 avg	100	29.0	0.4	28.6
Blackberries, raw	1 cup	144	18.6	5.9	12.7
Blueberries, raw	1 cup	140	21.4	2.1	19.3
Boysenberries, canned, water pack, solids & liquid	1 cup	140	12.7	2.7	10.0
Cantaloupe, raw	1 whole	770	57.8	2.3	55.5
Cherries, sweet, raw	1 cup	200	34.8	0.8	34.0
Cranberries, raw	1 cup	100	10.8	1.4	9.4
Dates, domestic, natural, dry	1 cup	178	128.5	4.1	124.4
Elderberries, raw	1 cup	458	75.1	32.1	43.0
Figs, raw	1 med	41	8.3	0.5	7.8
Figs, dry, uncooked	1 med	20	13.5	0.9	12.6
Gooseberries, raw	1 cup	150	14.6	2.8	11.8
Grapefruit, all varieties	1 whole	482	51.1	1.0	50.1

Food	Amount	Weight (g)	Carbohydrate (g)	Fibre (g)	Usable Carbohydrate (g)
Granadilla, purple (passion fruit) pulp & seeds, raw	1 avg	18	3.8	-	3.8
Grapes	1 cup	153	24.0	0.9	23.1
Honeydew melon	1 whole	900	69.3	5.4	63.9
Lemons, pulp without peel, raw	1 med	100	8.2	0.4	7.8
Lemon peel, candied	1 oz	28	22.6	0.6	22.0
Loganberries, raw	1 cup	150	22.4	4.5	17.9
Lychees, raw	1 avg	9	1.5	trace	1.5
Mangoes, raw	1 whole	200	33.6	1.8	31.8
Nectarine, raw	1 med	50	8.6	0.2	8.4
Oranges, raw, without peel	1 sm	100	12.2	0.5	11.7
Papayas, raw	1 med	300	30.0	2.7	27.3
Passion fruit, raw	1 oz	28	1.7	4.4	-
Peaches, raw	1 med	100	9.7	0.6	9.1
Pears, raw, w/skin	1 avg	200	30.6	2.8	27.8
Persimmons, native, raw	1 med	100	33.5	1.5	32.0
Pineapple, raw	1 cup	132	18.1	0.5	17.7
Pineapple, canned, light syrup	1 lg	100	15.4	0.3	15.1
Plums, prune type, raw	1 med	50	9.9	0.2	9.7
Prunes, dried, ready-to-eat	1 lg	10	6.3	0.2	6.1
Pumpkin, canned	1 cup	250	19.8	3.3	16.5
Raisins, California, Thompson seedless	1 tbsp	10	7.7	0.1	7.6
Raspberries, black, raw	1 cup	123	19.3	6.3	13.0
Raspberries, red, raw	1 cup	132	18.0	4.0	14.0
Rhubarb, raw	1 cup	117	4.3	0.8	3.5
Strawberries, raw	1 cup	150	12.6	2.0	10.6
Tangelos, raw	1 med	170	9.2	-	9.2

Food	Amount	Weight (g)	Carbohydrate (g)	Fibre (g)	Usable Carbohydrate (g)
Watermelon, raw	1 cup	200	12.8	0.6	12.2
GRAVIES & SAUCES					
Gravy, beef	1 tbsp	18	2.0	0	2.0
Gravy, chicken	1 oz	28	3.1	0	3.1
Sauce, barbecue	1 tbsp	16	1.3	0.1	1.2
Sauce, Hollandaise	1 tbsp	13	0.1	-	0.1
Sauce, tartar	1 tbsp	20	11.6	0.8	10.8
JUICES					
Apple, cider	1 cup	249	34.3	0	34.3
Apricot juice, unsweetened	1 cup	250	29.3	-	29.3
Apricot nectar, with vitamin C added	1 cup	247	36.1	0.5	35.6
Grapefruit juice	1 cup	250	23.0	-	23.0
Grape juice, canned or bottled	1 cup	250	41.5	-	41.5
Lemon juice, fresh	1 tbsp	15	1.2	-	1.2
Lime juice, fresh	1 tbsp	15	1.4	-	1.4
Orange juice, fresh, all varieties	1 cup	250	26.0	0.3	25.7
Peach nectar, canned, 40% fruit	1 cup	250	31.0	0.3	30.7
Pineapple juice, canned, unsweetened	1 cup	250	33.8	0.3	33.5
Prune juice, canned or bottled	1 cup	250	47.5	-	47.5
Tomato juice, canned or bottled	1 cup	200	8.7	0.4	8.3
Vegetable juice cocktail	1 cup	200	7.2	0.6	6.6
LEGUMES & PULSES					
Adzuki bean, boiled sweetened	1 oz	28	14.2	0.2	14.0
Beans, lima, mature seeds, dry, cooked	1 cup	169	43.3	2.9	40.4

Food	Amount	Weight (g)	Carbohydrate (g)	Fibre (g)	Usable Carbohydrate (g)
Lentils, dry, whole, cooked	1 cup	150	29.0	1.8	27.2
Peas, mature seeds, dry, split, without seed coat, cooked	1 cup	200	41.6	0.8	40.8
Soy beans, mature, dry, cooked	1 cup	180	19.4	2.9	16.5
Miso, fermented, cereal and soybeans	1 oz	28	6.6	0.6	6.0
Soya protein	1 oz	28	4.2	0.1	4.1
Tofu (bean curd)	1 oz	28	0.7	trace	0.7
MEATS					
Bacon, cured, fried, drained, sliced medium	1 slice	7	0.2	0	0.2
Porterhouse steak, choice, total edible, broiled, 57% lean, 43% fat, with bone	1 oz	28	0	0	0
Stew beef, choice, 90% lean, 10% fat, cooked	1 oz	28	0	0	0
T-bone steak, choice, total edible, broiled, 56% lean, 44% fat, with bone	1 oz	28	0	0	0
Frog legs, fried	1 lg	24	2.0	0	2.0
Duck, domestic, flesh only, roasted	1 oz	28	0	0	0
Duck, wild, total edible, raw	1 oz	28	0	0	0
Roast chicken, flesh & skin	1 oz	28	0	0	0
Goat meat (Chevon) carcass	1 oz	28	0	-	0
Lamb, leg, choice, total edible, roasted, 83% lean, 17% fat without bone	1 oz	28	0	0	0

Food	Amount	Weight (g)	Carbohydrate (g)	Fibre (g)	Usable Carbohydrate (g)
Calves' liver	1 oz	28	1.1	0	1.1
Cured ham or shoulder, chopped, canned	1 slice	28	0.4	0	0.4
Salami, dry	1 slice	28	0.3	0	0.3
Pork, fresh, all cuts, medium fat, total edible, cooked, 77% lean, 23% fat	1 oz	28	0	0	0
Ham, dry, long-cure, country style, medium fat	1 oz	28	0.1	0	0.1
Rabbit, domesticated, flesh only, stewed	1 oz	28	0	0	0
Veal, chop	1 oz	28	0	0	0
Venison, lean only, cooked	1 oz	28	0	-	0
MILK PRODUCTS					
Butter, regular, salted	1 tbsp	5	0	0	0
Butter, whipped	1 tbsp	9	0	0	0
Buttermilk, fluid, made from skim milk	1 cup	244	11.7	0	11.7
Cheese, blue	1 oz	28	0.7	0	0.7
Cheese, Brie	1 oz	28	0.1	0	0.1
Cheese, Camembert	1 oz	28	0.1	0	0.1
Cheese, Cheddar	1 oz	28	0.4	0	0.4
Cheese, cottage, large or small curd, uncreamed, 2% fat	1 cup	226	8.2	0	8.2
Cheese, cream	1 tbsp	15	0.4	0	0.4
Cheese, cottage, large or small curd, creamed	1 cup	225	6.0	0	6.0
Cheese, Edam	1 oz	28	0.4	0	0.4

Food	Amount	Weight (g)	Carbohydrate (g)	Fibre (g)	Usable Carbohydrate (g)
Cheese, goat's milk	1 oz	28	1.0	-	1.0
Cheese, Gouda	1 oz	28	0.6	0	0.6
Cheese, Gruyère	1 oz	28	0.1	0	0.1
Cheese, mozzarella	1 oz	28	0.6	0	0.6
Cheese, Parmesan, grated	1 tbsp	5	0.2	0	0.2
Cheese, ricotta, part skim	1 oz	28	1.4	0	1.4
Cheese, Roquefort	1 oz	28	0.6	0	0.6
Cream, whipping 31.3% fat	1 cup	248	7.1	0	7.1
Cream, coffee or table, light, 20.6% fat	1 cup	248	8.8	0	8.8
Cream, whipped topping, pressurised	1 oz	28	3.5	0	3.5
Icecream, regular, 12% fat	1 cup	135	27.8	0	27.8
Icecream, choc	1 cup	133	32.8	-	32.8
Icecream, strawb'y	1 cup	133	31.3	-	31.3
Milk, cows', 3.7% fat	1 cup	244	11.3	0	11.3
Milk, skimmed	1 cup	246	11.8	0	11.8
Milk, canned, evaporated, unsweetened	1 cup	256	25.7	0	25.7
Milk, goats'	1 cup	244	11.2	0	11.2
Milkshake, chocolate, thick	1 cup	345	58.0	0.3	57.7
Sour cream	1 tbsp	12	0.5	0	0.5
Yoghurt, plain, made with whole milk	1 cup	227	10.7	0	10.7
Yoghurt, plain, lowfat, made with lowfat milk and nonfat milk solids	1 cup	227	15.9	0	15.9

Food	Amount	Weight (g)	Carbohydrate (g)	Fibre (g)	Usable Carbohydrate (g)
Yoghurt, fruit varieties, lowfat, made with nonfat milk solids	1 cup	227	43.4	0	43.4
NUTS & SEEDS					
Alfalfa seeds	1 oz	28	-	2.2	-
Almonds, shelled	1 cup	142	27.7	20.3	7.4
Brazil nuts, shelled	1 cup	140	15.3	4.3	11.0
Cashew nuts, shelled	1 cup	140	41.0	2.0	39.0
Coconut, meat, fresh, grated	1 cup	130	12.2	5.2	7.0
Coconut, meat, dried, sweetened, shredded	1 cup	130	69.2	5.3	63.9
Flaxseed, dried	1 oz	28	10.4	2.5	7.9
Hazelnuts	1 oz	28	1.9	1.1	0.8
Peanuts, raw, with skins	1 cup	150	27.9	3.6	24.3
Peanuts, roasted, salted	1 cup	144	27.1	3.4	23.7
Pecans, unsalted	1 cup	108	15.8	2.5	13.3
Pistachio nuts, shelled	1 cup	125	23.8	2.4	21.4
Sesame seeds, dry, whole	1 oz	28	6.0	1.8	4.2
Walnuts, black, shelled, chopped	1 cup	125	18.5	2.1	16.4
PICKLES & RELISHES					
Olives, green	1 med	5	0.1	0.1	0
Olives, ripe	1 lge	5	0.2	0.1	0.1
Pickle, relish, sour	1 tbsp	15	0.4	0.2	0.2
Pickle, relish, sweet	1 tbsp	15	0.4	0.2	0.2
Pickle, cucumber, dill	1 lge	135	3.0	0.7	2.3
SALADS					
Carrot and raisin	1 oz	28	4.5	0.2	4.3

Food	Amount	Weight (g)	Carbohydrate (g)	Fibre (g)	Usable Carbohydrate (g)
Coleslaw	1 oz	28	1.6	0.2	1.4
Coleslaw with salad dressing	1 cup	120	8.5	0.8	7.7
Lettuce and tomato	1 serv	100	4.5	0.7	3.8
Macaroni salad, with onion and mayonnaise	1 cup	190	48.5	0	48.5
Potato salad	1 oz	28	4.6	1.5	3.1
Potato salad, with mayonnaise, French dressing, hardcooked egg and seasoning	1 cup	250	33.5	1.0	32.5
SALAD DRESSINGS					
Blue and Roquefort, regular, with salt	1 French	14	1.0	0	1.0
French (vinaigrette), regular	1 French	14	2.5	0.1	2.4
Italian, regular	1 French	14	1.4	0	1.4
Mayonnaise, regular	1 French	14	3.3	0	3.3
Thousand Island, regular	1 French	14	2.1	0.3	1.8
Vinegar and oil, homemade	1 French	16	0.4	-	0.4
SNACK FOODS					
Bacon rinds	1 serv	28	0	-	-
Corn chips	1 cup	40	20.9	0.4	20.5
Sour cream	1 French	15	1.1	-	1.1
Popcorn, popped with oil and salt	1 cup	9	5.3	0.2	5.1
Potato crisps	1 cup	20	10.0	0.3	9.7
Pumpkin and squash seed kernels, dry	1 cup	140	21.0	2.7	18.3
Sunflower seed kernels, dry, hulled	1 cup	145	28.9	5.5	23.4

Food	Amount	Weight (g)	Carbohydrate (g)	Fibre (g)	Usable Carbohydrate (g)
VEGETABLES					
Alfalfa sprouts, raw	1 cup	38	-	0.6	-
Artichokes, globe or French, boiled, drained	1 lge	100	5.8	1.9	3.9
Artichokes, Jerusalem, raw	1 sml	25	4.2	0.2	4.0
Asparagus, fresh, cooked, drained	1 spear	20	0.7	0.1	0.6
Aubergine, boiled, drained	1 cup	200	8.2	1.8	6.4
Bamboo shoots, canned	1 cup	133	3.5	0.9	2.6
Beans, green, boiled in small amount of water, drained	1 cup	125	6.8	1.3	5.5
Broccoli, spears, cooked	1 cup	150	6.8	2.4	4.4
Beans, frozen, cut, boiled, drained	1 cup	161	9.2	1.6	7.6
Beans, mung, sprouted seeds, uncooked	1 cup	210	13.9	1.3	12.6
Brussels sprouts, cooked	1 cup	150	9.6	2.4	7.2
Carrots, raw	1 lge	100	9.7	1.0	8.7
Cabbage, common, shredded, cooked in small amount of water	1 cup	145	6.2	1.2	5.0
Carrots, boiled, drained	1 cup	100	7.1	1.0	6.1
Cauliflower, raw	1 cup	100	5.2	1.0	4.2
Cauliflower, boiled, drained	1 cup	120	4.9	1.2	3.7
Celery, raw	1 sm	20	0.8	0.1	0.7
Chives, raw	1 tbsp	10	0.6	0.1	0.5

Food	Amount	Weight (g)	Carbohydrate (g)	Fibre (g)	Usable Carbohydrate (g)
Collards, leaves with stems, cooked in small amount of water	1 cup	200	9.8	1.6	8.2
Corn, sweet, fresh, white and yellow, cooked on cob	1 med	140	29.4	1.0	28.4
Cress, garden, raw	1 avg	2	0.1	0	0.1
Cucumbers, raw, peeled	1 med	100	3.2	0.3	2.9
Dandelions, boiled, drained	1 cup	200	12.8	2.6	10.2
Endive (curly and escarole), raw	1 med	7	0.3	0.1	0.2
Fennel, common, leaves, raw	1 cup	60	3.1	0.3	2.8
Garlic, clove, raw	1 avg	3	0.9	0	0.9
Horseradish, prepared	1 tbsp	15	1.4	trace	1.4
Kale, boiled, drained, leaves with stems	1 cup	110	4.4	1.2	3.2
Kohlrabi, boiled, drained	1 cup	200	7.9	1.5	6.4
Lambs' lettuce, boiled, drained	1 cup	200	10.0	3.6	6.4
Leeks, raw	1 avg	25	2.8	0.3	2.5
Lentil sprouts, raw	1 cup	130	-	1.1	-
Lettuce, raw, butterhead (Boston or Bibb)	1 cup	66	1.7	0.3	1.4
Lettuce, raw, Cos	1 cup	66	2.3	0.5	1.8
Mushrooms, *Agaricus campestris*, raw	1 sml	10	0.4	0.1	0.3
Mushrooms, *Agaricus campestris*, sautéed	1 cup	270	10.8	2.7	8.1

Food	Amount	Weight (g)	Carbohydrate (g)	Fibre (g)	Usable Carbohydrate (g)
Mustard greens, raw	1 cup	200	8.0	1.8	6.2
Parsley, raw	1 Tbls	4	0.3	0.1	0.2
Onions, young green, bulb & white portion of top	1 cup	8	0.8	0.1	0.7
Onions, young, green, raw, bulb & entire top	1 avg	20	1.6	0.2	1.4
Onions, mature (dry), yellow, boiled, drained	1 cup	210	13.7	1.2	12.5
Parsnips, boiled, drained	1 cup	200	29.8	4.0	25.8
Peas, podded, boiled, drained	1 cup	150	14.8	1.8	13.0
Peas, green, immature, sweet, boiled, drained	1 cup	150	18.2	3.0	15.2
Peas, green, immature, frozen, boiled, drained	1 med	40	1.9	0.8	1.1
Peppers, green, immature, raw	1 oz	28	1.1	0.4	0.7
Peppers, immature, green, boiled , drained	1 med	40	2.3	0.2	2.1
Peppers, hot, chilli, immature, green pods, no seeds, raw	1 avg	74	6.7	1.3	5.4
Peppers, hot, chilli, mature, red, raw pods, no seeds	1 oz	28	4.4	0.6	3.8
Pimentoes, canned, solids and liquid	1 med	40	2.3	0.2	2.1
Potatoes, baked in skin	1 med	100	21.1	0.6	20.5
Radishes, raw, common	1 sml	10	0.4	0.1	0.3

Food	Amount	Weight (g)	Carbohydrate (g)	Fibre (g)	Usable Carbohydrate (g)
Potatoes, boiled, peeled before cooking	1 med	100	14.5	0.5	14.0
Swede	1 cup	200	16.4	2.2	14.2
Sauerkraut, canned, solids and liquid	1 cup	150	6.0	1.1	4.9
Soybean sprouts, raw	1 cup	105	5.6	0.8	4.8
Spinach, raw	1 cup	100	4.3	0.6	3.7
Spinach, boiled, drained	1 cup	180	6.5	1.1	5.4
Sweet potato, baked in skin	1 sml	100	32.5	0.9	31.6
Swiss chard, boiled, drained	1 cup	166	5.5	1.2	4.3
Tapioca, minute	1 tbsp	10	8.9	trace	8.9
Tomato, paste, canned	1 cup	249	46.2	2.2	44.0
Tomatoes, ripe, raw	1 sm	100	4.7	0.5	4.2
Tomatoes, ripe, boiled	1 cup	240	13.2	1.4	11.8
Turnip greens, boiled in small amount of water, drained	1 cup	150	5.4	1.1	4.3

* 1oz equals approximately 28g.

Conversion Tables

Measurement Conversions

US	British	Metric
1 teaspoon	= 1 teaspoon	= 5 ml
2 teaspoons	= 1 dessertspoon	= 10 ml
1 tablespoon	= 1 tablespoon	= 15 ml
½ cup	= 4 fluid ounces	= 112.5 ml
1 cup	= 1 teacup	= 225 ml
2 cups (1 pint)	= ⅘ imperial pint	= 450 ml
1 quart	= ⅘ imperial quart	= 900 ml
1 gallon	= ⅘ imperial gallon	= 3.6 litres
1 pound	= 1 pound	= 454g

Note: 1 US pint = 16 ounces and 1 US gallon = 8 pounds
1 imperial pint = 20 ounces and 1 imperial gallon = 10 pounds

Oven Temperatures

Fahrenheit	Celsius	Heat	Gas No
150	65	Warm	Pilot light
225	107	Very Slow	
250	121	Very Slow	–
275	135	Very Slow	1
300	149	Slow	2
325	163	Slow	3
350	177	Moderate	4
375	191	Moderate	5
400	204	Hot	6
425	218	Hot	7

FURTHER READING

Allan, Christian B., and Lutz, Wolfgang, *Life Without Bread: How a Low-Carbohydrate Diet Can Save Your Life*. Los Angeles: Keats Publishing, 2000.

Atkins, Robert C., *Dr Atkin's Vita-Nutrient Solution*. New York: Simon & Schuster, New York, 1998.

Audette, R., *Neanderthal*. Dallas: Paleolithic Press, 1996.

Barnes, Broda, MD and Gayton, Lawrence *Hypothyroidism: The Unsuspected Illness*. Boston: Little, Brown, 1997.

Batmanghelidj, Fereydoon, *Your Body's Many Cries for Water*. Global Health Solutions, 1992; 800/759-3999.

Beachel, Thomas and Westcott, Wayne, *Strength Training Past 50*. Leeds: Human Kinetics, 1998.

Beutler, Jade, and Murray, Michael, *Understanding Fats and Oils: Your Guide To Healing With Essential Oils*. Vancouver: Apple Publishing Company, 1996.

Brand-Miller, Jennie, *et al.*, *The Glucose Revolution*. New York: Marlowe, 1999.

Budwig, Johanna, *Flax Oil as a True Aid Against Arthritis, Heart Infarction, Cancer and Other Diseases*. Vancouver: Apple Publishing Company, 1994.

Budwig, Johanna, *The Oil-Protein Diet*. Vancouver: Apple Publishing Company, 1994.

Challem, Jack *et al.*, *Syndrome X: The Complete Nutritional Program to Prevent and Reverse Insulin Resistance*. New York: John Wiley & Sons, 2000.

Colgan, Michael, *Anti-oxidants: The Real Story*. One in the Progressive Health Series, Colgan Institute. Vancouver: Apple Publishing Company, 1998.

Colgan, Michael, *Beat Arthritis*. Vancouver: Apple Publishing Company, 2000.

Colgan, Michael, *Hormonal Health: Nutritional and Hormonal Strategies for Emotional Well-Being and Intellectual Longevity*. Vancouver: Apple Publishing Company, 1996.

Colgan, Michael, *The New Nutrition: Medicine for the Millennium*. Vancouver: Apple Publishing Company, 1995.

Colgan, Michael, *The Right Protein for Muscle and Strength*. One in the Progressive Health Series, Colgan Institute. Vancouver: Apple Publishing Company, 1998.

Colgan, Michael, *Win the War Against Arthritis*. One in the Progressive Health Series, Colgan Institute. Vancouver: Apple Publishing Company, 1999.

Colgan, Michael with Colgan, Lesley, *The Flavonoid Revolution: Grape Seed Extract and Other Flavonoids Against Disease*. Vancouver: Apple Publishing Company, 1997.

Crayhon, Robert, *The Carnitine Miracle*. New York: M.Evans & Co. Inc, 1998.

Eades, Michael, and Eades, Mary Dan, *The Protein Power Lifeplan*. New York: Warner Books, 2000.

Eades, Michael, and Eades, Mary Dan, *Protein Power*. New York: Bantam Books, 1996.

Gittleman, Louise Ann, with Nunziato, Dina, R., *Eat Fat, Lose Weight: How the Right Fats Can Make You Thin for Life*. Los Angeles: Keats Publishing, 1999.

Goettemoeller, Jeffrey, *Stevia Sweet Recipes: Sugar Free Naturally.* Bloomingdale, Illinois: Vital Health Publishing, 1998.

Heinrich, Richard, L., *Starch Madness: Paleolithic Nutrition for Today.* Nevada City, California: Blue Dolphin Publishing, 1999.

Kenton, Leslie, and Kenton, Susannah, *The New Raw Energy.* London: Vermilion, 1994.

Kirkland, James, *Low-Carb Cooking with Stevia: The Naturally Sweet & Calorie-Free Herb.* Arlington, Texas: Crystal Health Publishing, 2000.

Mackarness, R., *Eat Fat and Grow Slim.* Garden City, New York: Doubleday & Co., 1959.

McCullough, Fran, *Living Low-Carb: The Complete Guide to Long-Term Low-Carb Dieting.* New York: Little, Brown, 2000.

McCullough, Fran, *The Low-Carb Cookbook.* New York: Hyperion, 1997.

McDonald, Lyle, *The Ketogenic Diet.* Kearney, Nebraska: Morris Publishing, 1998.

Montignac, Michel, *Dine Out and Lose Weight.* Montignac USA, Inc., 1991; 800/932-3229.

Montignac, Michel, *Eat Yourself Slim.* Translated by Daphné Jones, 5th edition, London: Montignac Publishing, 1996.

Morgenthaler, John and Simms, Mia, *The Low-Carb Anti-Aging Diet.* Petaluma, California: Smart Publications, 2000.

Murray, Michael, T., *Encyclopedia of Nutritional Supplements: The Essential Guide for Improving Your Health Naturally.* USA: Prima Publishing, 1996.

Nelson, Miriam, *Strong Women Stay Young.* New York: Bantam, 2000.

Ornstein, Robert, and Sobel, David, *Healthly Pleasures: Discover the Proven Medical Benefits of Pleasure and Live a Longer, Healthier Life.* Cambridge, Massachusetts: Perseus Books, 1989.

Pauling, Linus, *How to Live Longer and Feel Better.* New York: Avon Books, 1986.

Price, Weston, *Nutrition and Physical Degeneration.*, 6th edition., New Canaan, Connecticut: Keats Publishing Inc., 1997.

Sahelian, Ray, and Gates, Donna, *The Stevia Cookbook: Cooking with Nature's Calorie-Free Sweetner.* Garden City, New York: Avery Publishing, 1999.

Sears, Barry, *Enter the Zone.* New York: HarperCollins, 1995.

Sears, Barry with Bill Lawren, *The Zone, A Dietary Road Map.* New York: Regan Books, 1995.

Simms, Mia, *The Smart Guide to Low-Carb Cooking.* Petaluma, California: Smart Publications, 2000.

Simontacchi, Carol, *Your Fat Is Not Your Fault.* New York: Tarcher, 1997.

Schmidt, Michael, *Smart Fats: How Dietary Fats and Oils Affect Mental, Physical and Emotional Intelligence.* Berkeley, California: Frog Ltd, 1997.

Stefánsson, V., *The Fat of the Land.* New York: Hill and Wang, 1957.

Steffánson, V., *Cancer, Disease of Civilization.* New York: Hill and Wang, 1960.

Wharton, Jim and Phil, *The Wharton's Strength Book.* New York: Random House, 1999.

References

Part One: Wake-up Call
High Carbs Madness

Allan, Christian, B., and Lutz, Wolfgang, *Life Without Bread: How a Low-carbohydrate Diet Can Save Your Life.* Los Angeles: Keats Publishing, 2000.

Allred, J. B. 'Too much of a good thing? An overemphasis on eating low-fat foods may be contributing to the alarming increase in overweight among US adults.' In the *Journal of the American Dietetic Association,* April 1995, 95 (4): 417-18.

Banting, W., 'Letter on corpulence, addressed to the public.' In *Obesity Research,* March 1993, 1 (2): 153-63 (reprinted from the December 1863 third edition).

Berkson, Burton, Challem, Jack, and Smith, Melissa Diane, *Syndrome X: The Complete Nutritional Program to Prevent and Reverse Insulin Resistance.* Canada: John Wiley & Sons, 2000.

Eades, Michael,and Eades, Mary Dan, *The Protein Power Lifeplan.* New York: Warner Books, 2000.

Farquhar, J. W. *et al.,* 'Glucose, insulin and triglyceride responses to high and low carbohydrates diets in man.' In the *Journal of Clinical Investigation,* 1966, 45 (10): 1648-56.

Hainer, V. *et al.,* 'Body fat distribution, metabolic and hormonal indices in obese patients, treated initially by very low calorie diet.' In Obesity: Dietary Factors and Control, edited by Romsos, Himms-Hagan, and Suzuki. Tokyo: Japan Scientific Societies Press, 1991, pages 215-226.

Inoue, S. *et al.,* 'Effects of high sucrose diet and its components on glucose tolerance and serum lipids.' In *Obesity: Dietary Factors and Control,* edited by Romsos *et al.* Tokyo: Japan Scientific Societies Press, 1991, pages 159-67.

Kant, A. K., and Schatzkin, A., 'Consumption of energy-dense, nutrient-poor foods by the US population: effect on nutrient profiles.' In the *Journal of American College of Nutrition,* 1994, 13 (3): 285-91.

LeBlanc, J., 'Hormonal and metabolic responses to meals of various composition.' In *Obesity: Dietary Factors and Control,* edited by Romsos, *et al.* Tokyo: Japan Scientific Societies Press, 1991, pages 59-66.

O'Dea, K., 'Glucose and insulin responses to carbohydrate ingestion: acute and long-term consequences.' In *Obesity: Dietary Factors and Control,* edited by Romsos *et al.* Tokyo: Japan Scientific Societies Press, 1991, pages 47-57.

Williamson, D. F. *et al.,* 'The 10-year incidence of overweight and major weight gain in US adults.' In A*rchives of Internal Medicine,* March 1990, 150: 665-72.

Syndrome X – Fatmaker

Bevilacqua, S. *et al.,* 'Operation of Randle's cycle in patients with NIDDM.' In *Diabetes,* March 1990, 39: 383-9.

Bliss, M., 'The history of insulin.' In *Diabetes Care,* December 1993, 2 (suppl 3): 4-7.

Boden, G., Chen, X. and Ruiz, J., 'Mechanisms of fatty acid-induced inhibition of glucose uptake.' In *Journal of Clinical Investigation*, 1994; 93: 2438-2446.

Bukowieki, L. J. *et al.*, 'Insulin resistance and defective thermogenesis.' In *Obesity: Dietary Factor and Control*, edited by Romsos *et al.* Tokyo: Japan Scientific Societies Press, 1991, pages 107-117.

Cahill, G. F., 'Physiology of insulin in man.' In *Diabetes*, 1971, 20 (12): 785-99.

Carantoni M. *et al.*, 'Relationship between insulin resistance and partially oxidised LDL particles in healthy non-diabetic volunteers.' In *Arteriosclerosis, Thrombosis and Vascular Biology*, 1998, 18: 762-767.

Cermani *et al.*, 'Glucose and aging.' In *Scientific American*, May 1987, 90-6.

Challem, Jack *et al.*, *Syndrome X – The Complete Nutritional Program to Prevent and Reverse Insulin Resistance*. New York: John Wiley & Sons, 2000.

Chen, Y-D. *et al.*, 'Why do low-fat high-carbohydrate diets accentuate postprandial lipemia in patients with NIDDM?' In *Diabetes Care*, January 1995, 18: 10-16.

DeFronzo, R. A., and Ferrannini, E., 'Insulin resistance: A multifaceted syndrome responsible for NIDDM, obesity, hypertension, dyslipidemia, and atherosclerotic cardiovascular disease.' In *Diabetes Care*, March 1991, 14 (3): 173-94.

Dilman, V., and Dean, W., *The Neuroendocrine Theory of Aging and Degenerative Disease*. Pensacola, Florida: The Center for Bio-Gerontology, 1992.

Eades, Michael, and Eades, Mary Dan, *Protein Power*, New York: Bantam Books, 1996.

Everson, S. A. *et al.*, 'Weight gain and the risk of developing insulin resistance syndrome.' In *Diabetes Care*, 1998, 21 (10): 1637-1643.

Facchini, F. S. *et al.*, 'Enhanced sympathetic nervous system activity: The linchpin between insulin resistance, hyperinsulinemia, and heart rate.' In the *American Journal of Hypertension*, 1996, 9: 1013-1017.

Fontbonne, A. *et al.*, 'Body fat distribution and coronary heart disease mortality in subjects with impared glucose tolerance or diabetes mellitus: The Paris Prospective Study, 15-year follow-up.' In *Diabetologia*, 1992, 35 (5): 464-8.

Gaziano, J. M. *et al.*, 'Fasting triglycerides, high-density lipoprotein, and risk of myocardial infarction.' In *Circulation*, 1997, 96: 2520-2525.

Lee, B. M., and Wolever, T. M. S., 'Effect of glucose, sucrose and fructose on plasma glucose and insulin responses in normal humans; comparison with white bread.' In *European Journal of Clinical Nutrition*, 1998, 52: 924-928.

Maheux, P. *et al.*, 'Additive effects of obesity, hypertension and Type 2 diabetes on insulin resistance.' In *Hypertension*, 1994, 24: 695-698.

McDonald, L., The Ketogenic Diet – *A Complete Guide for the Dieter and Practitioner*. Kearney, Nebraska: Morris Publishing, 1998.

Modan, M. *et al.*,'Hyperinsulinemia: A link between hypertension, obesity and glucose intolerance.' In the *Journal of Clinical Investigation*, 1985, 75: 809-17.

Mooradian, A. D., and Thurman, J. E., 'Glucotoxicity – potential mechanisms.' In *Clinics in Geriatric Medicine*, 1999, 15 (2): 255-263.

Morgenthaler, J., and Simms, M., *The Smart Guide to the Low-Carb Anti-Aging Diet*. Petaluma, California: Smart Publications, 2000.

Raitakari, O. T. *et al.*, 'The role of insulin in clustering of serum lipids and blood pressure in children and adolescents.' In *Diabetologia*, 1995, 38: 1042-50.

Reaven, G. , 'Role of insulin resistance in human disease.' In *Diabetes*, 1988, 37: 1595-1607.

Reaven, G., 'Syndrome X.' In *Clinical Diabetes*, 1994, 3-4, 32-52.

Reaven, G., 'Syndrome X: 6 Years Later.' In the *Journal of Internal Medicine Supplement*, 1994, 736: 13-22

Schoen, R. E. *et al.*, 'Increased blood glucose and insulin, body size, and incident colorectal cancer.' In the *Journal of the National Cancer Institute*, 1999, 91 (13): 1147-1154.

Swislocki, A. L. M. *et al.*, 'Insulin resistance, glucose intolerance and hyperinsulinemia in patients with hypertension.' In the *American Journal of Hypertension*, May 1989, 2 (5 part 1): 419-23.

Torjeson, P. A. *et al.*, 'Lifestyle changes may reverse development of the insulin resistance syndrome.' In *Diabetes Care*, 1997, 20:26-31.

Trevisan, M. *et al.*, 'Syndrome X and mortality: A population-based study.' In the *American Journal of Epidemiology*, 1998, 148: 958-966.

Wells, A. S. *et al.*, 'Alterations in mood after changing to a low-fat diet.' In the *British Journal of Nutrition*, 1998, 79:23-30.

Zavoroni, I. *et al.*, 'Risk factors for coronary artery disease in healthy persons with hyerinsulinemia, and normal glucose tolerance.' In *The New England Journal of Medicine*, 1989, 320: 702-6.

Forgotten Magic

Allan, Christian, B., and Lutz, Wolfgang, *Life Without Bread: How a Low-carbohydrate Diet Can Save Your Life*. Los Angeles: Keats Publishing, 2000.

Atkins, Robert, *Dr Atkins' Diet Revolution*. New York: David McKay, 1972 (reissued 1989).

Cleave, T. L., *The Saccharine Disease*. New Canaan, Connecticut: Keats Publishing, 1978.

Eades, Michael, and Eades, Mary Dan, *Protein Power*. New York: Bantam Books, 1997.

Eaton, S. B., Eaton, S. B. III, and Konner, M. J., 'Paleolithic nutrition revisited: A twelve-year retrospective on its nature and implications.' In the *European Journal of Clinical Nutrition*, 1997, 51:207-216.

Eaton, S. B. *et al.*, 'An evolutionary perspective enhances understanding of human nutritional requirements.' In the *Journal of Nutrition*, 1996, 126:1732-1740.

Eaton, S. B., Shostak, M., and Konner, M., *The Paleolithic Prescription*. New York: Harper & Row, 1988.

Foster, D. W., 'The Banting Lecture 1984: From glycogen to ketones – and back.' In *Diabetes*, 1984, 33: 1188-99.

Herodotus, *The Histories (III/2)*, translated by Aubrey de Selincourt. Penguin Classics, 1954.

Lieb, C. W., 'The effects of an exclusive, long-continued meat diet.' In *Journal of the American Medical Association*, 1926, 87 (1): 25-26.

Lieb, C. W., 'The effects on human beings of a twelve-month exclusive meat diet.' In *Journal of the American Medical Association*, 1929, 93 (1): 20-22.

Mackarness, R., *Eat Fat and Grow Slim*. Garden City, New York: Doubleday, 1959.

Price, W., *Nutrition and Physical Degeneration*, 6th edition. New Canaan, Connecticut: Keats Publishing, 1997.

Savarin, A. B., *Physiologie du goût*. Munich: Bruckmann Querschnitte, 1962.

Schwartz, H., *Never Satisfied: The Cultural History of Diets, Fantasies, and Fat*. New York: The Free Press, 1986.

Stefánsson, V., *Cancer, Disease of Civilization*. New York: Hill & Wang, 1960.

Stefánsson, V., *The Fat of the Land.* New York: Macmillan Publishing, 1956.

Yudkin, J., *Sweet and Dangerous.* New York: Van Rees Press, 1972.

Back to the Future

Aiello, L. C. and Wheeler, P., 'The expensive-tissue hypothesis: The brain and the digestive system in human and primate evolution.' In *Current Anthropology,* April 1995, 36 (2): 199-221.

Ames, B. N., 'Paleolithic diet, evolution, and carcinogens.' In *Science,* 1987, 238: 1633-4.

Angel, J. L., 'Health as a crucial factor in the changes from hunting to developed farming in the Eastern Mediterranean.' In *Paleopathology at the Origins of Agriculture,* edited by M. N. Cohen and G. J. Armelagos. New York: Academic Press, 1984, pages 51-73.

Berkson, Burton, Challem, Jack, and Smith, Melissa Diane, *Syndrome X: The Complete Nutritional Program to Prevent and Reverse Insulin Resistance.* Canada: John Wiley & Sons, 2000.

Bower, B., 'The two-million-year-old meat and marrow diet resurfaces.' In *Science News,* 3 January 1987, page 7.

Carpenter, K. J., 'Protein requirements of adults from an evolutionary perspective.' In the *American Journal of Clinical Nutrition,* 1992, 55: 913-7.

Cassidy, C. M., 'Nutrition and health in agriculturalists and hunter-gatherers: A case study of two prehistoric populations.' In *Nutritional Anthropology: Contemporary Approaches to Diet and Culture,* edited by Jerome, N. M., Kandel, R. F., and Felto, G. H. Pleasantville, New York: Redgrave Publishing Company, 1980, pages 117-45.

Cohen, M. N., *Health and the Rise of Civilization.* New Haven: Yale University Press, 1989.

Eades, Michael, and Eades, Mary Dan, *Protein Power.* New York: Bantam Books, 1996.

Eaton, S. B., and Konner, M. J., 'Paleolithic nutrition: A consideration of its nature and current implications.' In the *New England Journal of Medicine,* 1985, 312: 283-9.

Eaton, S. B. *et al.,* 'Stone agers in the fast lane: Chronic degenerative diseases in evolutionary perspective.' In the *American Journal of Medicine,* 1988, 84: 739-49.

Eaton, S. B., *et al., The Paleolithic Prescriptions.* New York: Harper & Row, 1988.

Eaton, S. B., 'Humans, lipids and evolution.' In *Lipids,* 1992, 27 (10): 814-9.

Gordon, K. D., 'Evolutionary perspectives on human diet.' In *Nutritional Anthropology,* edited by F. E. Johnston. New York: Alan R. Liss, 1987, pages 3-39.

Klurfeld, D. M., and Kritchevsky, D., 'The Western diet: An examination of its relationship with chronic disease.' In the *Journal of American College of Nutrition,* 1986, 5: 477-85.

Neel, J. V., 'Diabetes mellitus: A 'thrifty' genotype rendered detrimental by progress?' In the *American Journal of Human Genetics,* 1963, 14: 353-62.

O'Dea, K., 'Westernization, insulin resistance and diabetes in Australian Aborigines.' In the *Medical Journal of Australia,* 19 August 1991, 155: 258-65.

Prive, Weston, *Nutrition and Physical Degeneration,* 6th edition. New Canaan, Connecticut: Keats Publishing, 1997.

Yudkin, J., 'Evolutionary and historical changes in dietary carbohydrates.' In the *American Journal of Clinical Nutrition,* 1967, 20: 108-15.

Yudkin, J., 'Medical problems from modern diet'. In the *Journal of the Royal College of Physicians of London,* January 1975, 9 (2): 161-4.

Part Two: Inside Story

Colour of Energy

Becker, Robert, O., 'Electromagnetic forces and life processes.' *Technological Review,* December 1972.

Bircher, Ralph, *A Turning Point in Nutritional Science* (speech, ca. 1950). Milwaukee, Wisconsin: Lee Foundation for Nutritional Research, Reprint No. 80.

Bircher-Benner, M., *The Essential Nature and Organization of Food Energy and the Application of the Second Principle of Thermo-Dynamics to Food Value and its Active Force.* London: John Bale & Sons & Curnow, 1949.

Bircher-Benner, M., *The Prevention of Incurable Disease.* Cambridge, England: James Clarke, 1981.

Bray, H. G., and White, K., *Kinetics and Thermodynamics in Biochemistry.* London: J. & A. Churchill, 1957.

Brekhman, I., *Man and Biologically Active Substances.* Oxford: Pergamon Press, 1980.

Burr, Harold Saxton, *Blueprint for Immortality: The Electric Patterns of Life.* London: Neville Spearman, 1952.

Crile, George, *The Bipolar Theory of Living Processes.* New York: Macmillan, 1926.

Crile, George, *The Phenomena of Life: A Radio-Electrical Interpretation.* New York: W. W. Norton, 1936.

Goulart, Frances Sheridan, *Super Healing Foods.* West Nyack, New York: Parker Publishing Company, 1995.

Hauschka, Rudolph, *The Nature of Substance.* London: Vincent Stuart, 1966.

Heinerman, John, *Heinermans's Encyclopaedia of Fruits, Vegetables, and Herbs.* West Nyack, New York: Parker Publishing Company, 1998.

Katahn, Martin, *The Tri-Colour Diet: A Miracle Breakthrough in Diet and Nutrition for a Longer, Healthier Life.* New York: W. W. Norton, 1996.

Margen, Sheldon, and the editors of the *University of California at Berkeley Wellness Letter, The Wellness Encyclopedia of Food and Nutrition.* New York: Health Letter Associates, 1992.

Morgan, Brain L., *Nutrition Prescription.* New York: Crown Publishers, 1987.

Murray, Michael, *Encyclopedia of Nutritional Supplements: The Essential Guide for Improving Your Health Naturally.* Rocklin, California: Prima Publishing, 1996.

Pardee, A. D., and Ingraham, L. L., 'Free energy and entropy in metabolism.' In *Metabolic Pathways,* vol 1, edited by Greenberg, D.M.

Schrödinger, Erwin, *What is Life? And Mind and Matter?* Cambridge University Press, 1980.

Simoneton, A., *Radiations des aliments ondes humaines, et sante.* Paris: Le Courrier du Livre, 1971.

Williams, R., 'Renaissance of nutritional science is imminent.' In *Perspectives in Biology and Medicine,* Autumn 1973, 17: 1.

Winter, Ruth, *A Consumer's Guide to Medicines in Food.* New York: Crown Trade

Paperbacks, 1995.

Zukav, G., *The Dancing Wu Li Master.* New York: William Morrow, 1979.

Carbs in Close-up

Allan, Christian, B., and Lutz, Wolfgang, *Life Without Bread: How a Low-carbohydrate Diet Can Save Your Life.* Los Angeles: Keats Publishing, 2000.

Behal, K. M., Howe, J. C., 'Effect of long-term consumption of amylose vs. amylopectin starch on metabolic variables in human subjects.' In the *American Journal of Clinical Nutrition,* 1995; 61: 334-340.

Berkson, Burton, Challem, Jack, and Smith, Melissa Diane, *Syndrome X: The Complete Nutritional Program to Prevent and Reverse Insulin Resistance.* Canada: John Wiley & Sons, 2000.

Brand-Miller, Jennie, *et al., The Glucose Revolution.* New York: Marlowe, 1999.

Chait, A., 'Dietary management of diabetes mellitus.' In *Contemporary Nutrition,* 1984, 9: 2.

De Wees, Allen, A., *The Glycemic Index: Glycemic Impact of Food.* At www.anndeweesallen.com/dal.gly2.htm.

Eades, Michael, and Eades, Mary Dan, *The Protein Power Lifeplan.* New York: Warner Books, 2000.

Eaton, S. B. and Konner, M., 'Paleolithic nutrition.' In the *New England Journal of Medicine,* 1985, 312 (5): 283-289.

Howe, J. C., Rumpler W. V., and Behall, K. M., 'Dietary starch composition and level of energy intake alter nutrient oxidation in 'carbohydrate-sensitive' men.' In the *Journal of Nutrition,* 1996, 126: 2120-2129.

Good, Bad and Ugly

Jenkins, D., and Wolever, T., 'Glycemic index of foods: a physiologic basis for carbohydrate exchange.' In *The American Journal of Clinical Nutrition,* 1981, 34: 362-366.

Landin, K. *et al.,* 'Guar gum improves insulin sensitivity, blood lipids, blood pressure, and fibrinolysis in healthy men.' In the *American Journal of Clinical Nutrition,* 1992, 56: 1061-1065.

Leclere, C. J. *et al.,* 'Viscous guar gums lower glycemic responses after a solid meal: Mode of action.' In the *American Journal of Clinical Nutrition,* 1994, 59 (supplement): 776S.

Ludwig, D. S. *et al.,* 'High Glycemic Index foods, overeating and obesity.' In *Pediatrics,* 1999, 103 (3): E26.

Lyons, T. J. *et al.,* 'Decrease in skin collagen glycation with improved glycemic control in patients with insulin-dependent diabetes mellitus.' In the *Journal of Clinical Investigation,* 1991, 87 (6): 1910-1915.

Odetti, P. *et al.,* 'Good glycemic control reduces oxidation and glycation end-products in collagen of diabetic rats.' In *Diabetologia,* 1996, 39 (12): 1440-1447.

Philipson, H., 'Dietary fibre in the diabetic diet.' In *Acta Medica Scandinavica,* 1983, 671 (supplement): 91-93.

Podell, R., *The G-Index Diet.* New York: Warner Books, 1993.

Rivellese, A., *et al.,* 'Effect of dietary fibre on glucose control and serum lipoproteins in diabetic patients.' In the *Lancet,* 1980, 2: 447.

Salmeron, J., *et al.*, 'Dietary fiber, glycemic load, and the risk of non-insulin-dependent diabetes mellitus in women.' In the *Journal of the American Medical Association*, 1997, 277: 472-477.

Stock, A., and Yudkin, J., 'Nutrient intake of subjects on low carbohydrate diet used in treatment of obesity.' In the *American Journal of Clinical Nutrition*, 1970, 23:948-952.

Wolever, T. M., *et al.*, 'Beneficial effect of low-Glycemic Index diet in overweight NIDDM subjects.' In *Diabetes Care*, 1992, 15 (4): 562-564.

Yudkin, J., 'The low-carbohydrate diet in the treatment of obesity.' In *Postgraduate Medicine*, 1972, 51: 151-154.

Protein Power

Allan, Christian, B., and Lutz, Wolfgang, *Life Without Bread: How a Low-carbohydrate Diet Can Save Your Life*. Los Angeles: Keats Publishing, 2000.

Barth, C. A. *et al.*, 'Endocrine response to animal and vegetable protein.' In Barth, C. A., and Schlimme, E., editors, *Milk Proteins*. New York: Springer Verlag, 1989: 62-67.

Berkson, Burton, Challem, Jack, and Smith, Melissa Diane, *Syndrome X: The Complete Nutritional Program to Prevent and Reverse Insulin Resistance*. Canada: John Wiley & Sons, 2000.

Budwig, Johanna, *The Oil-Protein Diet*. Vancouver: Apple Publishing Company, 1996.

Douglass, J. M., and Rasgon, I., 'Diet and diabetes.' In the *Lancet*, December 1976.

Douglass, J. M., *et al.*, 'Nutrition, non-thermally prepared food and nature's message to man.' In the *Journal of the International Academy of Preventative Medicine*, July 1982, 7: 2.

Eades, Michael, and Eades, Mary Dan, *Protein Power*. New York: Bantam Books, 2000.

FAO/WHO Expert Committee, *Protein Quality Evaluation. Report of a Joint FAO/WHO Expert Committee: Food and Nutrition Paper No 51*. Rome: FAO/WHO, 1990.

Henley, E. C., 'Food and Drug Administration's proposed labelling rules for protein.' In the *Journal of the American Dietetic Association*, 1992, 92:293-296.

Landau, R. L., *et al.*, 'The protein-sparing action of protein feeding: absence of relationship to insulin secretion.' In the *American Journal of Clinical Nutrition*, 1981, 34:1300-04.

Leichti-von Brasch, D., '70 Jahre Erfahrungsgut der Bircher-Benner Ordnungstherapie.' *Erfahrungsheilkunde*, Band XIX, Heft 6/7/8, 1970.

Lemon, P. W., 'Protein and exercise: Update 1987.' In *Medicine and Science in Sports and Exercise*, 1987, 5: S179-S190.

Livingstone, Virginia, and Wheeler, Owen, *Food Alive*. San Diego: The Livingston Wheeler Medical Clinic, 1977.

Remner, E., *Milk And Dairy Products in Human Nutrition*. Munich: Volswirtschaftlicher Verlag, 1983.

Young, V. R., and Pellet, P. L., 'Protein evaluation, amino acid scoring and the Food and Drug Administration's proposed food labelling regulations.' In the *Journal of Nutrition*, 1991, 121:145-150.

The Right Stuff

Barth, C. A. *et al.*, 'Endocrine response to animal and vegetable protein.' In Barth, C. A., and Schlimme, E., editors, *Milk Proteins*. New York: Springer Verlag, 1989: 62-67.

Bounous, G. *et al.*, 'The immunoenhancing property of dietary whey protein concentrate.' In *Clinical and Investigative Medicine*, 1988, 11: 271-278.

Bounous, G. *et al.*, 'The biological activity of undenatured dietary whey proteins: Role of glutathione.' In *Clinical and Investigative Medicine*, 1991, 14: 296-309.

Chandler, R. M. *et al.*, 'Cabohydrate-protein complex increases the rate of muscle glycogen storage after exercise.' In the *Journal of Applied Physiology*, 1992, 72: 1854-1859.

Colgan, Michael, *Optimum Sports Nutrition*. New York: Advanced Research Press, 1993.

Colgan, Michael, *The New Nutrition: Medicine For the Millennium*. Vancouver: Apple Publishing Company, 1994.

Colgan, Michael, *The Right Protein for Muscle and Strength*. One in the Colgan Institute's Progressive Health Series. Vancouver: Apple Publishing Company, 1998.

Di Pasquale, M., 'Dietary protein: The anabolic edge.' In *Anabolic Research*, 1996, 1:1-3.

Lemon, P. W., *et al.*, 'Protein requirements and muscle mass/strength changes during intensive training in novice bodybuilders.' In the *Journal of Applied Physiology*, 1992, 73:767-775.

Poullain, M. G. *et al.*, 'Effect of whey proteins: Their oligopeptide hydrolystates and free-amino acid mixtures on growth and nitrogen retention in fed and starved rats.' In the *Journal of Parenteral and Enteral Nutrition*, 1989, 13: 382-386.

Recommended Dietary Allowances, 10th edition. Washington DC: National Academy Press, 1989.

Sadler, R., 'The benefits of dietary whey protein concentrate on the immune response and health.' In the *South African Journal of Dairy Science*, 1992, 24: 2.

Young, V. R., and Pellet, P. L., 'Protein evaluation, amino acid scoring and the Food and Drug Administration's proposed food labelling regulations.' In the *Journal of Nutrition*, 1991, 121:145-150.

Young, V. R. *et al.*, 'A theoretical basis for increasing current estimates of the amino acid requirements in adult man with experimental support.' In the *American Journal of Clinical Nutrition*, 1989, 50:80-92.

Eat Fat

Capone, S. I., and Glaspy, J. A., 'Relationship between omega-3 and omega-6 fatty acid ratios and breast cancer.' In *Nutrition*, 1997, 13 (9): 822-23.

Beutler, Jake, and Murray, Michael, T., *Understanding Fats and Oils: Your Guide To Healing With Essential Oils*. Vancouver: Apple Publishing Company, 1996.

Budwig, Johanna, *The Oil-Protein Diet*. Vancouver: Apple Publishing Company, 1994.

Crawford, M. A., 'Fatty-acid ratios in free-living and domestic animals: Possible implications for atheroma.' In the *Lancet*, 1968, 13: 29-33.

Dorver, K. K., 'Dietary fish oil alters specific and inflammatory immune responses in chicks.' In the *Journal of Nutrition*, 1997,127: 2039-46.

Eades, Michael, and Eades, Mary Dan, *Protein Power: The Metabolic Breakthrough*. New York: Bantam Books, 1996.

Eaton, S. B., and Konne, Melvin, 'Paleolithic nutrition: A consideration of its nature and current implications.' In the *New England Journal of Medicine*, 1985, 312 (5): 283-89.

Eaton, S. B., Shostak, M., and Konner, M., *The Paleolithic Prescription*. New York: Harper & Row, 1998.

Enig, Mary, *Trans Fatty Acids in the Food Supply: A Comprehensive Report Covering 60 Years of Research*. Silver Spring, Maryland: Enig Associates, 1993.

Gittleman, Ann Louise, with Nunziato, Dina R., *Eat Fat, Lose Weight: How the Right Fats Can Make You Thin for Life*. Keats Publishing, 1999.

Golomb, B., 'Dietary fat and heart disease – dogma challenged?' In the *Journal of Clinical Epidemiology*, 1998, 51 (0): 461-64.

Harris, W. S. *et al.*, 'Dietary omega-3 fatty acids prevent carbohydrate-induced hypertriglyceridemia.' In *Metabolism*, November 1984, 33 (11): 1016-19.

Harris, William, *Fish Oils, Omega-3 Polyunsaturated Fatty Acids, and Coronary Heart Disease*. The PUFA Information Backgrounder, July 1997.

Holman, R. T., 'The slow discovery of the importance of omega-3 essential fatty acids in human health.' In the *Journal of Nutrition*, 1998, 128: 427S-33S.

Holman, R. T., 'Significance of essential fatty acids in human nutrition.' In *Lipids* 1, 1976: 215.

Horribin, D. F., 'Fatty acid metabolism in health and disease: The role of delta-6-desaturase.' In the *American Journal of Clinical Nutrition*, 1993, 57 (supplement): 732S-7S.

Kritchevsky, D., 'History of recommendations to the public about dietary fat.' In the *Journal of Nutrition*, 128: 449S-52S.

Lardinois, C. K., 'The role of omega-3 fatty acids on insulin secretion and insulin sensitivity.' In *Medical Hypotheses*, 1987, 24: 243-8.

Mowrey, Daniel B., *Fat Management! The Thermogenic Factor*. Lehi, Utah: Victory Publications, 1994.

Murray, Michael, T., and Beutler, Jade, *Understanding Fats and Oils*. Encinitas, California: Progressive Health Publishing, 1996.

Nordoy, A. *et al.*, 'Individual effects of dietary saturated fatty acids and fish oil on plasma lipids and lipoproteins in normal men.' In the *American Journal of Clinical Nutrition*, 1993, 57: 634-9.

Pariza, M. *et al.*, *Conjugated Linoleic Acid (CLA) Reduces Body Fat*. Abstract for Experimental Biology Conference, 1996.

Phillipson, B., *et al.*, 'Reduction of plasma lipids, lipoproteins, and apoproteins by dietary fish oils in patients with hypertriglyceridemia.' In the *New England Journal of Medicine*, 1985, 312: 1210-16.

Prince, M. J., 'Do n-3 fatty acids improve glucose tolerance and lipemia in diabetics?' *Lipidology*, 1997, 8: 7-11.

Radack, K. *et al.*, 'The effects of low doses of n-3 fatty acid supplementation on blood pressure in hypertensive subjects: A randomized controlled trial.' In the *Archives of Internal Medicine*, June 1991, 151: 1173-80.

Ravnskov, U., 'Questionable role of saturated and polyunsaturated fatty acids in cardiovascular disease.' In the *Journal of Clinical Epidemiology*, 1998, 51 (6): 443-60.

Raz, A., and Przeecki, N. N., 'Fish oil inhibits 6 desaturase activity in vivo: Utility in a dietary program.' In the *Journal of Nutritional Biochemistry*, 8: 558-65.

Rudkin, Donald, and Felix, Clara, *Omega-3 Oils. Garden City Park*, New York: Avery, 1996.

Schmidt, Michael, A., *Smart Fats: How Dietary Fats and Oils Affect Mental, Physical and Emotional Intelligence*. Berkeley, California: Frog Ltd, 1997.

Siguel, E. N., 'Altered fatty acid metabolism in patients with angiographically documented coronary artery disease.' In *Metabolism*, 1994, 43 (8): 982-993.

Valdini, A. F., *et al.*, 'Efficacy of fish oil supplementation for treatment of moderate elevation of serum cholesterol.' In the *Journal of Family Practice*, 1990, 30 (10): 55-9.

Willet, W. C. *et al.*, 'Intake of trans-fatty acids and risk of coronary heart disease among women.' In the *Lancet*, 1993, 341: 581-85.

Lean Means Energy

Anderson, R. E. *et al.*, 'Effects of lifestyle activity vs. structured aerobic exercise in obese women.' In the *Journal of the American Medical Association*, 1999, 281: 335-340.

Cappon, J. P. *et al.*, 'Acute effects of high fat and high glucose meals on the growth hormone response to exercise.' In the *Journal of Clinical Endocrinology and Metabolism*, 1992, 76 (6): 1418-22.

Colgan, Michael, *The New Power Program: Protocols for Maximum Strength*. Vancouver: Apple Publishing Company, 2001.

Crist, D. M. *et al.*, 'Body composition response to exogenous GH during training in highly conditioned adults.' In the *Journal of Applied Physiology*, 1988, 65:579-84.

Cutler, D. L., Gray, C. *et al.*, 'Low-carbohydrate diet alters intracellular glucose metabolism but not overall glucose disposal in exercise-trained subjects.' In *Metabolism*, October 1995, 44 (10): 1264-70.

Depres, J. P., 'Obesity, regional adipose tissue distribution, and metabolism: Effect of exercise.' in *Obesity: Dietary Factors and Control*, edited by Romsos, Himms-Hagan, and Suzuki. Tokyo: Japan Scientific Societies Press, 1991, pp 251-9.

DiPasqulae, M., 'High fat, high protein, low carbohydrate diet: Part I.' In *Drugs in Sports*, 1992, (4): 8-9.

DiPietro, L. *et al.*, 'Moderate-intensity aerobic training improves glucose tolerance in aging independent of abdominal adiposity.' In the *Journal of the American* Geriatrics Society, 1986; 46 (7): 875-879.

Dunn, A. L. *et al.*, 'Comparison of lifestyle and structured interventions to increase physical activity and cardiovascular fitness.' In the *Journal of the American Medical Association*, 199, 281: 327-334.

Flatt, J., 'Integration of the overall response to exercise.' In the *International Journal of Obesity and Related Disorders*, 1995 (supplement), 4: 31-40.

Henriksson, J., 'Influence of exercise on insulin sensitivity.' In the *Journal of Cardiovascular Risk*, 1995, 4: 303-309.

Hersey, W. C. III *et al.*, 'Endurance exercise training improves body composition and plasma insulin responses in 70 to 79 year old men and women.' In *Metabolism*, July 1994, 43 (7): 847-54.

Kraemer, W. J., 'Influence of the endocrine system on resistance training adaptations.' In the *National Strength and Conditioning Association Journal*, 1992, 14 (2): 47-54.

Langfort, J., *et al.*, 'Effect of low carbohydrate diet on metabolic and hormonal responses to graded exercise in men.' In the *Journal of Physiology and Pharmacology*, 1996, 47 (2): 361-371.

Mayer-Davis, E. J. *et al.*, 'Intensity and amount of physical activity in relation to insulin sensitivity.' In the *Journal of the American Medical Association*, 1998, 279: 669-674.

Paffenbarger, R. S. *et al.*, 'Physical activity, other life-style patterns, cardiovascular disease and longevity.' In *Acta Medica Scandinavica*, 1986, 711 (supplement): 85-91.

Paffenbarger, R. S. *et al.*, 'The association of changes in physical activity and other lifestyle characteristics with mortality.' In the *New England Journal of Medicine*, 1993, 328 (8): 538-545.

Powel, K. E. *et al.*, 'Physical activity and chronic diseases.' In the *American Journal of Clinical Nutrition*, 1989, 49: 999-1006.

Racette, S. B. *et al.*, 'Effects of aerobic exercise and dietary carbohydrate on energy expenditure and body composition during weight reduction in obese women.' In the *American Journal of Clinical Nutrition*, 1995, 61: 468-94.

Rudman, D. *et al.*, 'Effect of growth hormone in men over 60 years old.' In the *New England Journal of Medicine*, 1990, 232: 1-6.

Scholfield, J. G., 'Prostaglandin E1 and the release of growth hormone in vitro.' Letter in *Nature,* 10 October 1970, 228: 179.

Somer, E., *Age Proof Your Body.* New York: William Morrow, 1998.

Takemura, Y. *et al.,* 'The protective effect of good physical fitness when young on the risk of impaired glucose tolerance when old.' In *Preventive Medicine,* 1999, 28 (1): 14-19.

Walberg, J. L. *et al.,* 'Exercise capacity and nitrogen loss during a high or low-carbohydrate diet.' In *Medicine and Science in Sports and Exercise,* 1988, 20 (1): 34-43.

Fat Burning Body

Beachel, Thomas and Westcott, Wayne, *Strength Training Past 50.* Leeds: Human Kinetics, 1998.

Chu, D., *Exercise Power & Strength: Complex Training for Maximum Results.* Champaign, Illinois: Human Kinetics, 1996.

Corpos, E. *et al.,* 'Human growth hormone and human aging.' In *Endocrine Reviews,* 1993, 14 (1): 20-39.

Fields, R., 'Effects of exercise training in the elderly: Impact of progressive-resistance training on skeletal muscle and whole body protein metabolism.' *Proceedings of the Nutrition Society,* 1995, 54: 665-75.

McDonald, Lyle, *The Ketogenic Diet.* Kearney, Nebraska: Morris Publishing, 1998.

Part Three: Path to Power

Miracle of Nature

Atkins, Robert, *Dr Atkins' New Diet Revolution.* New York: Avon, 1997.

Benoit, F. *et al.,* 'Changes in body composition during weight reduction in obesity.' In the *Archives of Internal Medicine,* 1965, 63: (4) 604-612.

Carroll, J., and Koenigsberger, D., 'The ketogenic diet: A practical guide for caregivers.' *Journal of the American Dietetic Association,* 1998, 98 (3): 316-321.

Council on Food and Nutrition, 'A critique of low-carbohydrate ketogenic weight reducing regimes.' In the Journal *of the American Medical Association,* 1973, 224: 1415-1419.

Devlin, Thomas, M., editor, *Textbook of Biochemistry with Clinical Correlations,* 4th edition. New York: Wiley-Liss, 1997.

Eades, Michael, and Eades, Mary Dan, *Protein Power.* New York: Bantam Books, 1996.

Eades, Michael, and Eades, Mary Dan, *The Protein Power Lifespan.* New York: Warner Books, 2000.

Evans, E., *et al.,* 'The absence of undesirable changes during consumption of the low-carbohydrate diet.' In *Nutrition and Metabolism,* 1974, 17: 360-367.

Fery, R. *et al.,* 'Hormonal and metabolic changes induced by an isocaloric isoproteinic ketogenic diet in healthy subjects.' In *Diabetes and Metabolism,* 1982, 8: 299-305.

Golay, A. *et al.,* 'Weight-loss with low or high carbohydrate diet?' In the *International Journal of Obesity and Related Metabolic Disorders,* 1996, 20 (12): 1067-1072.

Johnson, W. A., Weinger, M. W., 'Protective effects of ketogenic diets on signs of hypoglycaemia.' In *Diabetes,* 1978, 27 (11): 1087-1091.

McDonald, L., *The Ketogenic Diet – A Complete Guide for The Dieter and Practitioner.*

Kearney, Nebraska: Morris Publishing,1998.

Mitchell, G. A. *et al.*, 'Medical aspects of ketone body metabolism.' In *Clinical and Investigative Medicine*, 1995, 18: 193-216.

Montignac, Michel, *Eat Yourself Slim*, translated by Daphne Jones, 5th edition. London: Montignac Publishing, 1996.

Nebeleng, L. C., 'Implementing a ketogenic diet based on medium-chain triglyceride oil in paedriatic patients with cancer.' In the *Journal of the American Dietetic Association*, 1995; 95: 693-697.

Nosadini, R. *et al.*, 'Ketone body metabolism: A physiological and clinical overview.' *Diabetes/Metabolism Reviews*, 1989, 5: 299-319.

Phinney, S. D., *et al.*, 'The human metabolic response to chronic ketosis without calorie restriction: Physical and biochemical adaptation.' In *Metabolism*, 1983, 32: (8): 757-768.

Simontacchi, Carol, *Your Fat is Not Your Fault.* New York: Tarcher, 1997.

Spring, B. *et al.*, 'Effects of protein and carbohydrate meals on mood and performance: Interaction with sex and age.' In the *Journal of Psychiatric Research*, 1983, 17 (2): 155-167.

Let It Burn

Atkins, Robert, *Dr Atkins' Diet Revolution.* New York: David McKay, 1972.

Atkins, Robert, *Dr Atkins' New Diet Revolution.* New York: Avon, 1992.

Benoit, F. *et al.*, 'Changes in body composition during weight reduction in obesity.' In the *Archives of Internal Medicine*, 1965, 63: (4) 604-612.

Berryman, M. S., 'The ketogenic diet revisited.' In the *Journal of the American Dietetic Association*, 1997, 97: S192-S194.

Blackburn, G. *et al.*, *Preservation of the Physiological Responses in a Protein Sparing Modified Fast.* Boston: MIT Cent Nut Res, NEDH and the Department of Nutrition and Food Science,

Cahill, G., 'Ketosis.' In *Kidney International*, 1981, 20: 416-425.

Cahill, G., 'Starvation in man.' In the *New England Journal of Medicine*, 1970, 282: 668-675.

Carlson, M G, *et al*, *Fuel and Energy Metabolism in Fasting Humans.*, J Clin Nutr, 1994; 60: 29-36.

Carroll, J. and Koenigsberger, D., 'The ketogenic diet: A practical guide for caregivers.' In the *Journal of the American Dietetic Association*, 1998, 98(3): 316-321.

Council on Foods and Nutrition, 'A critique of low-carbohydrate ketogenic weight reducing regimes.' In the *Journal of the American Medical Association*, 1973, 224: 1415-1419.

Devlin, Thomas, M., editor, *Textbook of Biochemistry with Clinical Correlations*, 4th edition. New York: Wiley-Liss, 1997.

Eades, Michael, and Eades, Mary Dan, *The Protein Power Lifeplan.* New York: Warner Books, 2000.

Eades, Michael, and Eades, Mary Dan, *Protein Power.* New York: Bantam Books, 1996.

Elia, M., *et al.*, 'Ketone body metabolism in lean male adults during short-term starvation, with particular reference to forearm muscle metabolism.' In *Clinical Science*, 1990, 78: 579-584.

Evans, E., *et al.*, 'The absence of undesirable changes during consumption of the low carbohydrate diet.' In *Nutrition and Metabolism*, 1974, 17: 360-367.

Flatt, J. P., 'Glycogen levels and obesity.' In the *International Journal of Obesity*, 1996, 20 (supplement): S1-S11.

Foster, D. W., 'The Banting Lecture 1984: From glycogen to ketones – and back.' In *Diabetes*, 1984, 33: 1188-99.

Freeman, Jennifer B., Freeman, John M., and Kelly, M. T., *The Epilepsy Diet Treatment: An Introduction to the Ketogenic Diet.* New York: Demos Vermade, 1996.

Golay, A., *et al.*, 'Weight-loss with low or high carbohydrate diet?' *International Journal of Obesity and Related Medical Disorders*, 1996, 20(12): 1067-1072.

Guyton, A. C., 'Protein metabolism.' In the *Textbook of Medical Physiology*, 8th edition. Philadelphia: W. B. Saunders, 1991.

Guyton, A. C., *Textbook of Medical Physiology*. Philadelphia: W. B. Saunders, 1996.

Johnson, W. A. and Weinger, M. W., 'Protective effects of ketogenic diets on signs of hypoglycaemia.' In *Diabetes*, 1978, 27 (11): 1087-1091.

Kwan, R. M. F. *et al.*, 'Effect of a low carbohydrate isoenergetic diet on sleep behaviour and pulmonary functions in healthy female adult humans.' In the *Journal of Nutrition*, 1986, 116: 2393-2402.

Magee, B. A. *et al.*, 'The inhibition of malignant cell growth by ketone bodies.' In the *Australian Journal of Experimental Biology and Medical Science*, 1979, 57(5): 529-239.

McDonald, L., *The Ketogenic Diet – A Complete Guide for The Dieter and Practitioner.* Kearney, Nebraska: Morris Publishing,1998.

Mitchell, G. A. e*et al.*, 'Medical aspects of ketone body metabolism.' In *Clinical and Investigative Medicine*, 1995, 18: 193-216.

Morgenthaler, J., and Simms, M., *The Smart Guide to the Low-Carb Anti-Aging Diet.* Petaluma, California: Smart Publications, 2000.

Nebeling, L. C., and Learner, E., 'Implementing a ketogenic diet based on medium-chain triglyceride oil in pediatric patients with cancer.' In the *Journal of the American College of Nutrition*, 1995, 95: 693-697.

Nebeling, L. C. *et al.*, 'Effects of a ketogenic diet on tumour metabolism and nutritional status in paediatric oncology patients: Two case reports.' In the *Journal of the American College of Nutrition*, 1995, 14: 202-208.

Nosadini, R. *et al.*, 'Ketone body metabolism: A physiological and clinical overview.' In *Diabetes/Metabolism Reviews*, 1989, 5: 299-319.

Owen, O. E. *et al.*, 'Brain metabolism during fasting.' In the Journal *of Clinical Investigation*, 1967, 10: 1589-1595.

Phinney, S. D., *et al.* 'The human metabolic response to chronic ketosis without caloric restoration: Physical and biochemical adaptation.' In *Metabolism*, 1983, 32(8): 757-768.

Sokoloff, L., 'Metabolism of ketone bodies by the brain.' In the *Annual Review of Medicine*, 1973, 24: 271-280.

Spring, B. *et al.*, 'Psycho-biological effects of carbohydrates.' In the *Journal of Clinical Psychiatry*, 50 (supplement), 1989.

Swink, T. D. *et al.*, 'The ketogenic diet: 1997.' In *Advances in Pediatrics*, 1997, 44: 297-239.

Walters, J. K. *et al.* 'The protein-sparing modified fast for obesity-related medical problems.' In *Cleveland Clinic Journal of Medicine*, 1997, 64: 242-243.

Willi, S. M. *et al.*, 'The effects of a high-protein, low-fat ketogenic diet on adolescents with morbid obesity: body composition, blood chemistries, and sleep abnormalities.' In *Pediatrics*, 1998, 101(1): 61-67.

Yudkin, J. and Carey, M., 'The low carbohydrate diet in the treatment of obesity.' In *Postgraduate Medicine*, 1972, 51: 151-154.

Part Four: New Life
21st-century Hunter Gatherer

Carroll, J., and Koenigsberger, D., 'The ketogenic diet: A practical guide for caregivers.' *Journal of the American Dietetic Association,* 1998, 98 (3): 316-321.

Cox, C., 'Effect of coconut butter and safflower oil on lipids and lipo-proteins in persons with moderately elevated cholesterol levels.' In the *Journal of Lipid Research,* 1995, 36; 1787-1795.

Kaunitz, H., 'Medium chain triglycerides (MCT) in aging and arteriosclerosis.' In the *Journal of Environmental Pathology, Toxicology and Oncology,* 1986, 6 (3-4): 115-121.

Nebeling, L. C., 'Implementing a ketogenic diet based on medium-chain triglyceride oil in pediatric patients with cancer.' In the *Journal of the American Dietetic Association,* 1995, 95: 693-697.

Peat, R., 'Coconut oil.' In the *Townsend Letter for Doctors and Patients,* 1995, 143: 152-156.

Portillo, M. P. *et al.,* 'Energy restriction with high-fat diet enriched with coconut oil gives higher UCP2 and lower white fat in rats.' In the *International Journal of Obesity and Related Metabolic Disorders,* 1998, 22 (10): 974-979.

Sweet Nothings

Bertorelli, A. M., 'Review of present and future use of non-nutritive sweeteners.' In *Diabetes Educator,* 1990; 16: 415-22.

Blundell, J. E., 'Effect of sucrose and sweeteners on appetite and energy intake.' In the *International Journal of Obesity and Related Metabolic Disorders,* 1996, 20 (2): S12-S17.

Curi, R. M. A. *et al.* 'Effect of Stevia rebaudiana on glucose tolerance in normal adult humans.' In the *Brazilian Journal of Medical and Biological Research,* 1986, 19: 71-4.

Hellekant, G. C. H., and Roberts, W., 'Sweet taste in the calf: 111 behavioural responses to sweeteners.' In *Physiology and Behaviour,* 1994, 56: 555-62.

Knight, I., 'The development and applications of sucralose, a new high-intensity sweetener.' In the *Canadian Journal of Physiology and Pharmacology,* 1994, 72: 435-9.

Lecos, C. W., 'Sweetness minus calories – Controversy.' In *The Consumer,* 1985, 85 (2205).

Rolls, B., 'Effects of intense sweeteners on hunger, food intake and body weight: A review.' In the *American Journal of Clinical Nutrition,* 1991, 53: 872-8.

Schifferstein, H., 'An equiratio mixture model for non-additive components: A case study for aspartame/acesulfame-K mixtures.' In *Chemical Senses,* 1996, 21: 1-11.

RESOURCES

Where to find help when you need it
Leslie Kenton's Website: **www.lesliekenton.com** Here you will find a mass of helpful tools, techniques, inspiration and resources for practitioners and products as well as links to other websites which Leslie has found valuable to people. The website is highly active and includes information about workshops and talks given by Leslie throughout the world. There you will find information that changes weekly including messages from Leslie, herbs of the week, recipes of the week, news about forthcoming events and workshops Leslie is doing throughout the world. There too you have the opportunity to **become a friend** and submit your questions. Those chosen each month will be answered personally by Leslie.

The Best Suppliers of Nutritional Supplements and Information
Unique in the world, **The NutriCentre** is not only the UK's leading supplier of supplements, it has also one of the finest collection of books on holistic health and nutrition including spiritual and psychological books related to health. This small shop in the basement of The Hale Clinic at 7 Park Crescent, London W1N 3HE is always at the cutting edge of what is happening in holistic health. Their products can be ordered easily on line from **www.nutricentre.com** or by telephone (44) 0207 436 5122 enq@nutricentre.com. Thanks to its brilliant and dedicated director, Rohit Mehta, who travels the world learning more about natural health care, The NutriCentre carries more than 20,000 health and natural beauty care products – those which are available in health food stores as well as those sold only through practitioners. What you order is dispatched within 24 hours throughout the world. They have become Britain's largest supplier of complementary medicine text books to British colleges and universities. They print an interesting newsletter on holistic health with extracts printed on line. The centre is dedicated to service. No order is too small or too large. Almost all of what you need for natural health and beauty you will find here. I can't recommend it highly enough.

Functional Medicine: If you want help in implementing either Ketogenic or Insulin Balance into your life, you can not do better than to work with a doctor or other health practitioner specifically trained in Functional Medicine. This is a cutting edge science-based healthcare approach to help a person establish the very highest level of health and vitality. It concerns assessing and treating underlying causes of illness using individually tailored therapies to restore and enhance health naturally as well as to improve whole-person functioning. Founded in 1993 by the highly respected American biochemist Jeffrey Bland, the Institute for Functional Medicine was established both to train doctors and other health-care professionals in this clinically proven, systematic approach to natural healing as well as to provide functional medicine products, publications and programmes to practitioners and their patients. To my knowledge the IFM is the only organisation in the world doing this. Their advanced understanding of health and healing is a good 30 years ahead of any other I have yet come across. Their products – most sold under the name of Metagenics – are the very best quality and the integrity of the organisation is the highest. These are distributed by various companies in different countries. If you wish to find a doctor or other health practitioner trained in functional medicine I suggest that you contact these companies direct and request from them a list of healthcare professionals in your area whom you may consult. In Britain the Metagenics products are also available from the Nutri Centre in London as well as by mail order from them and their website. (See below.)

Here is a list of Metagenics importers in various countries:

AUSTRALIA
Health World Ltd
8/663 Kingsford Smith Drive
Eagle Farm
Brisbane
Australia 4009
tel. 61 7 3260 330
fax 61 7 3260 3399
www.metagenics.co.z

NEW ZEALAND
J.M. Marketing Ltd
Unit 2 15 Parkway Drive
Mairangi Bay
Auckland, NZ
tel. 64 9 478 2540
fax 64 9 478 2740
www.metaganics.co.nz

REPUBLIC OF SOUTH AFRICA
Amino Research
Sharonne Gidish
PO Box 1827
2121 Parklands
Republic of South Africa
tel. 27 11 608 0280
fax: 27 11 608 0299

UNITED KINGDOM
Nutri Ltd
Buxton Road
New Mill
High Peak
Derbyshire SK22 3JU
tel. 44 166 3746 559
fax 44 166 3750 590

Metagenics UK
16A St Mary's Street
Wallingford
Oxfordshire OX10 OEW
tel. 44 149 1833 243
fax 44 149 1833 254
www.metaganics.co.uk

USA AND OTHER COUNTRIES
Visit the Metagenics website: www.metagenics.com

Other Products Mentioned in this Book

Flaxseed oil (Linseed oil): Is available in capsule form mail order from BioCare Ltd, Lakeside, 180 Lifford Lane, Kings Norton, Birmingham, West Midlands, B30 3NU. Tel: 0121 433 3727. Fax: 0121 433 3879. e-mail: biocare@biocare.co.uk. Vacuum-packed whole flaxseeds (linseeds) are available in most health-food stores. I use Linusit Gold as they are well packed and fresh, available from The Nutri Centre, 7 Park Crescent, London, W1N 3HE. Tel: 020 7436 5122. Fax: 020 7436 5171. Organic flaxseeds are also available from Higher Nature Limited, The Nutrition Centre, Burwash Common, East Sussex, TN19 7LX, Tel 01435 882 880. Keep them refrigerated.

Micro Filtered Whey Protein: Solgar produce Whey to Go Protein Powder in vanilla, chocolate, honeynut and mixed berry flavours. For stockists contact Solgar Vitamin & Herb Ltd, Aldbury, Tring, Herts HP23 5PT. Tel: 01442 890355. Fax: 01442 890366. Website: www.solgar.com.

Nutritional Supplements: Solgar produce excellent multiple vitamins and minerals – my favourite being their OMN1. For stockists contact Solgar Vitamin & Herb Ltd, Aldbury, Tring, Herts HP23 5PT. Tel: 01442 890355. Fax: 01442 890366. Website: www.solgar.com. BioCare and Higher Nature are also suppliers of good-quality nutritional supplements. Their contact details are: BioCare Ltd, Lakeside, 180 Lifford Lane, Kings Norton, Birmingham, West Midlands B30 3NU. Tel: 0121 433 3727. Fax: 0121 433 3879. E-mail: biocare@biocare.co.uk. Higher Nature Ltd, The Nutrition Centre, Burwash Common, East Sussex TN19 7LX. Tel: 01435 882 880. Fax: 01435 883 720.

Organic Foods: The Soil Association publishes a regularly updated national directory of farm shops and box schemes called Where to Buy Organic Foods that costs £5 including postage from: The Soil Association, Bristol House, 40-56 Victoria Street, Bristol BS1 6BY. Tel: 0117 929 0661. Fax: 0117 925 2504. e-mail: info@soilassociation.org. Website: www.soilassociation.org.

Organics Direct: Offers a nationwide home delivery service of fresh vegetables and fruits, delicious breads, juices, sprouts, fresh soups, ready-made meals, snacks and baby foods. They also sell the state-of-the-art 2001 Champion Juicers and the 2002 Health Smart Juice Extractor for beginners. They even sell organic wines – all shipped to you within 24 hours. Organics Direct, 1-7 Willow Street, London EC2A 4BH. Tel: 020 7729 2828. Fax: 020 7613 5800. Website: w.organicsdirect.com. You can order online.

Clearspring: Supply organic foods and natural remedies as well as macrobiotic foods by mail order. They have a good range of herbal teas, organic grains, whole seeds for sprouting, dried fruits, pulses, nut butters, soya and vegetable products, sea vegetables, drinks and Bioforce herb tinctures. Write to them for a catalogue: Clearspring, Unit 19a, Acton Park Estate, London W3 7QE. Tel: 020 8746 0152. Fax: 020 8811 8893. You can order by telephone, fax, post or shop online at www.clearspring.co.uk.

Longwood Farm Organic Meats: Good-quality organic beef, pork, bacon, lamb, chicken, turkey, duck and goose, a variety of types of sausage, all dairy products, vegetables and organic groceries (2000 lines), are available mail order from: Longwood Farm Organic Meats, Tudenham St Mary, Bury St Edmunds, Suffolk IP28 6TB. Tel: 01638 717120. Fax: 01638 717120.

Powdered Psyllium Husks: available from good health food stores or by mail order from The Nutri Centre, 7 Park Crescent, London W1N 3HE. Tel: 020 7436 5122. Fax: 0207 436 5171. E-mail: enq@nutricentre.com and Solgar Vitamin & Herb Ltd, Aldbury, Tring Herts HP23 5PT. Tel: 01442 890355. Fax: 01442 890366. Website: www.solgar.com.

Resistance Training: Michael Colgan, one of the most knowledgeable men in the world in the field of nutrition and weight training created a series of four videos for USANA called *The Get Lean Series*. Each video lasts about 30 minutes and trains a different body part using nothing more than dumbbells and leg weights which you can shove under the sofa when you are not using them. They are excellent. The best I have found. Seek out an independent USANA sales person in your area to order them.

Soya Milk: The best soya milk I have come across is called Bonsoy. It is a particularly good soya milk, unusual in that it is not packed in aluminium. It is organic and available from good health food stores. It does however contain malt extract so is not suitable for Ketogenics, only for Insulin Balance. Contact: Freshlands, 196 Old Street, London EC1V 9FR. Tel: 0207 250 1708 or Wild Oats, 210 Westbourne Grove, London, W11 2RH. Tel: 0207 229 1063.

Stevia: In most countries stevia is readily available in health food stores in a many different forms. It comes as clear liquid extract in distilled water, powered stevia leaf, as full strength (very sweet) stevioside extract. In shaker form you can use stevia as you would sugar to sprinkle on foods and drinks. It even comes in tiny single serving packets which you can carry around with you in your pocket or handbag. From the UK, where stevia is unfortunately not available, you can order it direct from Stevita Company in the USA. They will send it airmail. They do an enormous variety of different products including fruit flavoured stevia supplement drink mixes, powdered stevia leaf extract, pre-measured stevia packets, chocolate flavoured stevia and spoonable stevia blends. I have always found them an excellent source. The products themselves are not heavy and are therefore not enormously costly to send. Besides which even when you order a small quantity it literally lasts for months. Stevia is unquestionable the best form of sweetener in the world. Far from doing harm it actually has many beneficial properties. To order stevia contact: Stevita Company, 7650 US Hwy.287 #100, Arlington, Texas 76001, USA. Tel: +(1) 817 483 0044. Fax: +(1) 817 478 8891. Website: www.stevitastevia.com.

Udo's Choice: A perfect balance of both omega-3 and omega-6 essential fatty acids as well as other important fatty acids such as GLA. Available from good health food stores or by post from The Nutri Centre, 7 Park Crescent, London W1N 3HE. Tel: 020 7436 5122. Fax: 0207 436 5171. Keep refrigerated and do not heat.

Water As you know, getting pure water can be difficult. One in ten of us drink water which is contaminated with poisons above international standards. I have finally found a water purifier which I think is good – the Fresh Water 1000 Water Filter System. It removes more than 90 per cent of heavy metals, pesticides and hydrocarbons such as benzene, trihalmethanes, chlorine, oestrogen and bacteria without removing essential minerals like calcium. Available from The Fresh Water Filter Company, Carlton House, Aylmer Road, Leytonstone, London E11 3AD. Tel: 020 8558 7495. Fax: 020 8556 9270. Friends of the Earth have an excellent free booklet called *Water Pollution.* Contact: Friends of the Earth, 26-28 Underwood Street, London, NI 7JQ. Tel: 0207 490 1555. Fax: 0207 490 0881.

INDEX